Regulation of calcium transport in rat hippocampal mitochondria during development and following denervation
    Michel Baudry and Gary Lynch (Irvine, CA, USA) 107

Acid-base homeostasis in the brain: physiology, chemistry, and neurochemical pathology
    Bo K. Siesjö (Lund, Sweden) 121

Heterogeneous distribution of hydrogen and bicarbonate ions during complete brain ischemia
    Richard P. Kraig, William A. Pulsinelli and Fred Plum (New York, NY, USA) 155

Section III — Alterations in Protein and Lipid Metabolism

Calmodulin and protein phosphorylation: implications in brain ischemia
    Jerome Chin, Tom M. Buckholz and Robert J. DeLorenzo (New Haven, CT, USA) 169

Mechanisms underlying the neuronal response to ischemic injury. Calcium-activated proteolysis of neurofilaments
    William W. Schlaepfer and Un-Jin P. Zimmerman (Philadelphia, PA, USA) 185

Cerebral protein synthesis and ischemia
    W. Bodsch, K. Takahashi, A. Barbier, B. Grosse Ophoff and K.-A. Hossmann (Cologne, FRG) 197

Changes in lipid metabolism in traumatized spinal cord
    Paul Demediuk, Royal D. Saunders, Nancy R. Clendenon, Eugene D. Means, D.K. Anderson and L.A. Horrocks (Columbus and Cincinnati, OH, USA) 211

Cellular and molecular effects of polyunsaturated fatty acids in brain ischemia and injury
    Pak Hoo Chan, Robert A. Fishman, Susan Longar, Sylvia Chen and Albert Yu (San Francisco, CA, USA) 227

Free radical damage of the brain following ischemia
    Kyuya Kogure, Hiroyuki Arai, Koji Abe and Minory Nakano (Sendai and Maebashi, Japan) 237

Subject Index 261

SECTION I

Selective Neuronal Vulnerability

Post-ischemic resuscitation of the brain: selective vulnerability versus global resistance

K.-A. Hossmann

Max-Planck-Institute for Neurological Research, Department of Experimental Neurology, Ostmerheimer Str. 200, D-5000 Köln 91, FRG

Introduction

Despite considerable progress in the understanding of the pathophysiology of cerebral ischemia, the determination of the revival time of the brain remains a topic of great controversy. In the classic literature animal experiments and clinical observations of cardiac arrest suggested that cerebral ischemia of more than 4–5 minutes results in irreversible brain damage. This view was challenged by Hirsch et al. (1957) who observed recovery of EEG activity after 8–10 minutes of ischemia when cerebral blood flow was arrested without interfering with cardiac function, i.e. by inflating a pneumatic cuff around the animal's neck. They concluded that the shorter revival time of the brain after cardiac arrest was due to the fact that the recovery time of the heart had to be added to the ischemia of the brain. In 1968, Ames et al. discovered that even without cardiac insufficiency post-ischemic recirculation is a limiting factor of cerebral recovery. With the same tourniquet model as previously used by Hirsch and colleagues (1957), they noticed that after more than 7.5 minutes of ischemia a substantial volume of the brain was not recirculated, a phenomenon they called "no-reflow". They also observed that evoked potentials of isolated retina, maintained in vitro, recovered after much longer periods of oxygen and glucose deprivation than in the living animal after circulatory arrest (Ames and Gurian, 1963). They therefore speculated that recirculation disturbances may be responsible for the short revival time of the brain.

If this hypothesis is true, prolongation of the revival time of the brain should be possible under experimental conditions in which the no-reflow phenomenon is prevented. We have tested this hypothesis in our laboratory. It turned out in fact that appropriate treatment of post-ischemic recirculation disturbances led to recovery of energy metabolism and neuronal excitability after complete cerebro-circulatory arrest of as long as 1 hour at normal body temperature (Hossmann and Sato, 1970a,b). Systematic exploration of the limits of central nervous system revivability further revealed that functions of considerable complexity such as protein synthesis (Kleihues and Hossmann, 1971, 1973) or EEG activity (Hossmann and Zimmermann, 1974) returned, and that — occasionally — even restitution of neurological function occurred after these long periods of ischemia (Hossmann et al., in preparation).

However, neurological recovery is not predictable after prolonged ischemia, and an increasing number of delayed post-ischemic disturbances have been identified. These include post-ischemic hypoperfusion and dysregulation of blood flow (Hossmann et al., 1973; Nemoto et al., 1975), permeability changes of the blood-brain barrier (Ito et al., 1976; Petito et al., 1982), calcium-mediated processes (Hossmann et al., 1983; Dienel, 1984; Simon et al., 1984b), and even secondary depression of previously recovered metabolic activity (Mies et al., 1983; Pulsinelli and Duffy, 1983; Bodsch and Takahashi, 1984). Ito et al. (1975) coined the term "maturation phenomenon" for the gradual development of such disturbances. It was also pointed out that the delay of "maturation" increased inversely with the duration of ischemia (Ito et al., 1975), and that in certain "selectively vulnerable areas" of hippocampus delayed neuronal death could occur as long as 4 days after an ischemic period of as short as 5 minutes (Kirino, 1982; Suzuki et al., 1983a).

These observations caused the pendulum to swing back, and focus interest more and more on the deleterious effects of short-lasting ischemia. However, in many recent studies little attention has been given to post-ischemic complicating side factors, and methods are again being used for the production of ischemia which previously have been shown to delay or prevent the post-ischemic recovery process. These include tourniquet ischemia or severe incomplete ischemia. Studying mechanisms of ischemic brain damage in such models makes it extremely difficult to differentiate between phenomena caused by the primary ischemic impact from those resulting from unsuccessfully treated post-ischemic complicating side effects. Similarly, the mechanisms responsible for selective vulnerability should be clearly differentiated from those occurring in the more resistant parts of the brain. This differentiation is of particular importance for the establishment of therapeutic procedures because the same approach which may help to ameliorate damage in the selectively vulnerable areas might further impair the lesion in the resistant regions, and vice versa. At the present, many of the mechanisms discussed are controversial, and there are few studies in which a distinct differentiation between vulnerable and resistant areas has been made. In the following, the available information is reviewed and discussed with respect to this particular problem.

Limits of reversibility

(a) Selectively vulnerable areas

The topographical pattern and the morphological, biochemical and functional processes associated with selective vulnerability are discussed in detail in this volume by several authors (Bodsch et al., 1985; Kirino et al., 1985; Pulsinelli, 1985b; Wieloch, 1985; Siesjö, 1985; Suzuki et al., 1985). It is, therefore, sufficient to mention that the following regions are generally considered to be selectively vulnerable to ischemia: the limbic system, in particular pyramidal cells of CA1 subfield of hippocampus, Purkinje cells of cerebellum, small and medium-sized neurons of striatum, and layers 3, 5 and 6 of cortex. The lower limit of selective injury to CA1 neurons or Purkinje cells is less than 5 minutes (Kirino, 1982; Gurvitch et al., 1972); however, the phenomenon of selective vulnerability has also been studied after longer periods of ischemia such as 10 min tourniquet ischemia (Diemer and Siemkowicz, 1981a) or 30 min four-vessel occlusion in the rat (Pulsinelli et al., 1982a).

In acute experiments, identification of selective vulnerability requires certain methodological precautions. As pointed out by Klatzo and co-workers, the histological manifestation or "maturation" of cell damage may require up to several days, the shorter or milder the ischemia the longer the interval (Ito et al., 1975; Bubis et al., 1976). Similarly, certain epiphenomena of irreversible cell damage such as reduction of energy-producing metabolism (Mies et al., 1983) or breakdown of the blood-brain barrier (Ito et al., 1976) appear after a "maturation" interval which may be longer than the usual duration of an acute animal experiment. For this reason, failure to detect histological or biochemical lesions shortly after ischemia does not exclude the possibility that such changes may develop at a later time.

The clinical symptoms of injury to the selectively vulnerable brain regions have been poorly investigated. Isolated lesions of hippocampal subfield CA1 do not seem to provoke any major deficits, at least not in lower mammals such as gerbils and rats. Bothe et al. (1983) noticed a slight deterioration of avoidance reaction during the maturation phase which disappeared by the time although histological lesions became manifest. Similarly, Volpe et al. (1984) observed only a slight impairment of learning behavior after selective lesion of CA1 and striatum. Injury of the selectively vulnerable areas, in consequence, is compatible with life and seems to produce relatively mild neurological deficits.

(b) Resistant areas of the brain

All regions which are not selectively vulnerable, may be tentatively defined as "potentially resistant". As has been pointed out above, the no-reflow phenomenon may prevent recovery after ischemia as short as 7.5 min but appropriate treatment of this complication can result in progressive restoration of complex brain functions after complete cerebro-circulatory arrest of up to 1 hour. The limits of reversibility in resistant areas, in consequence, can only be explored after optimizing treatment of post-ischemic complicating side effects and, therefore, require special technical precautions (see below). Whenever these are taken, and when the core temperature and the density of ischemia are carefully documented to make sure that ischemia is complete and normothermic, positive evidence of post-ischemic recovery is more meaningful than demonstration of its absence.

Another factor which has to be taken into account, is the latency of the recovery. On the one hand, the latency of post-ischemic recovery depends on the duration of ischemia and, on the other, on the complexity of the biochemical or functional process. Shortlasting experiments, therefore, bear the risk that a lesion may be erroneously considered to be irreversible because the latency period for recovery has not elapsed. However, transient recovery during maturation of an irreversible lesion is also possible and in this case the demonstration of recovery may be erroneously interpreted as an indicator of post-ischemic revival, although the same function may disappear at a later time.

With these considerations in mind, it becomes understandable that the reported revival times of various brain functions may vary considerably from one laboratory to another, and that the discrepancies are more pronounced the more complex the function (Table 1). The most relevant observations are those in which the progression of clinical recovery has been followed, using intensive care for the prevention of complicating factors. In such studies complete neurological recovery consistently occurred after 12–15 min cerebro-circulatory arrest (Crowell and Smith, 1956; Safar et al., 1976; Nemoto et al., 1977). However, occasionally complete recovery or recovery with minor neurological deficits was reported after 15–18 min (Gilston, 1979), after 20–24 min (Miller and Myers, 1970), after 28 min (Makarenko, 1972), after 30 min (Volpe et al., 1984) or even after 60 min ischemia (Hossmann et al., in preparation). In the latter series of experiments the classical pattern of hippocampal injury was present but viable neurons were detected in most other regions of the brain including layers 3 and 5 of cortex and the Purkinje cell layer of cerebellum (Kleihues and Hossmann, 1973). Global resistance of the brain to ischemia, in consequence, exceeds by far the lower limits of damage in the selectively vulnerable regions. In the following, I shall discuss how far known mechanisms of ischemic brain damage may account for this difference.

Mechanisms of ischemic brain damage

(a) Factors related to disturbances of recirculation

Following a period of ischemia two types of recirculation disturbances can be distinguished: the no-reflow phenomenon and the (delayed) post-ischemic hypoperfusion syndrome. The *no-reflow phenomenon* (Ames et al., 1968) is the combined result of increased viscosity of (stagnant) blood (Fischer, 1973), microcirculatory compression by swollen perivascular glial cells (Arsenio-Nunes et al., 1973), formation of endothelial microvilli (Dietrich et al., 1984), increased intracranial pressure (Zimmermann et al., 1975), post-ischemic hypotension (Cantu et al., 1969) and disseminated intravascular coagulopathy (Hossmann and Hossmann, 1977). No-reflow is a limiting factor for post-ischemic resuscitation in most regions of the brain, as evidenced by the close correlation of this disturbance with histological lesions (Ginsberg and

TABLE 1

Revival times* of brain functions after complete ischemia in normothermia

Function	Method	Species	Duration (min)	Reference
Energy-producing metabolism	4-vessel occlusion	rat	30	Naruse et al., 1984
	CSF compression	rat	30	Nordström et al., 1978
	decapitation	guinea pig	45	Okada, 1974
	decapitation	rat	60	Ikrényi et al., 1976
	arterial inflow occlusion	cat	60	Hossmann et al., 1976
Protein biosynthesis	isolated retina	rabbit	20	Ames and Nesbett, 1983a
	4-vessel occlusion	rat	30	Dienel et al., 1980
	arterial inflow occlusion	cat	60	Kleihues and Hossmann, 1971
Evoked potentials	decapitation	guinea pig	45	Okada, 1974
	compression ischemia retina	rabbit	60	Foulds and Johnson, 1974
	isolated head	dog	60	Sobotka and Gebert, 1971
	arterial inflow occlusion	cat	60	Hossmann et al., 1983
EEG activity	occlusion aorta	cat	15	Ten Cate and Horsten, 1952
	cardiac arrest	cat	30	Hossmann and Hossmann, 1973
	isolated head	dog	30	Hirsch et al., 1975
	arterial inflow occlusion	monkey	60	Hossmann and Zimmermann, 1974
Clinical recovery	cardiac arrest	dog	10–15	Crowell and Smith, 1956
	cardiac arrest	dog	12	Safar et al., 1976
	tourniquet ischemia	monkey	15	Nemoto et al., 1977
	exsanguination	man	15–18	Gilston, 1979
	systemic circulatory arrest	monkey	20–24	Miller and Myers, 1970
	drowning	dog	28	Makarenko, 1972
	4-vessel occlusion	rabbit	30	Kolata, 1979
	arterial inflow occlusion	cat	60	Hossmann et al., in preparation

* Revival time is defined as the longest duration of ischemia compatible with recovery of the function under investigation.

Myers, 1972). The extent of no-reflow depends on the type and duration of ischemia. It increases with time, and seems to be most pronounced when brain vessels are filled with blood, i.e. after incomplete ischemia or when the venous outflow is obstructed. This is the reason that after only 15 min of tourniquet ischemia recirculation may fail in up to 95% of brain volume (Ames et al., 1968) — because this type of ischemia is both incomplete and stagnant. However, even without venous obstruction small areas of no-reflow are a consistent finding when ischemia is longer than 10 min (Kågström et al., 1983).

In our experience homogeneous blood reperfusion after prolonged ischemia is possible only when special methodological requirements are fulfilled. Ischemia must be induced by arterial inflow occlusion and it must be complete. In large laboratory animals like cats and monkeys, intrathoracal clamping of innominate, left subclavian and both mammary arteries under induced hypotension is best suited for this purpose (Hossmann and Zimmermann, 1974). Furthermore, recirculation must be initiated by a hypertensive "flush" in order to reach the critical capillary opening pressure (Fischer et al., 1979), and osmolality of blood must be increased for prevention of osmotic influx of fluid from the blood into the brain (Hossmann and Takagi, 1976). In our experiments of up to 1-h ischemia we raise systolic arterial pressure with catecholamines to about 180 mm Hg immediately *before* releasing the vessel clamps, and increase blood osmolality by about 30 mOsm with hypertonic solutions, also *before* the beginning of recirculation. Finally, because disseminated post-ischemic coagulation and post-ischemic hypotension are enhanced at low arterial pH, the acid equivalents released during the early recirculation period must be buffered by controlled infusion of Tris buffer or sodium bicarbonate, and arterial pCO_2 must be kept close to normal by controlled ventilation. For this reason blood gas analyses must be carried out at short intervals, and endtidal CO_2 must be monitored continuously. With this procedure recirculation rates up to 350% of control have been observed after 30 min and up to 250% of control after 60 min global ischemia (Hossmann et al., 1973). After shorter periods of ischemia adequate recirculation may be obtained with less drastic therapy but it is unlikely that a no-reflow phenomenon can be prevented without vigorous prophylaxis when ischemia exceeds a duration of more than 10 min.

Once the circulation has been reinitiated, reactive hyperemia continues at normal blood pressure because the blood viscosity of streaming blood abruptly decreases (Schmid-Schönbein, 1977) and because vascular tone is temporarily reduced after ischemia (Takagi et al., 1977). Reoxygenation of the brain results in rapid resolution of post-ischemic brain swelling and normalization of intracranial pressure (Hossmann, 1976). However, since the no--reflow phenomenon is heterogenous, postischemic reactive hyperemia is heterogenous as well (Ginsberg and Myers, 1972; Kågström et al., 1983). Measurement of global cerebral blood flow after ischemia, in consequence, may reveal normal or even increased flow rates although focal areas of no-reflow are still present. This may explain why several authors have observed irreversible brain damage although blood flow was not reduced (Harrison et al., 1975; Levy et al., 1975). On the other hand, the degree of hyperemia is a function of vascular patency; it is therefore not surprising that functional recovery after ischemia proceeds most rapidly in those cases in which reactive hyperemia is most pronounced (Hossmann et al., 1973).

It should be noted that prevention of no-reflow promotes recovery only in the resistant but *not* in the selectively vulnerable areas of the brain. The no-reflow phenomenon, in consequence, is not a limiting factor for ischemic damage in these regions. This conclusion is supported by the observation that selective vulnerability is seen after ischemia of only 5 min, i.e. after a period which is too short to evoke a no-reflow phenomenon.

The *post-ischemic hypoperfusion syndrome* is a consistent complication of post-ischemic recirculation even under those conditions in which a no-reflow phenomenon is absent or in which it has been successfully treated, and it develops after the phase of reactive hyperemia has ceased (Hossmann et al., 1973; Nemoto et al., 1975; Miller et al., 1980). The degree of post-ischemic hypoperfusion seems to be the more pronounced the shorter the duration of ischemia: after 5 min ischemia in gerbils flow decreased to about 30% (Cahn et al., 1985), after 30 min ischemia in rats to 50% (Pulsinelli et al., 1982b) and after 60 min ischemia in cats to 70% of control (Van den Kerckhoff et al., 1983). Post-ischemic hypoperfusion affects both the vulnerable and the resistant areas of the brain (Pulsinelli et al., 1982b). It is characterized by a dissociation between suppressed CO_2 reactivity and maintained autoregulation (Hossmann et al., 1973; Nemoto et al., 1975) leading to vascular constriction (Siemkowicz, 1980; White et al., 1983), and uncoupling of blood flow and metabolic activity (Levy and Duffy, 1977; Hossmann, 1979). Post-ischemic respiratory insufficiency aggravates the effects of hypoperfusion because it further reduces oxygen availability (Hossmann and Hossmann, 1977). It cannot be ameliorated by a variety of vasoactive substances but it diminishes after hemodilution (Hossmann et al., 1973). Some authors observed an improvement with calcium antagonists or a combination of indomethacin and prostacyclin (Hallenbeck and Furlow, 1979; White et al., 1982; Steen et al., 1983), but we did not (Van den Kerckhoff et al., 1983; Hossmann et al., 1983). Its significance for brain metabolic activity depends on the individual rate of oxygen consumption. At relatively low rates, i.e. when oxygen extraction from arterial blood is below 50%, the energy state of the brain is not affected, however, anaerobic glycolysis with tissue acidosis and subsequent metabolic disturbances develops at higher oxygen extraction rates (Hossmann, 1979). This is the reason that a vascular pattern of metabolic lesions may appear after global ischemia — such as cortical (vascular) columns of increased NADH fluorescence (Welsh and O'Connor, 1978), depletion of ATP in the borderzones of the main arterial territories (Paschen et al., 1983a), and even borderzone infarcts (Hossmann and Zimmermann, 1974).

It is likely that post-ischemic hypoperfusion limits the progression of global recovery after prolonged ischemia but it is less clear whether it is also of importance for the maturation of lesions in the selectively vulnerable areas after short-lasting ischemia. Most of the available evidence suggests that after brief periods of ischemia the degree of hypoperfusion is similar in all regions of the brain although only the vulnerable areas are damaged (Pulsinelli et al., 1982b). However, there are indications that in these regions functional activity is enhanced (Suzuki et al., 1983b), and since the resulting metabolic disturbances depend on the local metabolic activity, a focal disequilibration cannot be excluded. After a short-lasting period of severe ischemia deoxyglucose autoradiograms have demonstrated a selective increase of radioactivity in the hippocampus (Diemer and Siemkowicz, 1979; Suzuki et al., 1983a), and, although it still has to be clarified if this increase reflects enhanced metabolic activity or a Pasteur effect, the conclusion seems to be warranted that the preferential vulnerability of this area is associated with either an abnormality of blood flow or of metabolic activity.

(b) Factors related to disturbances of energy-producing metabolism

Failure of recovery or secondary suppression of energy-producing metabolism may be the consequence of circulatory impairment (see above) and/or disturbances of mitochondrial respiration (Rehncrona et al., 1979), reduced NADH production (Welsh et al., 1982) or "functional hypoxia" due to increased tissue glucose concentration (Siemkowicz et al., 1982). The degree of energy failure depends on one hand on the severity of hemodynamic and pulmonary dysfunction (see above) and on the other on specific biochemical disturbances induced by tissue acidosis (Hillered et al., 1984), free radical reactions (Yoshida et al., 1982; Watson et al., 1983), mitochondrial calcium overload (Simon et al., 1984b), etc. The duration of ischemia seems to be of lesser importance because there is positive evidence of restitution of energy-producing metabolism in the resistant areas of the brain after complete ischemia of 30 min (Nordström et al., 1978) or even 60 min (Kleihues et al., 1975; Paschen et al., 1983a).

The breakdown of energy-producing metabolism for whatever reason obviously results in irreversible brain damage; it is, therefore, not surprising that after prolonged ischemia electrophysiological recovery is closely associated with restitution of energy-producing metabolism (Hossmann et al., 1976; Schmidt-Kastner and Hossmann, in preparation). However, restoration of the energy state alone is not sufficient to prevent brain lesions, particularly not in the selectively vulnerable areas (Marshall et al., 1975; Welsh and O'Connor, 1978; Pulsinelli and Duffy, 1983). Despite normal levels of ATP for up to 2 days after 5 min severe ischemia (Mies et al., 1983), protein synthesis was irreversibly suppressed in the CA1 sector of hippocampus after 2 hours of recirculation (Bodsch and Takahashi, 1984), and tissue became necrotic after a few days (Kirino, 1982). Energy-producing metabolism, in consequence, is probably not the limiting factor in the pathogenesis of ischemic cell death (Farber, 1973; Siesjö, 1981).

(c) Factors related to hypermetabolism

Post-ischemic hypermetabolism has been described in various species after cerebro-circulatory arrest ranging between 10 and 60 min (Levy and Duffy, 1977; Diemer and Siemkowicz, 1979, 1981b; Nemoto et al., 1981; Choki et al., 1983). Although the methods used for measuring metabolic activity are not comparable in the different models, the reported data suggest that hypermetabolism is more pronounced after shorter than after longer periods of ischemia. Several factors may explain increased metabolic activity: post-ischemic functional hyperactivity (Suzuki et al., 1983b) — in gerbils occasionally even epileptic seizures (Brown et al., 1979), post-ischemic stimulation of repair processes (Levy and Duffy, 1977), and mitochondrial damage (Rehncrona et al., 1979). The latter results in an inhibition of state 3 respiration and hence increased glucose and oxygen consumption in order to yield a constant production of energy-rich phosphates. It should also be considered that increased cytosolic level of calcium (see below) stimulates mitochondrial Ca^{2+} sequestration at the expense of ATP production, and thus further enhances mitochondrial insufficiency (Nicholls, 1985).

It has not been established if post-ischemic hypermetabolism damages the brain *per se;* however, it is reasonable to assume that it may be deleterious during the phase of post-ischemic hypoperfusion, as described above. Considering the fact that both hypermetabolism and hypoperfusion may appear after very brief periods of ischemia, a relationship with the development of selective vulnerability cannot be excluded. This notion is supported by Kirino's finding, reported in this volume, that low dose of barbiturates given shortly after 5 min ischemia in gerbils reduces morphological lesions in hippocampus, presumably by inhibiting post-ischemic functional hyperactivity (Kirino et al., 1985). A similar mechanism could be responsible for the prevention of hippocampal lesions using other means of inhibiting functional hyperactivity, such as local injection of aspartate-antagonist (Simon et al., 1984a) or by deafferentation (Wieloch et al., 1985; Pulsinelli, 1985a). On the other hand, it should be remembered that barbiturates or other metabolic depressants do not ameliorate brain damage after prolonged ischemia (Pulsinelli et al., 1979; Gisvold et al., 1984). This difference can be explained by the fact that post-ischemic hyperactivity is most pronounced after brief episodes of ischemia, and that barbiturates inhibit metabolic activity indirectly by reducing functional activity. In fact, when thiopental was administered after 12–16 min cardiac arrest, an amelioration of ischemic brain lesions was observed in animals with epileptic but not with normal EEG pattern (Todd et al., 1982). The controversial results obtained by barbiturate treatment, therefore, do not refute post-ischemic hypermetabolism as a mechanism of ischemic brain damage in either selectively vulnerable or resistant brain regions.

(d) Factors related to tissue acidosis

The molecular mechanisms of tissue acidosis and ischemic brain lesions are discussed in detail by Siesjö in this volume, and therefore will be only briefly considered. During complete ischemia the degree of tissue acidosis depends mainly on the stores of glucose and glycogen because the production of lactate — in addition to hydrolysis of ATP — is the most important source of acid equivalents. Acidosis, therefore, is more severe in hyperglycemic than in starved animals. The duration of ischemia is of secondary importance because lactate reaches its maximum already within a few minutes after the onset of ischemia and does not further increase if ischemia is complete (Ljunggren et al., 1974).

During incomplete ischemia the situation is different. Continuous supply of glucose by a trickle of blood flow causes a gradual accumulation of lactate which increases over time, the final concentration depending both on the duration of ischemia and the glucose concentration of blood. Tissue acidosis, in consequence, may vary considerably in different ischemic models. This explains that in general complete ischemia is better tolerated than incomplete ischemia (Hossmann and Zimmermann, 1974; Nordström et al., 1976; Rehncrona et al., 1979), and that damage is less severe in hypoglycemic than in hyperglycemic animals (Myers and Yamaguchi, 1976; Siemkowicz and Hansen, 1978; Ginsberg et al., 1980; Pulsinelli et al., 1982c).

Although the general relationship between tissue acidosis and ischemic brain damage seems now to be well established, its particular role for selective vulnerability is less clear. It is unlikely that global ischemia produces more pronounced acidosis in the vulnerable than in other regions of the brain because the content of glucose and glycogen is relatively constant throughout the brain (Paschen et al., 1983a,b). On the other hand, the appearance of neuronal lesions in hippocampus after brief periods of ischemia is not an argument against the acidosis hypothesis because lactate reaches its peak concentration within a few minutes after circulatory arrest. Selective vulnerability, therefore, may be indirectly linked to acidosis in a similar way as to other global complicating events such as post-ischemic hypoperfusion or post-ischemic hypermetabolism.

(e) Factors related to disturbances of water and ion homeostasis

During and after cerebral ischemia severe disturbances of water and ion homeostasis occur. During complete ischemia, the brain is converted into a closed system, i.e. fluid and ion shifts occur between the various compartments of the brain with little changes of net water and electrolyte content (Hossmann, 1976). During incomplete ischemia or during the recirculation phase after ischemia, blood provides an almost unlimited reservoir for supply and/or removal of fluid and electrolytes, resulting in considerable net changes of tissue content. The most important factors responsible for edema formation are an increase in tissue osmolality (Hossmann and Takagi, 1976; Bandaranayake et al., 1978), inhibition of ion exchange pumps due to energy failure (Astrup, 1982), and permeability changes of cell membranes. The latter can be a functional change induced, for instance, by the release of glutamate which causes a transient increase in permeability of sodium and chloride (Van Harreveld, 1970). However, permeability changes of membranes may also be the consequence of structural lesions, e.g. due to peroxidation of phospholipids (Yoshida et al., 1982; Nemoto et al., 1983; Watson et al., 1983, 1984). The resulting fluid and electrolyte shifts are potentially reversible in all regions of the brain, even after complete ischemia of 1 hour (Hossmann, 1976). Prerequisite is rapid and homogeneous post-ischemic reperfusion because energy metabolism and hence the function of ion exchange pumps have to be restored before post-ischemic brain swelling becomes fatal. In cases of successful reperfusion, post-ischemic brain swelling is reversed within 2 to 3 hours after ischemia as long as 1 hour, and electrolytes return to or close to control levels after the same interval (Hossmann et al., 1977). Physical lesions of neuronal membranes, if any, are either reversible or of little functional significance because membranes recover their electrophysiological properties within 45 min after 1 hour ischemia (Hossmann and Sato, 1970a). The major physiological importance of water and electrolyte disturbances, in consequence, is the contribution to the development of the no-reflow phenomenon (see above) but it does not seem to appear to be a damaging factor per se.

This conclusion may not be true as far as disturbances of calcium homeostasis are concerned. As discussed by Wieloch in this volume, a considerable concentration gradient between extra- and intracellular calcium exists which is maintained by various pump mechanisms (Wieloch, 1985). During ischemia Ca^{2+} enters the intracellular compartment through voltage-dependent channels and accumulates in the cytoplasm because both mitochondrial sequestration and outward calcium transport are energy-consuming mechanisms. In vitro experiments suggest that this process is a mediator of ischemic cell death because irreversible changes can be delayed or prevented when calcium is removed from the incubation medium (Farber et al., 1981;

Ames and Nesbett, 1983b). However, in vivo studies of 60 min cerebral ischemia revealed progressive recovery of both metabolic and electrophysiological functions despite substantial increase of tissue calcium content (Hossmann et al., 1983), and there was no significant difference of calcium between vulnerable and resistant areas (Hossmann et al., in preparation). Electronmicroscopy demonstrated that calcium deposits were most conspicuous in damaged mitochondria but the occurrence of such mitochondria was the same in the hippocampus and cortex.

A similar observation was made after brief periods of ischemia in gerbils (Dux et al., in preparation). There was no difference between the resistant dentate gyrus and the vulnerable CA1 sector of hippocampus: in both areas relatively mild mitochondrial sequestration of calcium was noted 15 min after the beginning of recirculation which was reversible after 1 hour. However, massive uptake occurred in the selectively vulnerable CA1 sector of hippocampus after a few days, i.e. at a time when histological lesions had become manifest. These findings suggest that intracellular calcium accumulation after ischemia is neither a unique feature of selectively vulnerable neurons nor the primary reason for the development of ischemic cell damage but rather an unspecific accompaniment of manifested cell injury. This conclusion conforms to observations made in different experimental models of ischemia (Yanagihara and McCall, 1982; Dienel, 1984; Simon et al., 1984b) and is also corroborated by the recent observation of Dienel and Pulsinelli (1984) who observed that irreversibly damaged neurons incorporate not only Ca^{2+} but also a variety of other substances such as tetracycline, nickel, pertechnetate or sodium. It should be stressed, however, that selectively vulnerable neurons may react to the initial influx of calcium in a different way than resistant neurons, i.e. an unspecific event may provoke specific pathological reactions. This will be discussed in more detail in the following chapter.

(f) Factors related to disturbances of protein biosynthesis

Most of the biochemical studies which have been carried out during post-ischemic resuscitation have dealt with the energy-producing metabolism. However, restoration of the energy state of the brain is not equivalent to restoration of specific metabolic pathways. An example is protein biosynthesis. During complete ischemia, protein synthesis is inhibited because of energy failure but polyribosomes remain in an aggregated state (Kleihues and Hossmann, 1971; Kleihues et al., 1975; Morimoto and Yanagihara, 1981) and incubation of such ribosomes in vitro reveals that the protein synthetizing machinery remains intact (Cooper et al., 1977). Immediately after the beginning of recirculation, however, polyribosomes disaggregate and protein synthesis remains severely suppressed although energy-producing metabolism recovers. Presumably the reason for polyribosomal disaggregation is a selective inhibition of polypeptide chain initiation (Cooper et al., 1977), changes in RNA by either increased ribonuclease activity or reduced synthesis being of lesser importance (Kleihues and Hossmann, 1971; Yanagihara, 1976; Albrecht and Yanagihara, 1979; Bodsch and Takahashi, 1984).

The inhibition of protein synthesis is reversible provided a no-reflow phenomenon can be prevented: after 5 min ischemia it is normal after 1 hour (this was the earliest interval measured, Bodsch and Takahashi, 1984), after 10–15 min it recovers within 4 hours (Cooper et al., 1977; Dienel et al., 1980), and after 30 or 60 min ischemia within 1–2 days (Dienel et al., 1980; Bodsch et al., 1985).

In the selectively vulnerable areas protein synthesis initially recovers as fast as in the rest of the brain but after a delay which depends on the duration of ischemia it is secondarily suppressed: after 5 min ischemia delayed suppression occurs after 2 hours (Bodsch and Takahashi, 1984), and after 1 hour ischemia after 12 hours (Bodsch et al., 1985). The mechanisms responsible for the delayed suppression are still under investigation. As discussed in detail by Bodsch et al., in this volume,

Ca^{2+}-calmodulin-dependent protein phosphorylation is disturbed in stratum radiatum of hippocampus 2 hours after 5 min ischemia, followed 2 hours later by abnormalities of the pattern of phosphoproteins. This finding may be a key for the understanding of selective vulnerability. Since the Ca^{2+}-calmodulin-dependent protein phosphorylation system provides the depolarization-induced trigger for the release of neurotransmitter molecules (DeLorenzo et al., 1979), its damage may be the link between increased post-ischemic functional activity and calcium fluxes on one hand, and permanent structural damage on the other. The delay between onset of these disturbances and cell death could be explained by the long half-life of proteins which would enable the cell to survive for some time despite this deficit. This interpretation would also conform to the fine-structural changes of hippocampal neurons which during the maturation phase exhibit changes uncommon for acute anoxia, such as accumulation of cisterns of endoplasmic reticulum (Kirino et al., 1985).

However, as attractive as this hypothesis may appear, it is still highly speculative. So far, measurements have only been carried out in stratum radiatum of CA1 sector in which the first morphological alterations appear (Von Lubitz and Diemer, 1983). However, it is not known if similar changes are present also in other layers of hippocampus or even in the resistant areas of the brain. Without this information it would be premature to conclude that post-ischemic phosphorylation disturbances are the first step in a chain of events leading eventually to cell death, and not one of the many epiphenomena of this process.

A puzzling observation in this context is the increasing delay of secondary suppression with increasing duration of ischemia (Bodsch et al., 1985). One might speculate that after prolonged ischemia the equally delayed primary recovery process reduces the production of non-functional proteins and that a critical level of such proteins is reached at a later time. Arguing further on this line, one might also speculate that the recovery of protein synthesis in resistant areas of the brain after prolonged ischemia may also be a transient phenomenon, followed by a secondary suppression after an even longer interval. However, all these considerations are purely speculative and not yet supported by experimental data.

Coordinating hypothesis of cerebral vulnerability to ischemia

The available experimental evidence clearly indicates that the vulnerability of the brain to ischemia is determined by both ischemic and post-ischemic events. *Ischemic alterations* obviously are a function of the duration of circulatory arrest, catabolic changes being more pronounced the longer ischemia lasts. However, there are at least two processes considered to be of particular importance for the development of ischemic brain lesions which are relatively independent of the duration of ischemia: tissue acidosis and intracellular flooding with calcium. Both events reach their peaks a few minutes after onset of ischemia and they do not progress further as ischemia continues, provided ischemia is complete. If these changes are responsible for ischemic cell death, it would be understandable that sensitive cells are irreversibly damaged within 5 minutes of ischemia whereas the resistant ones are left intact after ischemia up to 1 hour. However, the possibility of preventing irreversible injury of selectively vulnerable neurons by post-ischemic drug therapy clearly indicates that *post-ischemic changes* are equally important for the manifestation of irreversible injury. Among these, one has to differentiate between global (unspecific) disturbances and focal (specific) responses. The most important global disturbances are the no-reflow phenomenon and delayed post-ischemic hypoperfusion. The *no-reflow phenomenon* is a relevant factor only after ischemia of more than 10 minutes. It is, therefore, not responsible for selective vulnerability, but its prevention is the prerequisite for revival of the resistant areas of the brain after prolonged ischemia.

Delayed *post-ischemic hypoperfusion,* on the other hand, is of equal importance for vulnerable and resistant areas because it appears already after

5 minutes of ischemia and it affects all regions of the brain to a similar degree. The failure of metabolic regulation of blood flow during this phase bears the risk of post-ischemic relative hypoxia whenever local oxygen requirements exceed local oxygen availability. Similarly, blood flow may be too slow for adequate clearance of metabolic waste products, including carbon dioxide. Damage resulting from this disturbance, in consequence, depends on the post-ischemic functional or metabolic state of each individual region. There are good arguments discussed in this volume by a number of authors (Bodsch et al., 1985; Kirino et al., 1985; Pulsinelli, 1985b; Siesjö, 1985; Suzuki et al., 1985; Wieloch, 1985) that specific neuroanatomical connections, synaptic organization, membrane properties and the pattern of neurotransmitters and receptors are responsible for the fact that selectively vulnerable neurons in the hippocampus become hyperactive during post-ischemic recirculation, particularly after a preceding phase of disturbed ion homeostasis. This would explain why the hippocampus or other selectively vulnerable areas are more endangered than less active regions, and that this differential vulnerability is relatively independent of the duration of ischemia.

If the concept is true that ischemic and post-ischemic events concur in producing irreversible injury, it would have some interesting therapeutic consequences. Ischemic cell damage could then be ameliorated by interfering either with the ischemic molecular or with the post-ischemic hemodynamic and functional disturbances. Obviously, a combined approach would be most efficient for amelioration of post-ischemic brain damage. Establishment of such procedures in combination with measures to prevent a no-reflow phenomenon, therefore, could have a realistic chance to extend the limits of reversibility of ischemic brain damage to considerable length, not only in the resistant but equally in the selectively vulnerable areas.

References

Albrecht, J. and Yanagihara, T. (1979) Effect of anoxia and ischemia on ribonuclease activity in brain. *J. Neurochem.*, 32: 1131–1133.

Ames, A., III. and Gurian, B.S. (1963) Effects of glucose and oxygen deprivation on function of isolated mammalian retina. *J. Neurophysiol.*, 26: 617–634.

Ames, A., III. and Nesbett, F.B. (1983a) Pathophysiology of ischemic cell death: I. Time of onset of irreversible damage; importance of the different components of the ischemic insult. *Stroke*, 14: 219–226.

Ames, A., III. and Nesbett, F.B. (1983b) Pathophysiology of ischemic cell death: III. Role of extracellular factors. *Stroke*, 14: 233–240.

Ames, A., III., Wright, R.L., Kowada, M., Thurston, J.M. and Majno, G. (1968) Cerebral ischemia. II. The no-reflow phenomenon. *Am. J. Pathol.*, 52: 437–453.

Arsenio-Nunes, M.L., Hossmann, K.-A. and Farkas-Bargeton, E. (1973) Ultrastructural and histochemical investigation of the cerebral cortex of cat during and after complete ischaemia. *Acta Neuropathol.*, 26: 329–344.

Astrup, J. (1982) Energy-requiring cell functions in the ischemic brain. Their critical supply and possible inhibition in protective therapy. *J. Neurosurg.*, 56: 482–497.

Bandaranayake, N.M., Nemoto, E.M. and Stezoski, S.W. (1978) Rat brain osmolality during barbiturate anesthesia and global brain ischemia. *Stroke*, 9: 249–254.

Bodsch, W. and Takahashi, K. (1984) Selective neuronal vulnerability to cerebral protein- and RNA-synthesis in the hippocampus of the gerbil brain. In: A. Bes, P. Braquet, R. Paoletti and B.K. Siesjö (Eds.), *Cerebral Ischemia*. Excerpta Medica, Amsterdam, New York, Oxford, pp. 197–208.

Bodsch, W., Takahashi, K., Barbier, A., Grosse Ophoff, B. and Hossmann, K.-A. (1985) Cerebral protein synthesis and ischemia. *This volume*, pp. 197–210.

Bothe, H.W., Bosma, H.J., Hofer, H., Hossmann, K.-A. and Angermeier, W.F. (1983) Operant learning, cerebral blood flow and neurohistology in *Meriones unguiculatus* after unilateral carotid artery ligation. In: J.S. Meyer, H. Lechner, M. Reivich and E.O. Ott (Eds.), *Cerebral Vascular Disease 4*. Excerpta Medica, Amsterdam, Oxford, Princeton, pp. 250–255.

Brown, A.W., Levy, D.E., Kublik, M., Harrow, J., Plum, F. and Brierley, J.B. (1979) Selective chromatolysis of neurons in the gerbil brain: a possible consequence of "epileptic" activity produced by common carotid artery occlusion. *Ann. Neurol.*, 5: 127–138.

Bubis, J.J., Fujimoto, T., Ito, U., Mrsulja, B.J., Spatz, M. and Klatzo, I. (1976) Experimental cerebral ischemia in mongolian gerbils. V. Ultrastructural changes in H-3 sector of the hippocampus. *Acta Neuropathol.*, 36: 285–294.

Cahn, R., Martinez, H., Klatzo, I. and Mrsulja, B.B. (1985) Ischemic brain damage. II. Hemodynamic and energetic profile of hippocampal recovery from 5-minute carotid occlusion in young and adult gerbils. In: *Proceedings of the International Salzburg Conference on Cerebral Vascular Disease 1984.* Excerpta Medica, Amsterdam, in press.

Cantu, R.C., Ames, A., III., DiGiacinto, G. and Dixon, J. (1969) Hypotension: a major factor limiting recovery from cerebral ischemia. *J. Surg. Res.,* 9: 525–529.

Choki, J., Greenberg, J. and Reivich, M. (1983) Regional cerebral glucose metabolism during and after bilateral cerebral ischemia in the gerbil. *Stroke,* 14: 568–574.

Cooper, H.K., Zalewska, T., Kawakami, S., Hossmann, K.-A. and Kleihues, P. (1977) The effect of ischaemia and recirculation on protein synthesis in the rat brain. *J. Neurochem.,* 28: 929–934.

Crowell, J.W. and Smith, E. (1956) Effect of fibrinolytic activation on survival and cerebral damage following periods of circulatory arrest. *Am. J. Physiol.,* 186: 283–285.

DeLorenzo, R.J., Freedman, S.D., Yohe, W.B. and Maurer, S.C. (1979) Stimulation of Ca^{2+}-dependent neurotransmitter release and presynaptic nerve terminal protein phosphorylation by calmodulin and a calmodulin-like protein isolated from synaptic vesicles. *Proc. Natl. Acad. Sci. U.S.A.,* 76: 1838–1842.

Diemer, N.H. and Siemkowicz, E. (1979) Regional glucose metabolism in the rat brain after ischemia. *Neuropathol. Appl. Neurobiol.,* 5: 82–83.

Diemer, N.H. and Siemkowicz, E. (1981a) Regional neurone damage after cerebral ischaemia in the normo- and hypoglycaemic rat. *Neuropathol. Appl. Neurobiol.,* 7: 217–227.

Diemer, N.H. and Siemkowicz, E. (1981b) Postischemic changes in the rat brain glucose utilization in regions with and without nerve cell loss. *Acta Neurol. Scand.,* 63: 139–144.

Dienel, G.A. (1984) Regional accumulation of calcium in postischemic rat brain. *J. Neurochem.,* 43: 913–925.

Dienel, G.A. and Pulsinelli, W.A. (1984) Radioactive tracers to label selectively ischemic damaged brain. *Ann. Neurol.,* 16: 115–116.

Dienel, G.A., Pulsinelli, W.A. and Duffy, T.E. (1980) Regional protein synthesis in rat brain following acute hemispheric ischemia. *J. Neurochem.,* 35: 1216–1226.

Dietrich, W.D., Busto, R. and Ginsberg, M.D. (1984) Cerebral endothelial microvilli: Formation following global forebrain ischemia. *J. Neuropathol. Exp. Neurol.,* 43: 72–83.

Farber, E. (1973) ATP and cell integrity. *Fed. Proc.,* 32: 1534–1539.

Farber, J.L., Chien, K.R. and Mittnacht, S., Jr. (1981) The pathogenesis of irreversible cell injury in ischemia. *Am. J. Pathol.,* 102: 271–281.

Fischer, E.G. (1973) Impaired perfusion following cerebrovascular stasis. *Arch. Neurol.,* 29: 361–366.

Fischer, E.G., Ames, A., III. and Lorenzo, A.V. (1979) Cerebral blood flow immediately following brief circulatory stasis. *Stroke,* 10: 423–427.

Foulds, W.S. and Johnson, N.F. (1974) Rabbit electroretinogram during recovery from induced ischaemia. *Trans. Ophthalmol. Soc. U.K.,* 94: 383–393.

Gilston, A. (1979) Complete cerebral recovery after prolonged circulatory arrest. A report of 2 cases. *Intensive Care Med.,* 5: 193–198.

Ginsberg, M.D. and Myers, R.E. (1972) The topography of impaired microvascular perfusion in the primate brain following total circulatory arrest. *Neurology,* 22: 998–1011.

Ginsberg, M.D., Graham, D.I., Welsh, F.A. and Budd, W.W. (1979) Diffuse cerebral ischemia in the cat. III. Neuropathological sequelae of severe ischemia. *Ann. Neurol.,* 5: 350–358.

Ginsberg, M.D., Welsh, F.A. and Budd, W.W. (1980) Deleterious effect of glucose pretreatment on recovery from diffuse cerebral ischemia in the cat. I. Local cerebral blood flow and glucose utilization. *Stroke,* 11: 347–354.

Gisvold, S.E., Safar, P., Hendrickz, H.H.L., Rao, G., Moossy, J. and Alexander, H. (1984) Thiopental treatment after global brain ischemia in pigtailed monkeys. *Anesthesiology,* 60: 88–96.

Gurvitch, A.M., Romanova, N.P. and Mutuskina, E.A. (1972) Quantitative evaluation of brain damage resulting from circulatory arrest to the central nervous system or the entire body. I. Electroencephalographic and histological evaluation of the severity of permanent post-ischemic damage. *Resuscitation,* 1: 205–218.

Hallenbeck, J.M. and Furlow, T.W., Jr. (1979) Prostaglandin I_2 and indomethacin prevent impairment of post-ischemic brain reperfusion in the dog. *Stroke,* 10: 629–637.

Harrison, M.J.G., Sedal, L., Arnold, J. and Ross Russell, R.W. (1975) No-reflow phenomenon in the cerebral circulation of gerbil. *J. Neurol. Neurosurg. Psychiat.,* 38: 1190–1193.

Hillered, L., Ernster, L., Siesjö, B.K. (1984) Influence of in vitro lactic acidosis and hypercapnia on respiratory activity of isolated rat brain mitochondria. *J. Cereb. Blood Flow Metabol.,* 4: 430–437.

Hirsch, H., Euler, K.H. and Schneider, M. (1957) Über die Erholung und Wiederbelebung des Gehirns nach Ischämie bei Normothermie. *Pflügers Arch.,* 265: 281–313.

Hirsch, H., Oberdörster, G., Zimmer, R., Benner, K.U. and Lang, R. (1975) The recovery of electrocorticogram of normothermic canine brains after complete cerebral ischemia. *Arch. Psychiatr. Nervenkr.,* 221: 171–179.

Hossmann, K.-A. (1976) Development and resolution of ischemic brain swelling. In: H. Pappius and W. Feindel (Eds.), *Dynamics of Brain Edema,* Springer, Berlin, Heidelberg, New York, pp. 219–227.

Hossmann, K.-A. (1979) Cerebral dysfunction related to local and global ischemia of the brain. In: F. Hoffmeister and C. Müller (Eds.), *Brain Function in Old Age.* Springer, Berlin, Heidelberg, New York, pp. 385–393.

Hossmann, K.-A. (1982) Treatment of experimental cerebral ischemia. *J. Cereb. Blood Flow Metabol.,* 2: 275–297.

Hossmann, K.-A. and Hossmann, V. (1977) Coagulopathy fol-

lowing experimental cerebral ischemia. *Stroke,* 8: 249–254.
Hossmann, K.-A. and Sato, K. (1970a) The effect of ischemia on sensorimotor cortex of cat. Electrophysiological, biochemical and electronmicroscopical observations. *Z. Neurol.,* 198: 33–45.
Hossmann, K.-A. and Sato, K. (1970b) Recovery of neuronal function after prolonged cerebral ischemia. *Science,* 168: 375–376.
Hossmann, K.-A. and Takagi, S. (1976) Osmolality of brain in cerebral ischemia. *Exp. Neurol.,* 51: 124–131.
Hossmann, K.-A. and Zimmermann, V. (1974) Resuscitation of the monkey brain after 1 hour complete ischemia. I. Physiological and morphological observations. *Brain Res.,* 81: 59–74.
Hossmann, K.-A., Lechtape-Grüter, H. and Hossmann, V. (1973) The role of cerebral blood flow for the recovery of the brain after prolonged ischemia. *Z. Neurol.,* 204: 281–299.
Hossmann, K.-A., Sakaki, S. and Kimoto, K. (1976) Cerebral uptake of glucose and oxygen in the cat brain after prolonged ischemia. *Stroke,* 7: 301–305.
Hossmann, K.-A., Sakaki, S. and Zimmermann, V. (1977) Cation activities in reversible ischemia of the cat brain. *Stroke,* 8: 77–81.
Hossmann, K.-A., Paschen, W. and Csiba, L. (1983) Relationship between calcium accumulation and recovery of cat brain after prolonged cerebral ischemia. *J. Cereb. Blood Flow Metabol.,* 3: 346–353.
Hossmann, V. and Hossmann, K.-A. (1973) Return of neuronal functions after prolonged cardiac arrest. *Brain Res.,* 60: 423–438.
Ikrényi, K., Dóra, E., Hajós, F. and Kovách, A.G.B. (1976) Metabolic and electron microscopic studies post mortem in brain mitochondria. *Adv. Exp. Med. Biol.,* 75: 159–164.
Ito, U., Spatz, M., Walker, J.T., Jr. and Klatzo, I. (1975) Experimental cerebral ischemia in mongolian gerbils. I. Light microscopic observations. *Acta Neuropathol.,* 32: 209–223.
Ito, U., Go, K.G., Walker, J.T., Jr., Spatz, M. and Klatzo, I. (1976) Experimental cerebral ischemia in mongolian gerbils. III. Behaviour of the blood-brain barrier. *Acta Neuropathol.,* 34: 1–6.
Kågström, E., Smith, M.-L. and Siesjö, B.K. (1983) Local cerebral blood flow in the recovery period following complete ischemia in the rat. *J. Cereb. Blood Flow Metabol.,* 3: 170–182.
Kirino, T. (1982) Delayed neuronal death in the gerbil hippocampus following ischemia. *Brain Res.,* 239: 57–69.
Kirino, T., Tamura, A. and Sano, K. (1985) Selective vulnerability of the hippocampus to ischemia — reversible and irreversible types of ischemic cell damage. *This volume,* pp. 39–58.
Kleihues, P. and Hossmann, K.-A. (1971) Protein synthesis in the cat brain after prolonged cerebral ischemia. *Brain Res.,* 35: 409–418.
Kleihues, P. and Hossmann, K.-A. (1973) Regional incorporation of L-(3-^{3}H)-tyrosine into cat brain proteins after 1 hour of complete ischemia. *Acta Neuropathol.,* 25: 313–324.
Kleihues, P., Hossmann, K.-A., Pegg, A.E., Kobayashi, K. and Zimmermann, V. (1975) Resuscitation of the monkey brain after 1 hour complete ischemia. III. Indications of metabolic recovery. *Brain Res.,* 95: 61–73.
Kolata, R.J. (1979) Survival of rabbits after prolonged cerebral ischemia. *Stroke,* 10: 272–277.
Levy, D.E. and Duffy, T.E. (1977) Cerebral energy metabolism during transient ischemia and recovery in the gerbil. *J. Neurochem.,* 28: 63–70.
Levy, D.E., Brierley, J.B. and Plum, F. (1975) Ischaemic brain damage in the gerbil in the absence of "no-reflow". *J. Neurol. Neurosurg. Psychiat.,* 38: 1197–1205.
Levy, D.E., Pike, R.L. and Uitert, R.L. (1978) Delayed dissociation of cerebral blood flow and metabolism following stroke in gerbils. *Neurology,* 28: 378–379.
Ljunggren, B., Schutz, H. and Siesjö, B.K. (1974) Changes in the energy state and acid-base parameters of the rat brain during complete compression ischemia. *Brain Res.,* 73: 277–289.
Makarenko, N.V. (1972) Higher nervous activity in dogs revived following prolonged terms of clinical death from drowning or bloodletting. *Zh. Vyssh. Nervn. Deyat.,* 22: 82–88.
Marshall, L.F., Welsh, F., Durity, F., Lounsbury, R., Graham, D.I. and Langfitt, T.W. (1975) Experimental cerebral oligemia and ischemia produced by intracranial hypertension. Part 3. Brain energy metabolism. *J. Neurosurg.,* 43: 323–328.
Mies, G., Paschen, W., Hossmann, K.-A. and Klatzo, I. (1983) Simultaneous measurement of regional blood flow and metabolism during maturation of hippocampal lesions following short-lasting cerebral ischemia in gerbils. *J. Cereb. Blood Flow Metabol.,* 3, Suppl. 1: S329–330.
Miller, C.L., Lampard, D.G., Alexander, K. and Brown, W.A. (1980) Local cerebral blood flow following transient cerebral ischemia. I. Onset of impaired reperfusion within the first hour following global ischemia. *Stroke,* 11: 534–541.
Miller, J.R. and Myers, R.E. (1970) Neurological effects of systemic circulatory arrest in the monkey. *Neurology,* 20: 715–724.
Morimoto, K. and Yanagihara, T. (1981) Cerebral ischemia in gerbils: Polyribosomal function during progression and recovery. *Stroke,* 12: 105–110.
Myers, R.E. and Yamaguchi, M. (1976) Effects of serum glucose concentration on brain response to circulatory arrest. *J. Neuropathol. Exp. Neurol.,* 35: 301.
Naruse, S., Horikawa, Y., Tanaka, C., Hirakawa, K., Nishikawa, H. and Watari, H. (1984) In vivo measurement of energy metabolism and the concomitant monitoring of electroencephalogram in experimental cerebral ischemia. *Brain Res.,* 296: 370–372.
Nemoto, E.M., Snyder, J.V., Carroll, R.G. and Morita, H. (1975) Global ischemia in dogs: Cerebrovascular CO_2 reactivity and autoregulation. *Stroke,* 6: 425–431.

Nemoto, E.M., Bleyaert, A.L., Stezoski, S.W., Moossy, J., Rao, G.R. and Safar, P. (1977) Global brain ischemia. A reproducible monkey model. *Stroke*, 8: 558–564.

Nemoto, E.M., Hossmann, K.-A. and Cooper, H.K. (1981) Postischemic hypermetabolism in cat brain. *Stroke*, 12: 666–676.

Nemoto, E.M., Shiu, G.K., Nemmer, J.P. and Bleyaert, A.L. (1983) Free fatty acid accumulation in the pathogenesis and therapy of ischemic-anoxic brain injury. *Am. J. Emerg. Med.*, 2: 175–179.

Nicholls, D.G. (1985) A role for the mitochondrion in the protection of cells against calcium overload? *This volume*, pp. 97–106.

Nordström, C.-H., Rehncrona, S. and Siesjö, B.K. (1976) Restitution of cerebral energy state after complete and incomplete ischemia of 30 min duration. *Acta Physiol. Scand.*, 97: 270–272.

Nordström, C.-H., Rehncrona, S. and Siesjö, B.K. (1978) Restitution of cerebral energy state, as well as of glycolytic metabolites, citric acid cycle intermediates and associated amino acids after 30 minutes of complete ischemia in rats anesthetized with nitrous oxide or phenobarbital. *J. Neurochem.*, 30: 479–486.

Okada, Y. (1974) Recovery of neuronal activity and high-energy compound level after complete and prolonged brain ischemia. *Brain Res.*, 72: 346–349.

Paschen, W., Hossmann, K.-A. and van den Kerckhoff, W. (1983a) Regional assessment of energy-producing metabolism following prolonged complete ischemia of cat brain. *J. Cereb. Blood Flow. Metabol.*, 3: 321–329.

Paschen, W., Djuricic, B.M., Bosma, H.-J. and Hossmann, K.-A. (1983b) Biochemical changes during graded ischemia in gerbils. Part 2. Regional evaluation of cerebral blood flow and brain metabolites. *J. Neurol. Sci.*, 58: 37–44.

Petito, C.K., Pulsinelli, W.A., Jacobson, G. and Plum, F. (1982) Edema and vascular permeability in cerebral ischemia: comparison between ischemic neuronal damage and infarction. *J. Neuropathol. Exp. Neurol.*, 41: 423–436.

Pulsinelli, W.A. (1985a) Deafferentiation of the hippocampus protects CA_1 pyramidal neurons against ischemic injury. *Stroke*, 16: 144.

Pulsinelli, W.A. (1985b) Selective neuronal vulnerability: morphological and molecular characteristics. *This volume*, pp. 29–37.

Pulsinelli, W.A. and Duffy, T.E. (1983) Regional energy balance in rat brain after transient forebrain ischemia. *J. Neurochem.*, 40: 1500–1503.

Pulsinelli, W.A., Plum, F. and Brierley, J.B. (1979) Barbiturate exacerbation of ischemic brain damage following bilateral hemispheric ischemia in the rat. *Ann. Neurol.*, 6: 156.

Pulsinelli, W.A., Brierley, J.B. and Plum, F. (1982a) Temporal profile of neuronal damage in a model of transient forebrain ischemia. *Ann. Neurol.*, 11: 491–498.

Pulsinelli, W.A., Levy, D.E. and Duffy, T.E. (1982b) Regional cerebral blood flow and glucose metabolism following transient forebrain ischemia. *Ann. Neurol.*, 11: 499–509.

Pulsinelli, W.A., Waldman, St., Rawlinson, D. and Plum, F. (1982c) Moderate hyperglycemia augments ischemic brain damage: a neuropathologic study in the rat. *Neurology (N.Y.)*, 32: 1239–1246.

Rehncrona, S., Mela, L. and Siesjö, B.K. (1979) Recovery of brain mitochondrial function in the rat after complete and incomplete cerebral ischemia. *Stroke*, 10: 437–446.

Safar, P., Stezoski, W. and Nemoto, E.M. (1976) Amelioration of brain damage after 12 minutes' cardiac arrest in dogs. *Arch. Neurol.*, 33: 91–95.

Schmid-Schönbein, H. (1977) Microrheology of erythrocytes and thrombocytes, blood viscosity and the distribution of blood flow in the microcirculation. In: H.-W. Altmann, F. Büchner, H. Cottier et al. (Eds), *Handbuch der Allgemeinen Pathology III/7: Mikrozirkulation*. Springer, Berlin, Heidelberg, New York, pp. 289–384.

Siemkowicz, E. (1980) Cerebrovascular resistance in ischemia. *Pflügers Arch.*, 388: 243–247.

Siemkowicz, E. and Hansen, A.J. (1978) Clinical restitution following cerebral ischemia in hypo-, normo- and hyperglycemic rats. *Acta Neurol. Scand.*, 58: 1–8.

Siemkowicz, E., Hansen, A.J. and Gjedde, A. (1982) Hyperglycemic ischemia of rat brain: the effect of post-ischemic insulin on metabolic rate. *Brain Res.*, 243: 386–390.

Siesjö, B.K. (1981) Cell damage in the brain: a speculative synthesis. *J. Cereb. Blood Flow Metabol.*, 1: 155–185.

Siesjö, B.K. (1985) Acid-base homeostasis in the brain: physiology, chemistry, and neurochemical pathology. *This volume*, pp. 121–154.

Simon, R.P., Swan, J.H., Griffith, T. and Meldrum, B.S. (1984a) Pharmacological blockade of excitatory amino acid neurotransmission attenuates the neuropathological damage of ischemia. *Ann. Neurol.*, 16: 112.

Simon, R.P., Griffiths, T., Evans, M.C., Swan, J.H. and Meldrum, B.S. (1984b) Calcium overload in selectively vulnerable neurons of the hippocampus during and after ischemia: an electron microscopy study in the rat. *J. Cereb. Blood Flow Metabol.*, 4: 350–361.

Sobotka, P. and Gebert, E. (1971) The effect of local application of strychnine and acetylcholine on the brain cortex after complete ischemia. *Pflügers Arch.*, 326: 142–151.

Suzuki, R., Yamaguchi, T., Kirino, T., Orzi, F. and Klatzo, I. (1983a) The effects of 5-minute ischemia in Mongolian gerbils. I. Blood-brain barrier, cerebral blood flow, and local cerebral glucose utilization changes. *Acta Neuropathol.*, 60: 207–216.

Suzuki, R., Yamaguchi, T., Li, C.-L. and Klatzo, I. (1983b) The effects of 5-minute ischemia in Mongolian gerbils. II. Changes of spontaneous neuronal activity in cerebral cortex and CA1 sector of hippocampus. *Acta Neuropathol.*, 60: 217–222.

Suzuki, R., Yamaguchi, T., Inaba, Y. and Wagner, H.G. (1985) Microphysiology of selectively vulnerable neurons. *This volume*, pp. 59–86.

Steen, P.A., Newberg, L.A., Milde, J.H. and Michenfelder, J.D. (1983) Nimodipine improves cerebral blood flow and neurologic recovery after complete cerebral ischemia in the dog. *J. Cereb. Blood Flow Metabol.,* 3: 38–43.

Takagi, S., Cocito, L. and Hossmann, K.-A. (1977) Blood recirculation and pharmacological responsiveness of the cerebral vasculature following prolonged ischemia of cat brain. *Stroke,* 8: 707–712.

Ten Cate, J. and Horsten, G.P.M. (1952) Sur l'influence de la ligature temporaire de l'aorte sur l'activité électrique de l'écorce cérébrale. *Arch. Int. Physiol.,* 60: 441–448.

Todd, M.M., Chadwick, H.S., Shapiro, H.M., Dunlop, B.J., Marshall, L.F. and Dueck, R. (1982) The neurologic effects of thiopental therapy following experimental cardiac arrest in cats. *Anesthesiology,* 57: 76–86.

Van den Kerckhoff, W., Hossmann, K.-A. and Hossmann, V. (1983) No effect of prostacyclin on blood flow, regulation of blood flow and blood coagulation following global cerebral ischemia. *Stroke,* 14: 724–730.

Van Harreveld, A. (1970) A mechanism for fluid shifts specific for the central nervous system. In: H.T. Wycis (Ed.), *Current Research in Neurosciences. Topical Probl. Psychiat. Neurol., Vol. 10.* Karger, Basel, New York, pp. 62–70.

Volpe, B.T., Pulsinelli, W.A., Tribuna, J. and Davis, H.P. (1984) Behavioral performance of rats following transient forebrain ischemia. *Stroke,* 15: 558–562.

Von Lubitz, D.K.J.E. and Diemer, N.H. (1983) Cerebral ischemia in the rat: ultrastructural and morphometric analysis of synapses in stratum radiatum of the hippocampal CA-1 region. *Acta Neuropathol.,* 61: 52–60.

Watson, B.D., Busto, R. and Goldberg, W.J. (1983) Direct evidence for lipid peroxidation induced by reversible global ischemia in rat brain. *Stroke,* 14: 127.

Watson, B.D., Busto, R., goldberg, W.J., Santiso, M., Yoshida, S. and Ginsberg, M.D. (1984) Lipid peroxidation in vivo induced by reversible global ischemia in rat brain. *J. Neurochem.,* 42: 268–274.

Welsh, F.A. and O'Connor, M.J. (1978) Patterns of microcirculatory failure during incomplete cerebral ischemia. *Adv. Neurol.,* 20: 133–139.

Welsh, F.A., O'Connor, M.J., Marcy, V.R., Spatacco, A.J. and Johns, R.L. (1982) Factors limiting regeneration of ATP following temporary ischemia in cat brain. *Stroke,* 13: 234–242.

White, B.C., Gadzinski, D.S., Hoehner, P.J. et al. (1982) Effect of flunarizine on canine cerebral cortical blood flow and vascular resistance post cardiac arrest. *Ann. Emerg. Med.,* 11: 119–126.

White, B.C., Winegar, C.P., Henderson, O. et al. (1983) Prolonged hypoperfusion in the cerebral cortex following cardiac arrest and resuscitation in dogs. *Ann. Emerg. Med.,* 12: 414–417.

Wieloch, T. (1985) Neurochemical correlates to selective neuronal vulnerability. *This volume,* pp. 69–85.

Wieloch, T., Lindvall, O., Blomquist, P and Gage, F. (1985) Evidence for amelioration of ischemic neuronal damage in the hippocampal formation by lesions of the perforant path. *Neurol. Res.,* in press.

Yanagihara, T. (1976) Cerebral ischemia in gerbils: differential vulnerability of protein, RNA and lipid syntheses. *Stroke,* 7: 260–263.

Yanagihara, R. and McCall, J.T. (1982) Ionic shift in cerebral ischemia. *Life Sci.,* 30: 1921–1925.

Yoshida, S., Abe, K., Busto, R., Watson, B.D., Kogure, K. and Ginsberg, M.D. (1982) Influence of transient ischemia on lipid-soluble anti-oxidants, free fatty acids and energy metabolites in rat brain. *Brain Res.,* 245: 307–316.

Zimmermann, V., Hossmann, V. and Hossmann, K.-A. (1975) Intracranial pressure after prolonged cerebral ischemia. In: N. Lundberg, U. Pontén and M. Brock (Eds.), *Intracranial Pressure II.* Springer, Berlin, Heidelberg, New York, pp. 177–182.

reperfusion impairments may strongly exacerbate ischemic injury. However, if care is taken to optimize the physiologic state during recirculation, then it appears that no-reflow is uncommon, even following prolonged periods of ischemia (Hossmann et al., 1973).

Others have argued that since a significant degree of tissue damage is sustained in the absence of impaired reperfusion, no-reflow is an epiphenomenon, occurring only in supra-maximal insults (Levy et al., 1975). Thus, ischemic neuronal damage has been demonstrated in several models which do not exhibit no-reflow (Levy et al., 1975; Marshall et al., 1975; Ginsberg et al., 1978; Pulsinelli et al., 1982a,b). While not disputing these results, it is clear that optimal reperfusion is required to minimize the degree of ischemic injury and neurologic dysfunction. Therefore, it is important to define the factors which may contribute to reperfusion deficits.

It may be helpful first to distinguish between (a) absolute failure to reperfuse following an ischemic interval and (b) transient reperfusion. Thus, Kågström et al. (1983a) described unequivocal "no-reflow" at 5 min of recirculation following 10–15 min of complete compression ischemia in the rat, despite immediate normalization of cerebral perfusion pressure. By 60 min of recirculation, however, flow had returned throughout the brain, indicating that the perfusion defects present at 5 min had been resolved. By contrast, extending the duration of compression ischemia to 30 min caused reperfusion defects which were observed at 30 min and 90 min of recirculation. Therefore, it is likely that these areas of no-reflow represent regions in which perfusion was never re-established. However, it is apparent that the duration of ischemia must exceed 15 min before reflow was permanently impaired.

These results are similar to those reported for cat brain following 15 min or 30 min of severe oligemia (Ginsberg et al., 1978). Thus, impaired reperfusion, measured at 90 min of recirculation, occurred following ischemia of 30 min, but not 15 min duration. However, regional levels of NADH, measured in animals subjected to 30 min of oligemia and 90 min recirculation, indicated that reperfusion had occurred to some degree (Welsh et al., 1978a). NADH levels will remain high for many hours as long as there is no delivery of oxygen to the tissue. Therefore, regions which fail to reflow will exhibit high levels of NADH and, thus, are easily detectable in sections of frozen brain using NADH fluorometry. Areas exhibiting the high levels of NADH characteristic of no-reflow were not detected in postischemic cat brain (Welsh et al., 1978a, 1980, 1982a). Rather, areas with impaired recovery of high energy phosphates typically contained a normal content of NADH, while the tissue sections exhibited a diminution of NADH fluorescence in the regions with energy failure (Fig. 5). Therefore, following 30 min of severe oligemia in cat brain, regions showing impaired flow and metabolite levels must have undergone reperfusion to some degree.

Because of the regional variation of postischemic reperfusion, it is helpful to employ methods capable of serial measurements of local blood flow. Using the hydrogen clearance method we investigated re-

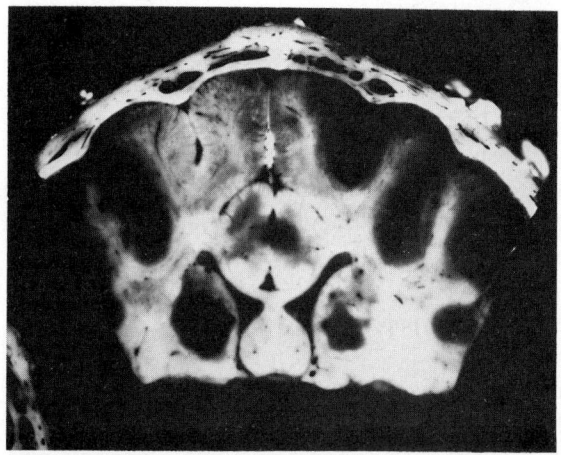

Fig. 5. Focal diminution of NADH fluorescence during postischemic recirculation. Severe cerebral oligemia in cat brain was produced using simultaneous occlusion of the basilar and common carotid arteries and arterial hemorrhage to a mean pressure of 80 mm Hg. After a 15-min insult, the brain was reperfused for 90 min and frozen in situ using liquid nitrogen. The brain was sectioned and fluoresced for NADH at low temperature. Regions exhibiting diminished NADH contained the lowest concentrations of ATP and phosphocreatine. (Data modified from Welsh et al., 1980.)

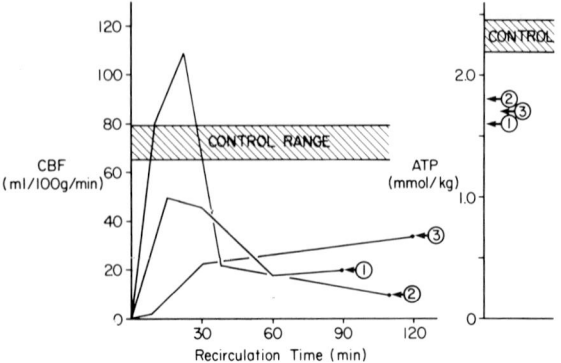

Fig. 6. Recovery of postischemic blood flow. Local cerebral blood flow (CBF) was measured in cerebral cortex using hydrogen electrodes during recirculation from 30 min of tourniquet-induced ischemia in cat brain. Each line (1–3) represents a single electrode in a separate animal. At 120 min, the brains were frozen in situ and samples adjacent to the electrode were analyzed for ATP content. (Data from Marcy and Welsh, 1984.)

covery of blood flow following severe oligemia in cat brain (Marcy and Welsh, 1984). Following an insult of 30 min duration, restoration of blood flow occurred in all cases, although in some instances there was a delay of 5–10 min (Fig. 6). However, following longer periods of ischemia (60 min), blood flow either did not resume or returned only briefly before subsiding again to immeasurable levels. Interestingly, reflow failure following a 60-min insult could be prevented by prior craniectomy, suggesting that increased intracranial pressure may be a major factor limiting postischemic restoration of cerebral blood flow.

Secondary hypoperfusion

In many experimental models of temporary cerebral ischemia, recirculation is initially characterized by a brief period of hyperemia, but is then followed by a reduction of blood flow, sometimes to levels below 50% of control. The central question is: does this secondary reduction in flow contribute in any way to the genesis of ischemic injury? Alternatively, the hypoperfusion may be a consequence of the re-establishment of the normal coupling between flow and metabolism, the rate of metabolism being lower than normal. The distinction between these possi-

bilities is not easily made. To evaluate the adequacy of perfusion, both the rate of blood flow and the rate of energy metabolism is required. In addition, since the energy state of the tissue is a sensitive index of the balance between flow and metabolism, it is useful to determine the levels of high energy phosphates and lactate. A further complication results from regional heterogeneities in flow, metabolism, and tissue energy state during the postischemic period. Thus, it is essential to measure these variables using regional methods if meaningful results are to be obtained.

In a study of the effects of severe oligemia in cat brain, Ginsberg et al. (1978) reported that regional blood flow, measured after 90 min of recirculation following 15 min of ischemia, ranged from 22% of control in the mid-suprasylvian gyrus of cerebral cortex to 45% of normal in the caudate nucleus. Examination of the flow autoradiograms failed to reveal any foci of no-reflow following the 15-min insult. In a parallel series of animals, perfusion-fixed for neuropathologic assessment, the distribution of neurons showing ischemic alteration was rather diffuse (Ginsberg et al., 1979). Curiously, the degree of histopathologic alteration was slightly diminished in the mid-suprasylvian gyrus, relative to adjacent regions with greater amounts of blood flow. Thus, there was no evidence to indicate that the degree of histopathologic change correlated with the extent of postischemic hypoperfusion. Furthermore, tissue levels of ATP and phosphocreatine were restored nearly to normal in all regions analyzed in spite of the large reductions in postischemic blood flow (Welsh et al., 1978a). However, that levels of lactate and NADH remained elevated may be an indication that the level of reperfusion was not optimal.

More recently, Pulsinelli and coworkers investigated a model of severe forebrain ischemia in the rat (Pulsinelli and Brierley, 1979) and they have characterized the neuropathology (Pulsinelli et al., 1982a), regional flow and glucose metabolism (Pulsinelli et al., 1982b), and regional metabolite levels (Pulsinelli and Duffy, 1983). Following a 30-min insult, there was an initial hyperemia, but blood flow subsided by 30 min to 35% of normal in parietal cortex, 40% in striatum, 45% in hippocampus, and 50% in the diencephalon. Areas of no-reflow were not detected, although a recent report by Kågström et al. (1983b) noted the presence of perfusion deficits at 5 min of recirculation. Therefore, in this model, reperfusion may be delayed briefly in circumscribed regions. The duration of secondary hypoperfusion, noted above, varied from 3 h to 48 h in striatum and parietal cortex, respectively. By 48 h postischemia, blood flow was normal or above in all regions quantitated. Interestingly, hyperemia was present at 48 h in the striatum and hippocampus, regions in which histologic injury was most pronounced. Thus, the distribution of histopathology correlated with focal *hyper*-perfusion, rather than hypoperfusion. Further, during the early stages of recirculation (30 min), there was no correlation between the degree of hypoperfusion and regions in which neuronal injury ultimately occurred.

In this same model, the rate of energy metabolism was estimated using the deoxyglucose autoradiographic method. Generally, the metabolic rate was depressed in all structures during postischemic recirculation, although not to the same degree as blood flow. Thus, the ratio of flow to metabolism decreased toward the ischemic range in many regions. However, there was again no apparent correlation between the flow/metabolism ratio and the eventual appearance of histopathology. Further, the recovery of tissue levels of high energy phosphates and of lactate during the early stages of recirculation indicated that the level of perfusion was adequate for the metabolic demands of the tissue (Pulsinelli and Duffy, 1983). Thus it appears that the metabolic rate was sufficiently low to permit normalization of tissue metabolites in spite of the reduction in blood flow. However, it is conceivable that this degree of hypoperfusion might contribute to the injury of individual neurons. Measurement of tissue metabolites in samples several mg in weight would not detect changes occurring in a small fraction of the tissue. There are also uncertainties in the interpretation of the deoxyglucose method for estimating metabolic rate in damaged brain. However, in the model of forebrain ischemia, oxygen utilization was lower than normal during postischemic recirculation, thus supporting the finding of decreased glucose consumption (Pulsinelli et al., 1982b). Nevertheless, quantitation of alterations in metabolic rate, as determined with the deoxyglucose method, should be considered provisional.

Kågström et al. (1983b) also investigated the recovery of regional flow following forebrain ischemia in the rat. Recirculation for 90 min following a 15-min insult produced hypoperfusion of all brain structures analyzed, although the levels of flow ranged from 22% of control in cerebral cortex to 73% of control in substantia nigra. Again, there was no obvious association between regions with lower flows and "vulnerable" regions such as striatum and hippocampus, in which histopathologic change is most pronounced. Thus, in these models of severe cerebral oligemia, there is little evidence to indicate that secondary hypoperfusion contributes significantly to histologic injury.

One of the technical limitations inherent in many studies of ischemia is the necessity of using separate animals for measurements of flow, metabolism, and histopathology. Even the most reproducible experimental models are not without individual variability, which may obscure all but the most obvious correlations. Thus, we have attempted to use methods in which flow and metabolic state can be determined in the same region of the same animal in order to obtain a more direct correlation between these variables. Employing a cranial window to monitor cortical perfusion and NADH fluorescence, we reported a decline in the rate of formation of NADH early in postischemic recirculation period, at a time prior to the onset of secondary hypoperfusion (Welsh et al., 1982a). These results, along with the finding that there was a 40% decrease in the total pool of $NADH + NAD^+$, led us to speculate that there was a primary impairment in the metabolism of NADH and that the perfusion failure occurred secondarily. In a second series of experiments, we used the hydrogen clearance method in combination with metabolite measurements in samples adjacent to the hydrogen electrode (Marcy and Welsh, 1984). During recirculation from 30 min of cerebral ischemia, the initial restoration of cortical flow was followed by pronounced hypoperfusion to as low as 14% of control values (Fig. 6). However, this reduction in flow did not grossly compromise restoration of ATP levels in the tissue. Finally, in a model of unilateral hypoxia-ischemia in mouse brain, we measured the uptake of a diffusible flow tracer and the content of ATP in the same tissue sample (Welsh et al., 1983). At 15 min of recovery, there was a poor correlation between blood flow and ATP levels. Indeed, in one group of animals, regions with lower levels of ATP had higher blood flow. Thus, using combined measurements of blood flow and metabolite levels in several postischemic settings, we have been unable to obtain convincing evidence that secondary hypoperfusion plays a causative role in the irreversible failure of energy metabolism.

References

Adams, J.H., Brierley, J.B., Connor, R.C.R. and Treip, C.S. (1966) The effects of systemic hypotension upon the human brain. *Brain*, 89: 235–268.

Ames, A., III, Wright, R.L., Kowada, M., Thurston, J.M. and Majno, G. (1968) Cerebral ischemia. II. The no-reflow phenomenon. *Am. J. Pathol.*, 52: 437–453.

Brierley, J.B. and Excell, B.J. (1966) The effects of profound systemic hypotension upon the brain of *M. Rhesus*. Physiological and pathological observations. *Brain*, 89: 269–298.

Brierley, J.B., Brown, A.W., Excell, B.J. and Meldrum, B.S. (1969) Brain damage in the Rhesus monkey resulting from profound arterial hypotension. I. Its nature, distribution and general physiological correlates. *Brain Res.*, 13: 68–100.

Craigie, E.H. (1945) The architecture of the cerebral capillary bed. *Biol. Reviews*, 20: 133–146.

Folbergrová, J., Lowry, O.H. and Passonneau, J.V. (1970) Changes in metabolites of energy reserves in individual layers of mouse cerebral cortex and subadjacent white matter during ischemia and anesthesia. *J. Neurochem.*, 17: 1155–1162.

Gatfield, P.D., Lowry, O.H., Schultz, D.W. and Passonneau, J.V. (1966) Regional energy reserves in mouse brain and changes with ischemia and anesthesia. *J. Neurochem.*, 13: 185–195.

Ginsberg, M.D., Reivich, M., Giandomenico, A. and Greenberg, J.H. (1977) Local glucose utilization in acute focal cerebral ischemia: local dysmetabolism. *Neurology (Minneap.)*, 27: 1042–1048.

Ginsberg, M.D., Budd, W.W. and Welsh, F.A. (1978) Diffuse cerebral ischemia in the cat. I. Local blood flow during severe ischemia and recirculation. *Ann. Neurol.*, 3: 482–492.

Ginsberg, M.D., Graham, D.I., Welsh, F.A. and Budd, W.W. (1979) Diffuse cerebral ischemia in the cat. III. Neuropathological sequelae of severe ischemia. *Ann. Neurol.*, 5: 350–358.

Hossmann, K.-A., Lechtape-Grüter, H. and Hossmann, V. (1973) The role of cerebral blood flow for the recovery of the brain after prolonged ischemia. *Z. Neurol.*, 204: 281–299.

Kågström, E., Smith, M.-L. and Siesjö, B.K. (1983a) Local cerebral blood flow in the recovery period following complete cerebral ischemia in the rat. *J. Cereb. Blood Flow Metabol.*, 3: 170–182.

Kågström, E., Smith, M.-L. and Siesjö, B.K. (1983b) Recirculation of the rat brain following incomplete ischemia. *J. Cereb. Blood Flow Metabol.*, 3: 183–192.

Kennedy, C., Des Rosiers, M.H., Sakurada, O. et al. (1976) Metabolic mapping of the primary visual system of the monkey by means of the autoradiographic [^{14}C]deoxyglucose technique. *Proc. Natl. Acad. Sci. (USA)*, 73: 4230–4234.

Lesnick, J.E., Michele, J.J., Simeone, F.A., DeFeo, S. and Welsh, F.A. (1984) Alteration of somatosensory evoked potentials in response to global ischemia. *J. Neurosurg.*, 60: 490–494.

Levy, D.E., Brierley, J.B. and Plum, F. (1975) Ischemic brain damage in the gerbil in the absence of "no-reflow". *J. Neurol. Neurosurg. Psychiat.*, 38: 1197–1205.

Marcy, V.R. and Welsh, F.A. (1984) Correlation between cerebral blood flow and ATP content following tourniquet-induced ischemia in cat brain. *J. Cereb. Blood Flow Metabol.*, 4: 362–367.

Marshall, L.F., Durity, F., Lounsbury, R., Graham, D.I., Welsh, F. and Langfitt, T.W. (1975) Experimental cerebral oligemia and ischemia produced by intracranial hypertension. Part 1: Pathophysiology, electroencephalography, cerebral blood flow, blood-brain barrier, and neurological function. *J. Neurosurg.*, 43: 308–317.

McIlwain, H. (1966) *Biochemistry and the Central Nervous System*, 3rd edn. Little, Brown and Company, Boston, p. 55.

Mueller, S.M., Heistad, D.D. and Marcus, M.L. (1977) Total and regional cerebral blood flow during hypotension, hypertension and hypocapnia. *Circ. Res.*, 41: 350–356.

Paschen, W., Hossmann, K.-A. and van den Kerckhoff, W. (1983) Regional assessment of energy-producing metabolism following prolonged complete ischemia of cat brain. *J. Cereb. Blood Flow Metabol.*, 3: 321–329.

Pasztor, E., Symon, L., Dorsch, N.W.C. and Branston, N.M.

(1973) The hydrogen clearance method in assessment of blood flow in cortex, white matter and deep nuclei of baboons. *Stroke*, 4: 556–567.

Pulsinelli, W.A. and Brierley, J.B. (1979) A new model of bilateral hemispheric ischemia in the unanesthetized rat. *Stroke*, 10: 267–272.

Pulsinelli, W.A. and Duffy, T.E. (1983) Regional energy balance in rat brain after transient forebrain ischemia. *J. Neurochem.*, 40: 1500–1503.

Pulsinelli, W.A., Brierley, J.B. and Plum, F. (1982a) Temporal profile of neuronal damage in a model of transient forebrain ischemia. *Ann. Neurol.*, 11: 491–498.

Pulsinelli, W.A., Levy, D.E. and Duffy, T.E. (1982b) Regional cerebral blood flow and glucose metabolism following transient forebrain ischemia. *Ann. Neurol.*, 11: 499–509.

Reivich, M., Jehle, J., Sokoloff, L. and Kety, S.S. (1969) Measurement of regional cerebral blood flow with antipyrine-C^{14} in awake cats. *J. Appl. Physiol.*, 27: 296–300.

Rice, J.E., Vannucci, R.C. and Brierley, J.B. (1981) The influence of immaturity on hypoxic-ischemic brain damage in the rat. *Ann. Neurol.*, 9: 131–141.

Sokoloff, L., Reivich, M., Kennedy, C et al. (1977) The ^{14}C-deoxyglucose method for the measurement of local cerebral glucose utilization: theory, procedure, and normal values in the conscious and anesthetized albino rat. *J. Neurochem.*, 28: 897–916.

Welsh, F.A. and O'Connor, M.J. (1978) Patterns of microcirculatory failure during incomplete cerebral ischemia. *Advances in Neurol.*, 20: 133–139.

Welsh, F.A., Durity, F. and Langfitt, T.W. (1977) The appearance of regional variations in metabolism at a critical level of cerebral oligemia. *J. Neurochem.*, 28: 71–79.

Welsh, F.A., Ginsberg, M.D., Rieder, W. and Budd, W.W. (1978a) Diffuse cerebral ischemia in the cat: II. Regional metabolites during severe ischemia and recirculation. *Ann. Neurol.*, 3: 493–501.

Welsh, F.A., O'Connor, M.J. and Marcy, V.R. (1978b) Effect of oligemia on regional metabolite levels in cat brain. *J. Neurochem.*, 31: 311–319.

Welsh, F.A., Ginsberg, M.D., Rieder, W. and Budd, W.W. (1980) Deleterious effect of glucose pretreatment on recovery from diffuse cerebral ischemia in the cat. II. Regional metabolite levels. *Stroke*, 11: 355–363.

Welsh, F.A., O'Connor, M.J., Marcy, V.R., Spatacco, A.J. and Johns, R.L. (1982a) Factors limiting regeneration of ATP following temporary ischemia in cat brain. *Stroke*, 13: 234–242.

Welsh, F.A., Vannucci, R.C. and Brierley, J.B. (1982b) Columnar alterations of NADH fluorescence during hypoxia-ischemia in immature rat brain. *J. Cereb. Blood Flow Metabol.*, 2: 221–228.

Welsh, F.A., Sims, R.E. and McKee, A.E. (1983) Effect of glucose on recovery of energy metabolism following hypoxia-oligemia in mouse brain: dose-dependence and carbohydrate specificity. *J. Cereb. Blood Flow Metabol.*, 3: 486–492.

Wolf, A. and Siris, J. (1937) Acute non-traumatic encephalomalacia complicating neurosurgical operations in the sitting position. *Bull. Neurol. Inst. N.Y.*, 6: 42–61.

Zülch, K.J. (1953) Neue Befunde und Deutungen aus der Gefässpathologie des Hirns und Rückenmarks. *Zentralbl. Allg. Pathol. Pathol. Anat.*, 90: 402.

Selective neuronal vulnerability: morphological and molecular characteristics*

William A. Pulsinelli

Cerebrovascular Disease Research Center and Department of Neurology, Cornell University Medical College, 1300 York Avenue, New York, NY 10021, USA

Historical introduction

Twenty-five years ago, a group of 34 international experts met in Baden, FRG to discuss "Selective Vulnerability of the Brain in Hypoxemia" (Schadé and McMenemy, 1963). The Chairmens' opening remarks for that conference indicate that the prevailing views on the pathogenesis of selective neuronal vulnerability were still in the "Gestalt" stage (Haymaker and McMenemy, 1963). Substantial progress has been made in uncovering the mechanisms of ischemic brain injury during the past two decades, but more importantly very recent results, some of which will be reported at this meeting, give promise that the next 5 years will be an exciting period in this clinically important area of brain research.

A large proportion of the 1961 meeting in Baden was dedicated to defining the morphological characteristics of ischemic damage to the brain. It is fitting, therefore, that this symposium begin with a review of the characteristics and definitions of the various types of ischemic brain injury. It is crucial that we keep constant sight of these neuropathological patterns as we discuss the underlying molecular mechanisms of ischemic brain damage. In keeping with this theme, the goals of this presentation are two-fold: first to define the distinct morphological patterns of ischemic brain injury and second to discuss possible pathogenesis of ischemic damage to selectively vulnerable brain neurons.

Historically, the notion that the brain could be easily damaged by relatively brief periods of hypoxia-ischemia was well known by the turn of the century. The work of individuals like Spielmeyer (1925), Meyer (1936), C. and O. Vogt (1937), and Scholz (1953) is responsible for the concept that specific brain regions may be more vulnerable to ischemic injury than others. Spielmeyer (1925) suggested that peculiarities of the local vascular supply facilitated vascular insufficiency to regions like hippocampus. In contrast, the Vogts (1937) hypothesized that the physico-chemical properties of specific neurons made them more susceptible to hypoxia-ischemia and for this they coined the term "topistic" lesions. Scholz (1953, 1963), in an attempt to unify these views, recapitulated the evidence which demonstrated that under specific pathophysiological conditions focal ischemic brain injury could be attributed primarily to the vascular peculiarities of the anatomy while under other conditions the pattern of brain damage could only be explained by the unique properties of the cells themselves.

Morphological patterns of ischemic brain damage

Vascular patterns

Boundary zone or watershed lesions (Meyer, 1953; Zülch, 1953) are the best examples of focal ischemic

---

* Presented at the Sendai Forum '84 on Cerebrovascular Accidents.

brain injury caused by the vascular anatomy. In such lesions, ischemic necrosis occurs in the watershed zones between major arterial territories and is best exemplified by infarction of the boundary zone between the anterior and middle cerebral arteries. Such boundary zone lesions typically occur in episodes of severe hypotension and have been reported in both clinical and experimental animal material (Brierley and Excell, 1966; Bricrley, 1977).

Micro-watershed lesions were reported by Rice et al. (1981) in immature rats subjected to unilateral common carotid artery ligation and simultaneous hypoxia. Animals treated in this manner developed collumnar zones of neuronal damage in the neocortex. The pathogenesis of these microlesions was thought to reflect micro-boundary zones between the arteries and veins which penetrate the neocortex in a highly organized perpendicular arrangement. Further evidence that this anatomical configuration will lead to gradations of tissue hypoxia with a collumnar geometry is evidenced by the collumnar pattern of tissue NADH fluorescence (Welsh et al., 1982) and 2-deoxyglucose metabolism (Pulsinelli and Duffy, 1979) seen in animals subjected to a similar hypoxic insult.

Topistic patterns

There are a variety of highly focal ischemic lesions of brain which are clearly independent of the vascular distribution and which can only be explained by the unique physical and chemical properties of the affected cells. Neurons are the most sensitive cells in brain followed in order by the oligodendroglia, astroglia, and finally endothelial cells (Jacob, 1963). This order of vulnerability is not specific for hypoxia-ischemia since it can be seen in various intoxications, in hyperthermia and in post-mortem brains undergoing autolysis (Jacob, 1963). The presence of ordered cell damage in post-mortem brain could be the result of agonal changes since Kalimo et al. (1977) report uniform disruptions of all brain cells with terminal ischemia in well-controlled experimental animal studies.

Among neurons there is a further hierarchy of susceptibility to ischemic injury (Brierley, 1977; Brown, 1977). The CA1 pyramidal cells in hippocampus and the cerebellar Purkinje cells appear to be the most highly vulnerable neurons in brain followed in order by striatal medium-sized neurons and then neocortical neurons in layers 3, 5, and 6. Within the hippocampus, cerebellum, striatum, and neocortex there is a further order of sensitivity to ischemia which is presented in Table 1. An example of selective neuronal necrosis is presented in Fig. 1 which demonstrates a normal-appearing large striatal neuron surrounded by irreversibly damaged small and medium-sized striatal neurons in a rat subjected to transient (30 min) forebrain ischemia and then survival for several days. This pattern of vulnerability to ischemia has been documented in a variety of experimental animal models (Brown, 1977) and also in conditions of human global ischemia (Graham, 1977).

Pathological definitions

The neuropathologists have defined at least three morphologically distinct varieties of ischemic brain damage which include autolysis, infarction, and selective neuronal necrosis (SNN). To this list a fourth pattern may be added which we will term

TABLE 1

	Order of neuronal vulnerability
Decreasing vulnerability	Hippocampus — CA1, CA4 > CA3 > granule cells Cerebellum — Purkinje > stellate and basket > granule > Golgi cells Striatum — small and medium-sized > large neurons Neocortex — layers 3,5,6, > layers 2,4

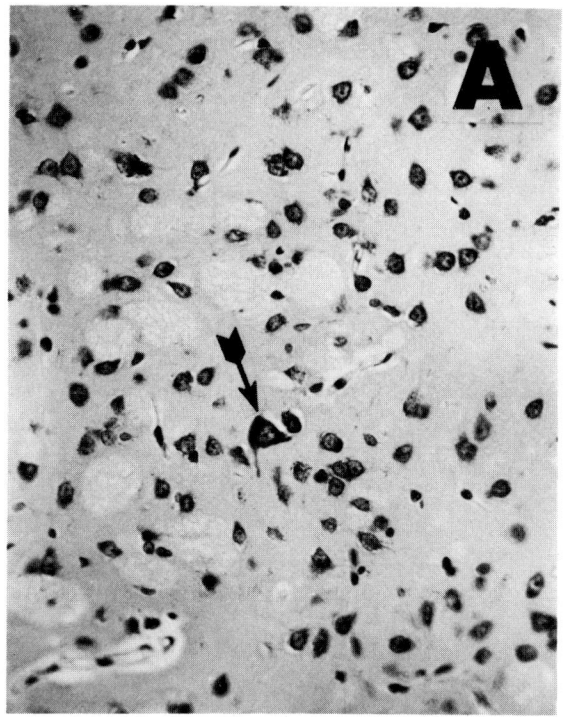 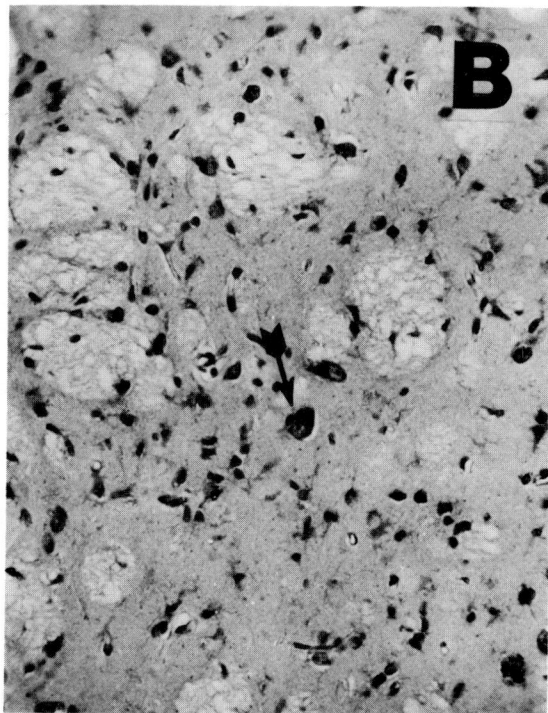

Fig. 1. Photomicrographs of normal rat striatum (A) and rat striatum taken from an animal at 7 days after 30 min of forebrain ischemia (B). The arrows point to normal large striatal neurons in both rats. Note the normal medium-sized neurons throughout the field in A and the shrunken damaged neurons throughout the field in B. (Data from Francis and Pulsinelli, 1982.)

generalized neuronal necrosis (GNN). Autolytic brain damage is characterized by chromatin clumping, mitochondrial swelling and dispersion of ribosomes uniformly throughout all brain cells (Kalimo et al., 1977). Such changes are the consequence of terminal ischemia of the brain without reperfusion and is seen in post-mortem brain tissue. Infarction has been defined by the neuropathologists as an area of pannecrosis, i.e. irreversible damage to all cell types, including astroglia and endothelial cells within a specific vascular territory of the brain. The transition zone between an area of cerebral infarction and entirely normal brain tissue frequently contains necrotic neurons but normal astroglia (Strong et al., 1983). Such border zone necrosis of neurons develops irrespective of the brain region and, therefore, differs from selective neuronal necrosis which occurs only in those populations of vulnerable neurons defined in Table 1.

The limitations on time and space do not allow for a detailed comparison of the factors involved in producing these different types of ischemic brain injury. However, we should bear in mind the distinct differences between cerebral infarction, general neuronal necrosis, and selective neuronal necrosis and consider the possibility that although all varieties of ischemic brain damage may share final common pathways of cell death, triggering mechanisms may differ for each of these entities. Since the topic of this specific session is "Selective Neuronal Vulnerability", the remainder of this presentation will focus on the pathogenesis of SNN.

Selective neuronal necrosis in the rat

Regional energy metabolism and selective neuronal necrosis

Severe but transient forebrain ischemia in rats for periods of 10–30 min results in ischemic damage to the highly sensitive neurons in the hippocampus (pyramidal cells in zones CA1 and CA3), to small and medium-sized striatal neurons and to neocortical neurons in layers 3, 5, and 6 (Pulsinelli and Brierley, 1979b). A remarkable feature of this damage is that the number of damaged cells progressively increases in several neuronal populations over a period of 24 to 72 hours following cerebral reperfusion (Fig. 2). In the striatum, the number of irreversibly damaged medium-sized neurons increased between 6 and 24 hours. In the hippocampus and neocortex, there was an increase in the number of injured neurons for up to 72 hours after cerebral reperfusion. Most surprising was the delay in the onset of damage to the majority of CA1 hippocampal pyramidal cells which did not show light (Pulsinelli and Brierley, 1979a; Pulsinelli et al., 1982a) or electron microscopic evidence (Petito and Pulsinelli, 1984) of damage until after 24 hours of cerebral reperfusion.

Kirino (1982) reported a similar delayed injury to CA1 hippocampal neurons beginning 2 days after 5 min of global ischemia in the gerbil. Ito et al. (1975) described a "maturational" aspect to neuronal injury in gerbils subjected to 15 min or longer of unilateral carotid artery occlusion. This maturation phenomenon, which was defined best in the H2 sector (Rose terminology, 1927) of the gerbil hippocampus, was characterized as a process which showed accentuation of neuronal staining at 20 hours of survival and then severe neuronal necrosis of this same population of neurons in animals surviving 1 week. This report provides no quantitative description of an increase in the numbers of neurons with irreversible damage versus time. Moreover, the process was found to occur principally in the H2 sector of the hippocampus, a region which corresponds to the CA2 or CA3 zone (Lorente de Nó terminology, 1934), an area known to be quite resistant to ischemic injury. Possibly this reflects a mislabeling by Ito et al. of the CA1 zone which Kirino (1982) found to develop a delayed variety of ischemic neuronal injury. Whether the results of Ito et al. are directly comparable to those of delayed neuronal injury reported in the rat (Pulsinelli et al., 1982a) or in the 5-min gerbil (Kirino, 1982) is further complicated by the fact that 15 min or longer of cerebral ischemia in the gerbil is quite likely to cause repetitive post-ischemic seizures and all of the associated systemic complications (hypotension, hypoxia) which may add further insult to the post-ischemic brain. Post-ischemic seizures were not a factor contributing to delayed neuronal injury in the rat since animals with convulsions following cerebral reperfusion were excluded from the study (Pulsinelli et al., 1982a).

Measurements of regional cerebral blood flow (rCBF) and regional glucose metabolism (rCGU) in the rat model of forebrain ischemia indicate that abnormalities in post-ischemic rCBF and rCGU could not explain the delayed onset and then progression of injury noted in these various neuronal populations (Pulsinelli et al., 1982b, 1984). In animals meeting the criteria of complete unresponsiveness throughout the duration of forebrain ischemia (Pulsinelli et al., 1982b, 1983) blood flow to the neocortex, striatum and hippocampus is severely reduced (Table 2). Post-ischemic CBF was similar in all forebrain regions regardless of the ultimate severity of neuronal injury and a dissociation between

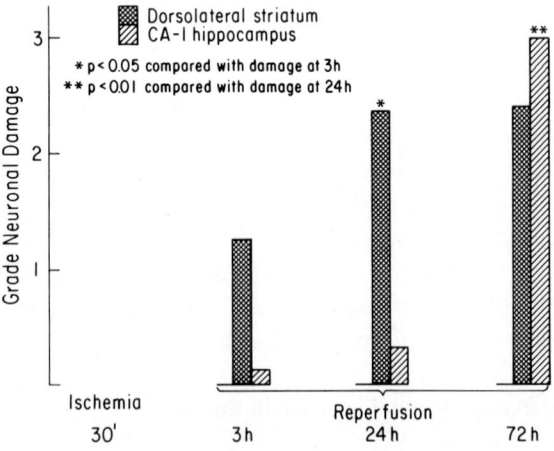

Fig. 2. Regional neuronal damage after ischemia. Time courses of neuronal damage in the striatum and CA1 hippocampus of rats subjected to 30 min of forebrain ischemia. Damage was graded on a scale of 0 representing no damaged neurons to 3 representing the majority of neurons with irreversible damage. (Data from Pulsinelli et al., 1982a.)

TABLE 2

Regional cerebral blood flow (CBF) (ml/100 g per min) in 4-vessel occlusion rat model

	Control (n = 6)	Ischemia			Post-ischemia		
		5 min (n = 5)	15 min (n = 5)	30 min (n = 5)	5 min (n = 5)	60 min (n = 6)	360 min (n = 5)
Parietal neocortex	140 ± 9	2 ± 0.5[a]	1 ± 0.1[a]	1 ± 0.2[a]	178 ± 26	45 ± 5[a]	65 ± 11[b]
Striatum	97 ± 3	2 ± 0.3[a]	1 ± 0.2[a]	1 ± 1[a]	141 ± 20	42 ± 3[a]	90 ± 11
Hippocampus	80 ± 4	8 ± 1[a]	3 ± 0.4[a]	2 ± 1[a]	151 ± 22[b]	32 ± 2[b]	57 ± 5

Values represent mean ± SEM.
[a] Values significantly different from control at $p < 0.01$ (ANOVA and Dunnett test).
[b] Values significantly different from control at $p < 0.05$ (ANOVA and Dunnett test).
Data from Pulsinelli et al., 1982b.

blood flow and glucose metabolism noted in these animals could not readily explain the temporal profile of neuronal damage (Pulsinelli et al., 1984).

Measurements of brain phosphocreatine, ATP, and lactate concentrations following transient forebrain ischemia demonstrated near-complete recovery of energy reserves in the striatum at 6 hours and complete recovery of energy stores in the CA1 zone of the hippocampus by 24 hours (Pulsinelli and Duffy, 1983; Pulsinelli et al., 1984). With survival periods beyond 24 hours, there was a secondary decline in energy reserves in striatum and hippocampus (Fig. 3) which coincided with the attainment of maximal neuronal damage in the respective brain areas. Electronmicroscopic studies in similarly treated animals demonstrated that neuronal mitochondria were swollen and vacuolated upon early recirculation of the brain. However, these mitochondria quickly recovered normal morphology even in brain regions which were destined to develop irreversible neuronal injury (Petito and Pulsinelli, 1983). The results suggest that neurons which will ultimately undergo ischemic necrosis in this animal model recover normal or near-normal mitochondrial function and are viable, in terms of high energy phosphate metabolism, for many hours before the onset of irreversible injury.

Neurotransmitters and selective neuronal necrosis

Local differences in the cerebral metabolic rate and blood flow do not readily explain the greater sensitivity of certain populations of neurons to tran-

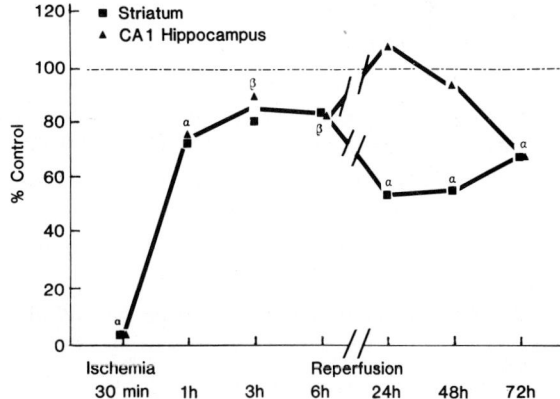

Fig. 3. Regional ATP concentration during and after ischemia. ATP concentration expressed as percent of control values in the striatum and CA1 hippocampus from rats subjected to 30 min of forebrain ischemia and then reperfusion. Control values for ATP were 2.74 × 0.08 μmol/g in the striatum and 2.25 × 0.03 μmol/g in the CA1 hippocampus. Significantly different from control values by ANOVA and Dunnett's test: [a] $p < 0.01$; [b] $p < 0.05$. [b] below the line indicates different only in the CA1 zone. (Data from Pulsinelli and Duffy, 1983.)

sient ischemia. One characteristic which separates neurons into subpopulations is their ability to synthesize, release, and respond to different neurotransmitters. Could specific neurotransmitter properties of select neuronal populations explain why some are more susceptible to ischemia than others? We addressed this question by measuring neurotransmitter synthetic enzyme activities in two brain regions with known populations of vulnerable neurons.

The sensitivity of GABAergic neurons to ischemia was assessed by measuring the activity of glutamic acid decarboxylase (GAD) and the sensitivity of cholinergic neurons was estimated by measuring choline acetyl transferase (CAT) (Francis and Pulsinelli, 1982). Following 30 min of severe forebrain ischemia in the rat and then recovery for approximately 7 days, GAD activity in the striatum was 50% of control values while CAT activity remained unchanged from control levels (Table 3). In hippocampus, forebrain ischemia had no effect on GAD or CAT activities. The results demonstrate that striatal GABAergic neurons are highly vulnerable to ischemia, but cholinergic neurons in this region are more resistant. In contrast, hippocampal GABAergic neurons, which are thought to represent hippocampal basket cells, were also resistant to ischemia. These data suggest that GABAergic neurons, as a neurotransmitter-defined population, are not equally sensitive throughout brain and, therefore, a single neurotransmitter cell type cannot explain the phenomenon of selective neuronal vulnerability.

Other neurotransmitter-related properties, namely the effect of excitatory neurotransmitter input onto sensitive neurons may be an important factor in determining the susceptibility of such neurons to ischemia (Francis and Pulsinelli, 1982). Intracerebral injections of glutamate (Van Harreveld and Fifkova, 1971) and amino acid analogs with excitatory properties (Olney, 1978) are toxic to neurons. Injection of low-dose kanic acid into the striatum of rats results in a lesion in which small and medium-sized neurons are damaged and the large neurons are spared (Coyle et al., 1978). This pattern of kainate-induced damage is identical to that caused by transient ischemia.

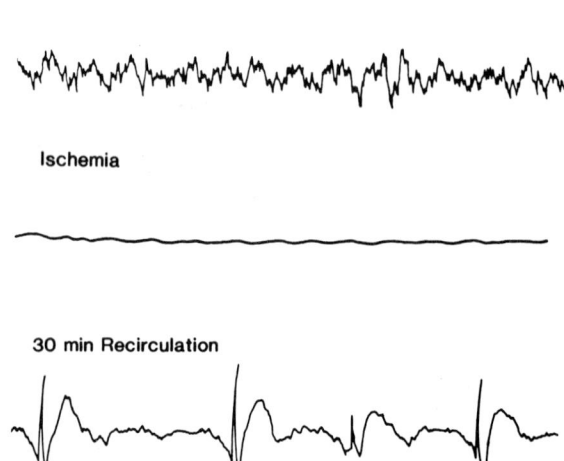
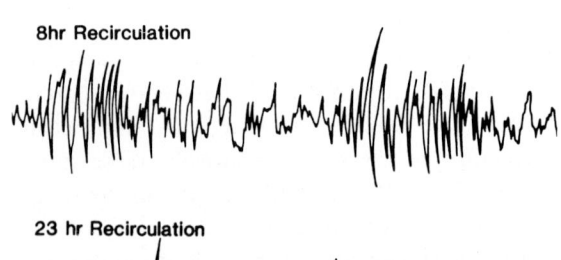
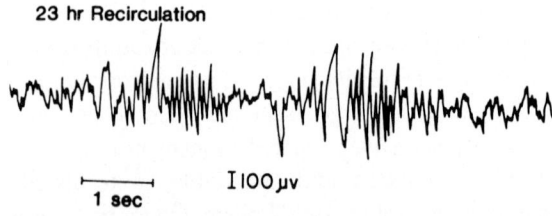

Fig. 4. Electroencephalographic activity recorded with depth electrodes placed in the dorsal-lateral striatum of a rat subjected to 30 min of forebrain ischemia and then reperfusion.

TABLE 3

Neurotransmitter enzyme activity (% control)

Striatum		Hippocampus	
GAD	CAT	GAD	CAT
54 ± 6[a]	114 ± 8	97 ± 15	113 ± 6

[a] Different from control values at $p < 0.001$.
Data from Francis and Pulsinelli, 1982.

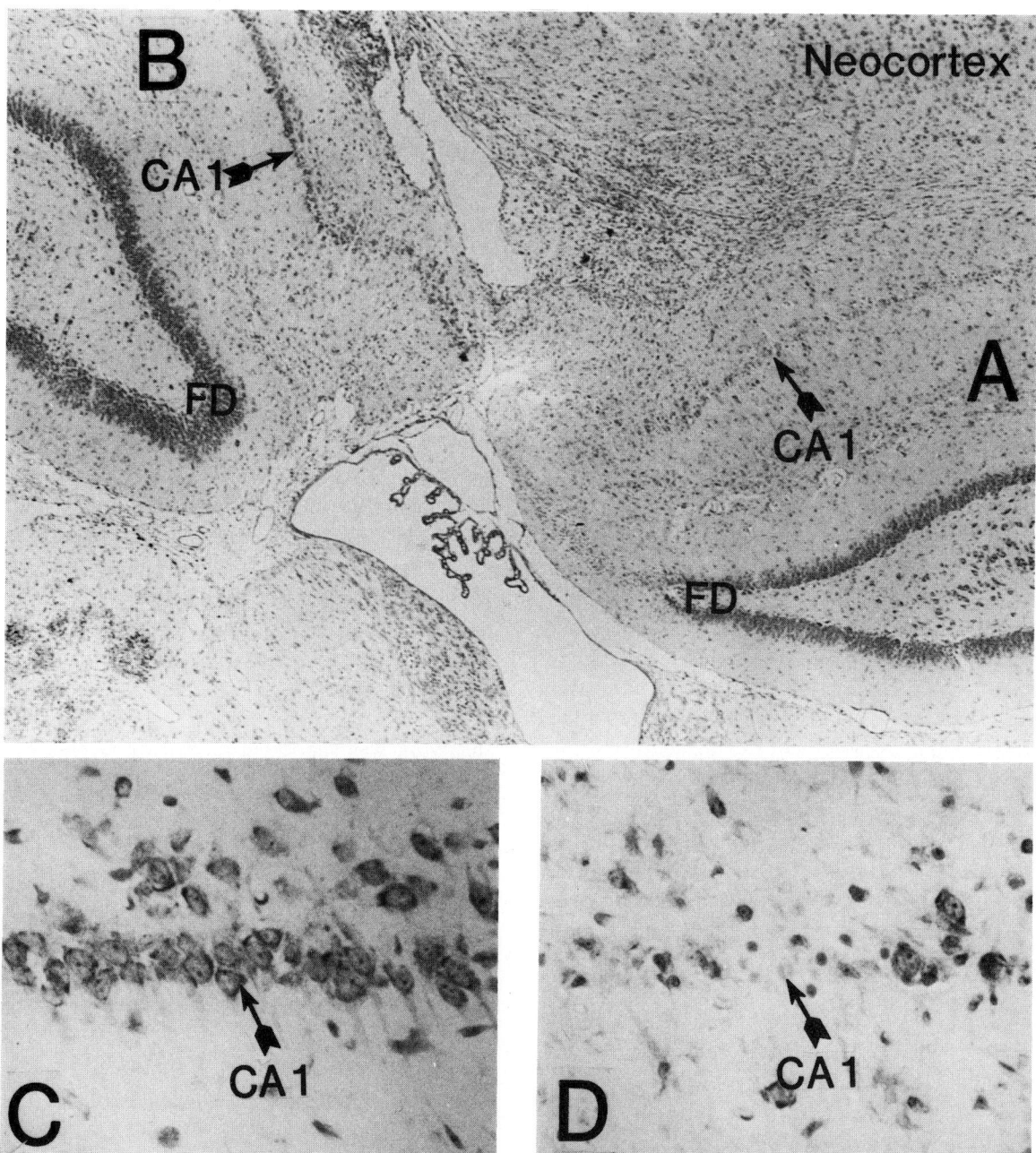

Fig. 5. Photomicrographs of CA1 pyramidal neurons from the intact hippocampus (A and D) and deafferented hippocampus (B and C); the rat was subjected to 30 min of forebrain ischemia and 3 days of postrecirculation survival. Note the preservation of CA1 neurons in the deafferented hippocampus (B and C) and the marked loss of CA1 neurons in the intact hippocampus (A and D). The deafferented hippocampus (B) is pushed above the horizontal plane when the overlying neocortex is removed at surgery. FD represents the fascia dentata. Cresyl violet. A and B × 25; C and D × 400.

To examine whether electrophysiological events and neurotransmitter input played a role in the process of selective neuronal vulnerability, we examined the electroencephalographic (EEG) activity from local electrodes placed in the striatum and CA1 zone of the hippocampus of rats subjected to transient forebrain ischemia. The EEG pattern presented in Fig. 4 demonstrates that activity in the form of spike and wave and burst-suppression patterns began by 18 min after cerebral reperfusion and persisted for at least 24 hours (Lacy and Pulsinelli, 1982). The Fig. presents data obtained from the striatum, but recordings from CA1 hippocampus were identical to these.

In more recent experiments, we have attempted to deafferent the CA1 zone of the hippocampus to determine whether depriving the hippocampus of extrahippocampal afferents could alter ischemic injury to the CA1 pyramidal neurons (Pulsinelli, 1985). To accomplish this, the neocortex and subcortical white matter overlying the right dorsal hippocampus were removed in anesthetized rats to expose the underlying hippocampus. An anterior transverse cut was made to sever the septal-hippocampal input. A lateral cut was made to interrupt the Schaffer collateral input to CA1 pyramidal cells. Finally a posterior transverse cut was made across the full extent of the hippocampus to sever the perforant pathway input from the entorhinal cortex. The surgically lesioned animals were allowed to survive for 5 to 7 days to attain full degeneration of afferent synapses. The animals were then subjected to 30 min of severe forebrain ischemia and allowed to recover for 3 days. The brains were examined with the light microscope for evidence of hippocampal injury. The results (Table 4) demonstrate that the CA1 pyramidal cells in the surgically deafferented hippocampus were protected from ischemic injury while the CA1 pyramidal cells in the intact contralateral hippocampus were irreversibly damaged (Fig. 5). These data suggest that neurotransmitter input may be an important determinant of selective ischemic injury to neurons. The biochemical mechanisms responsible for these neurotransmitter-related events are unknown but may be related to glutamate or other excitatory amino acid stimulated influx of calcium ions into postsynaptic cells. Such findings raise the strong possibility of influencing ischemic necrosis of neurons through the pharmacological modification of neurotransmitter receptors.

TABLE 4

Hippocampal injury

	Grade neuronal damage	
	Left hippocampus	Right hippocampus
Sham controls	2.3 ± 0.2	2.6 ± 0.2
Deaff. right hippocampus	3.0	1.1 ± 0.1[a]

[a] $p < 0.01$ compared to right hippocampus of sham controls or left hippocampus of deafferented rats. $n = 8$ for the sham controls and 7 for the deafferented group.

Acknowledgements

This work was supported in part by Grants NS-03346 and NS-07141. I thank E. Hoff for his technical assistance and C. Hopkins for assistance in manuscript preparation.

References

Brierly, J.B. (1977) Cerebral hypoxia. In: W. Blackwood and J.A.N. Corsellis (Eds.), *Greenfield's Neuropathology*. Year Book Medical Publishers, Edinburgh, pp. 43–85.

Brierley, J.B. and Excell, B.J. (1966) The effect of profound systemic hypotension upon the brain of *M. Rhesus*. Physiological and pathological observations. *Brain*, 89: 269–298.

Brown, A.W. (1977) Structural abnormalities in neurons. *J. Clin. Pathol.*, 30: Suppl. 11, 155–169.

Brown, A.W., Levy, D.E., Kublik, M., Harrow, J., Plum, F. and Brierley, J.B. (1979) Selective chromatolysis of neurons in the gerbil brain: a possible consequence of epileptic activity produced by common carotid artery occlusion. *Ann. Neurol.*, 5: 127–138.

Coyle, J., Molliver, M. and Kuhar, M. (1978) In situ injection of kainic acid: a new method for selectively lesioning neuronal cell bodies while sparing axons of passage. *J. Comp. Neurol.*, 180: 301–324.

Francis, A. and Pulsinelli, W.A. (1982) Response of GABAergic and cholinergic neurons to transient cerebral ischemia. *Brain Res.*, 243: 271–278.

Graham, D.I. (1977) Pathology of hypoxic brain damage in man. *J. Clin. Pathol.*, 30: Suppl. 11, 170–180.

Haymaker, W. and McMenemey, W.H. (1963) Chairman's Opening Remarks. In: J.P. Schadé and W.H. McMenemey (Eds.), *Selective Vulnerability of the Brain in Hypoxemia*. F.A. Davis Co., Philadelphia, pp. 1–3.

Ito, U., Spatz, M., Walker, J.T. and Klatzo, I. (1975) Experimental cerebral ischemia in Mongolian gerbils. *Acta Neuropathol.*, 32: 209–232.

Jacob, H. (1963) CNS tissue and cellular pathology in hypoxemic states. In: P. Schadé and W.P. McMenemey (Eds.), *Selective Vulnerability of the Brain in Hypoxemia*. F.A. Davis Co., Philadelphia, pp. 153–176.

Kalimo, H., Garcia, J.H., Kamijyo, Y., Tanaka, J. and Trump, B.F. (1977) The ultrastructure of brain death. Electronmicroscopy of feline cortex after complete ischemia. *Virchows Arch. B. Cell Pathol.*, 25: 207–220.

Kirino, T. (1982) Delayed neuronal death in the gerbil hippocampus following ischemia. *Brain Res.*, 239: 57–69.

Lacy, P. and Pulsinelli, W.A. (1982) Subclinical epileptiform activity and morphological damage in the striatum of rats after transient forebrain ischemia. *Soc. Neurosci. Abstr.*, 8: 88.

Lorente de Nó, R. (1934) Studies on the structure of the cerebral cortex. II. Continuation of the study of the ammonic system. *J. Psychol. Neurol.*, 46: 113–177.

Meyer, A. (1936) The selective regional vulnerability of the brain and its relation to psychiatric problems. *Proc. Roy. Soc. Med.*, 29: 1175–1181.

Meyer, J.E. (1953) Über die Lokalisation frühkindlicher Hirneschäden in arteriellen Grenzgebieten. *Arch. Psychiat. Nervenkr.* 190: 328–341.

Olney, J.W. (1978) Neurotoxicity of excitatory amino acids. In: E.G. McGeer, J.W. Olney and P.L. McGeer (Eds.), *Kainic Acid as a Tool in Neurobiology*. Raven Press, New York, pp. 37–70.

Petito, C. and Pulsinelli, W.A. (1983) Sequential development of reversible and irreversible neuronal damage following cerebral ischemia. *J. Neuropathol. Exp. Neurol.*, 43: 141–153.

Petito, C.K. and Pulsinelli, W.A. (1984) Delayed neuronal recovery and neuronal death in rat hippocampus following severe cerebral ischemia: Possible relationship to abnormalities in neuronal processes. *J. Cereb. Blood Flow Metabol.*, 4: 194–205.

Pulsinelli, W.A. (1985) Deafferentation of the hippocampus protects CA1 pyramidal cells against ischemic injury. *Stroke*, 16: 144.

Pulsinelli, W.A. and Brierley, J.B. (1979a) The temporal profile of ischemic neuronal damage in the four-vessel occlusion rat model (Abstract). *Stroke*, 10: 492.

Pulsinelli, W.A. and Brierley, J.B. (1979b) A new model of bilateral hemispheric ischemia in the unanesthetized rat. *Stroke*, 10: 267–272.

Pulsinelli, W.A. and Duffy, T.E. (1979) Local cerebral glucose metabolism during controlled hypoxemia in rats. *Science*, 204: 626–629.

Pulsinelli, W.A. and Duffy, T.E. (1983) Regional energy balance in rat brain after transient forebrain ischemia. *J. Neurochem.*, 40: 1500–1503.

Pulsinelli, W.A., Brierley, J.B. and Plum, F. (1982a) Temporal profile of neuronal damage in a model of transient forebrain ischemia. *Ann. Neurol.*, 11: 491–498.

Pulsinelli, W.A., Levy, D.E. and Duffy, T.E. (1982b) Regional cerebral blood flow in glucose metabolism following transient forebrain ischemia. *Ann. Neurol.*, 11: 499–505.

Pulsinelli, W.A., Duffy, T.E. and Levy, D.E. (1983) Cerebral blood flow in the four-vessel occlusion rat model. *Stroke*, 14: 832–833.

Pulsinelli, W.A., Duffy, T.E., Levy, D.E., Petito, C. and Plum, F. (1984) Ischemic injury to selectively vulnerable neurons in the rat. In: A. Bes, P. Braquet, R. Paoletti and B.K. Siesjö (Eds.), *Cerebral Ischemia, ICS 654*. Excerpta Medica, Amsterdam-New York-Oxford, pp. 35–44.

Rice, J.E., Vannucci, R.C. and Brierley, J.B. (1981) The influence of immaturity on hypoxic-ischemic brain damage in the rat. *Ann. Neurol.*, 9: 131–141.

Rose, M. (1927) Der Allocortex beim Tier und Mensch. *J. Psychol. Neurol.*, 34: 1–111.

Schadé, J.P. and McMenemey, W.H. (Eds.) (1963) *Selective Vulnerability of the Brain in Hypoxemia*. F.A. Davis Co., Philadelphia.

Scholz, W. (1953) Selective neuronal necrosis and its topistic patterns in hypoxemia and olegemia. *J. Neuropathol. Exp. Neurol.*, 12: 249–261.

Scholz, W. (1963) Topistic lesions. In: J.P. Schadé and W.H. McMenemey (Eds.), *Selective Vulnerability of the Brain in Hypoxemia*. F.A. Davis Co., Philadelphia, pp. 257–267.

Spielmeyer, W. (1925) Zur Pathogenese der örtlich elektiven Gehirnveränderungen. *Z. Neurol. Psychiat.*, 99: 756–777.

Strong, A.J., Tomlinson, B.E., Venables, G.S., Gibson, G. and Hardy, J.A. (1983) The cortical ischemic penumbra associated with occlusion of the middle cerebral artery in the cat. II. Studies of histopathology, water content, and in vitro neurotransmitter uptake. *J. Cereb. Blood Flow Metabol.*, 3: 97–108.

Van Harreveld, A. and Fifkova, E. (1971) Light- and electron microscopic changes in central nervous tissue after electrophoretic injection of glutamate. *Exp. Mol. Pathol.*, 15: 61–81.

Vogt, C. and Vogt, O. (1937) Sitz und Wesen der Krankheiten im Lichte der topistischen Hirnforschung und des Variierens der Tiere. *J. Psychol. Neurol.*, 47: 237–457.

Welsh, F.A., Vannucci, R.C. and Brierley, J.B. (1982) Collumnar alterations of NADH fluorescence during hypoxia-ischemia in immature rat brain. *J. Cereb. Blood Flow Metabol.*, 2: 221–228.

Zülch, K.J. (1953) Neue Befunde und Deutungen aus der Gefässpathologie des Hirns und Rückenmarks. *Z. Pathol. Pathol. Anat.*, 90: 402.

Selective vulnerability of the hippocampus to ischemia — reversible and irreversible types of ischemic cell damage

Takaaki Kirino, Akira Tamura and Keiji Sano

Department of Neurosurgery, Teikyo University School of Medicine, 2–11–1 Kaga, Itabashi-ku, Tokyo 173, Japan

Introduction

Biological organisms which live in an aerobic condition are destined to die when oxygen and metabolic substrates are withdrawn. Any type of cells forming our body cannot survive an extended period of ischemia. From this point of view, neuronal cell death due to ischemia may be nothing less than ischemic cell death in general. The underlying mechanism of cell damage may be identical and any superficial difference may be a reflection of the quantitative difference of individual cells.

The central nervous system (CNS) is one of the organs in the body most vulnerable to ischemia. In the CNS, certain areas are selectively damaged even by a transient, brief ischemic insult. Several layers of the cerebral cortex, certain subfields of the hippocampus, and the cerebellar cortex are among those known to be vulnerable regions (Brierley, 1976). The reason why CNS neurons die so easily after ischemia is still not completely understood. Furthermore, we have only limited knowledge regarding the question why restricted regions of the brain are especially vulnerable to ischemia. The phenomenon of selective vulnerability may be the result of regional, quantitative differences in the CNS. The regional blood flow, the regional metabolic rate, or the regional amount of metabolic substrates stored may be among such factors. These factors play, without doubt, essential roles in the pathogenesis of ischemic brain damage.

There remains, however, the possibility that there are a number of different mechanisms which, triggered by brief ischemia, cause neuronal damage. In other words, ischemia, if it is mild, may not necessarily kill neurons directly but may reset or deviate the metabolic state of neurons to a certain degree and in a certain direction. The workings of this reset or deviation may completely depend on the biological characteristics of each neuron. The influence of brief ischemia on neurons may differ from neuron to neuron, rather than from region to region in the brain.

Provided that this hypothesis is correct, it reminds us of the fact that each neuron is different and unique in its circuit formation and its signal processing. This difference seems to be based upon the uniqueness of the surface membrane receptors or neurotransmitters which combine with those receptors. This implies that the information on the characteristics of each neuronal group is of paramount importance in clarifying the mechanism of ischemic neuronal damage. The hippocampus, among those vulnerable regions, is the area where anatomic, physiologic and behavioral investigations have been copiously documented (Isaacson and Pribram, 1975; O'Keefe and Nadel, 1978; Isaacson, 1982). It is advantageous, therefore, to conduct further research using the available knowledge of this structure. Also, if this hypothesis is valid, neurons, following ischemia, are left in an unstable state between death and survival. As a consequence, there is the possibility of salvaging dying neurons following ischemia. What we are required to find is, probably, how to restore the metabolic state of neurons, which has been disturbed by transient ischemia. We hope that, in the future, neurons in those vulnerable areas will be saved from the dying process, at least following transient, brief ischemia.

Ischemic neuronal damage

Experimental studies on the morphological changes in neurons resulting from ischemia critically depend upon satisfactory fixation of the brain tissue. Without an adequate fixation procedure, certain types of ischemic neuronal damage can be confused with artifacts. This problem can be avoided, for the most part, by intravascular perfusion fixation and the proper handling of fixed brains (Brierley, 1976). Brierley and his colleagues extensively researched the neuronal changes that follow ischemia or anoxia and they emphasized the rapid progression of ischemic cell damage (McGee-Russel et al., 1970; Brown and Brierley, 1972; Brierley, 1976). They observed that, when brains were appropriately perfusion-fixed, ischemic neuronal injury appears rapidly enough to be observed by light microscopy within a few hours following ischemia. Affected neurons at first displayed vacuoles in their perikarya (microvacuolation), then became shrunken and darkly stained with displaced nuclei (ischemic cell change), and later on showed incrustation around the cell bodies. Finally, the stage of homogenizing cell change followed until neurons were disintegrated and absorbed completely. The whole process of ischemic cell injury is believed to evolve through well-defined, predictable stages. The temporal course of the change is said to depend only on the size of individual neurons, not on the magnitude of the ischemia (Salford et al., 1973). This hypothesis means that one can predict the course of change for each neuron at a relatively early period after ischemia.

The change observed in neurons following ischemia, previously believed to evolve in a single, well-defined pattern, is not simple. Kalimo et al. (1981) observed rat brains following ischemia and found that there are two types, dark type and pale type, of ischemic nerve cell injury, and thus proved that the pathogenesis of ischemic neuronal damage is more complex.

A different view of ischemic neuronal alteration was reported by Ito et al. (1975) who observed brains of the Mongolian gerbil following unilateral occlusion of the carotid artery. They noticed that, when the duration of ischemia is short, ischemic neuronal damage progresses slowly, but, as ischemia lasts longer, the changes occurred faster after recirculation. This phenomenon is now known as the "maturation phenomenon". The implication of their observations is that the pattern of ischemic neuronal damage depends on the magnitude of the ischemia. In addition, Ito et al. (1975) and Bubis et al. (1976) reported that, in a restricted area of the hippocampus, a novel type of cell change occurs in the gerbil. They called this "reactive change".

Morphological research of ischemic brain has revealed many aspects of the phenomenon of ischemic neuronal damage. We should, however, realize that there are limitations to this method. Although structural observation has an enormous spatial resolution, it is not usually effective in detecting the underlying pathogenetic mechanisms. One should await further studies on mechanisms mediated by certain biochemical or physiological factors. Moreover, even if one can find one specific structural abnormality, it does not necessarily mean one specific pathomechanism. Another factor we have to consider is the problem of fixation. As was indicated by Brierley (1976), adequate fixation is a sine qua non for morphological study in experimental animals. However, even optimally accomplished perfusion fixation could be sometimes inadequate for certain purposes. It is known that aldehyde fixatives routinely used for electron microscopy cannot completely immobilize biomembranes. For example, the extracellular space of the CNS, even in normal condition, appears less prominent by electron microscopy than it actually is believed to be (Van Harreveld et al., 1965). There is no guarantee that perfusion fixation, a chemical process, works identically in ischemic brain as it does in normal animals.

In the case of extremely prolonged ischemia, perfusion of fixative solution through the vasculature becomes difficult and one has to abandon further precise morphological observation. The morphological method in this situation is, however, still useful in evaluating the regional pattern of brain damage.

Selective vulnerability of the hippocampus to ischemia

Normal hippocampus

In the rodent, the hippocampus (Ammon's horn) extends beneath the corpus callosum. The dorsal part of the hippocampus lying ventrally to the corpus callosum is referred to as the dorsal hippocampus. The hippocampus proper is roughly C-shaped, at the end of the curvature of the letter C lies a cell group assembled in the form of the letter V. This is the granule cell layer of the dentate gyrus. The hippocampus has been divided into several subfields based upon the morphology of the pyramidal cells. Lorente de Nó (1934) studied this region using the Golgi method and classified the hippocampus into four subfields: i.e., CA1, CA2, CA3, and CA4 (Fig. 1). Since his subdivision was based on the characteristics of neuronal processes, it is closely related to the pattern of neuronal circuitry. Although Sommer did not give any specific anatomical landmarks for the vulnerable part of the hippocampus (see the following), the CA1 is believed to correspond to Sommer's sector.

The hippocampus can be divided into two major functional modules; the CA1 and the CA3 (Shepherd, 1979). The CA3 subfield connects with mossy fiber terminals from the dentate granule cells and the CA3 neurons then send off Shaffer's collaterals to the CA1 pyramidal cells. The CA1 sector in turn receives fibers from the CA3 and has connections with the subiculum (see Fig. 2).

The apical dendrites of the CA1 pyramidal cells extend ventrally into the stratum radiatum, where the thick dendritic shafts give the appearance of *radiation*. The terminal ramification of dendrites is seen in the stratum lacunosum-moleculare. The molecular layer of the dentate gyrus is contiguous with this stratum lacunosum-moleculare, the fused hippocampal fissure being the border.

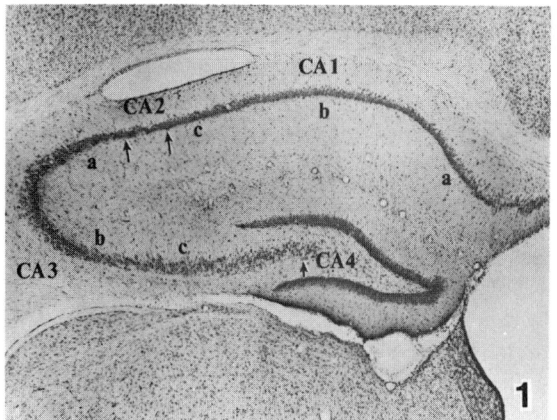

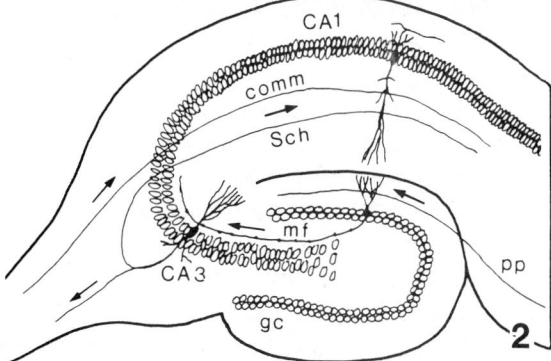

Fig. 1. Normal dorsal hippocampus of the gerbil. Subfields of the hippocampus (CA1–CA4) and their subdivisions (a, b etc.). Vibratome section, cresyl fast violet, × 22.

Fig. 2. Neuronal elements and interconnections in the hippocampus. (Cited from Bliss and Dolphin, 1982.)

Since the hippocampus, a structure within the rhinencephalon, has a very similar neuronal architecture from lower mammals on up to the human and since the susceptibility of the hippocampus to ischemic injury is known in various species, it seems reasonable to focus our attention on a restricted region of the brain, the hippocampus, to understand the more general problem of ischemic neuronal damage. For further information, several recent reviews or monographs are available (Isaacson and Pribram, 1975; O'Keefe and Nadel, 1978; Isaacson, 1982).

Hippocampal damage following ischemia

The hippocampus has attracted the interest of many pathologists for more than a century. At the beginning, the alteration was noticed in epileptic patients. The earliest description of the change in the hippocampus is credited to Bouchet and Cazauvieilh (1825) who found frequent changes in the consistency of the hippocampus, i.e. hardening or softening, in epileptic patients. The first microscopic observation on the hippocampal lesion was reported by Sommer (1880). He described that one-third of epileptic patients showed an extensive loss of neurons in a circumscribed portion of the hippocampus. This area of the hippocampus is now called Sommer's sector (CA1). The change in this area was attributed to repeated circulatory disturbances provoked by seizure attacks (Pfleger, 1880). Later, Bratz (1899) confirmed Sommer's findings, but noted also that the endfolium (CA4) was as often affected as Sommer's sector. The pathologic process in Sommer's sector has attracted clinical interest because it seemed to be related to secondary temporal lobe epilepsies in epileptic patients (Sano and Malamud, 1953).

The relationship between anoxia/ischemia and hippocampal damage has received particular attention especially since the works of Spielmeyer and his colleagues (Spielmeyer, 1925, 1927, 1929). His group laid emphasis on the role of the local circulatory factor. The length and tortuous course of the artery supplying Sommer's sector (Uchimura, 1928), the rake-like pattern of the terminal hippocampal arterioles (Scharrer, 1940), and the location of the hippocampal area in the watershed between the carotid and vertebrobasilar territories (Coceani and Gloor, 1966) were considered to be responsible for the hippocampal selective vulnerability. This hypothesis is known as the "vascular theory". Contrarily Vogt believed that the selective intolerance of the hippocampus to ischemia was due to a difference in the physical or chemical characteristics of individual neurons (Vogt and Vogt, 1922). He proposed a hypothetical term, "pathoclisis", to describe the difference in susceptibility to ischemic injury. In spite of the elaborate work by Spielmeyer and his associates, the "vascular theory" seems to be unsatisfactory to explain the cell damage in a circumscribed region of the hippocampus. In contrast, there is, as described later, increasing evidence that the ischemic damage to hippocampal neurons is related to the chemical characteristics and interconnection of individual neurons in the complex circuitry of the brain.

The problem of the hippocampal selective vulnerability to ischemia has in the past been studied in autopsy material. It was not usually a matter of experimental trial before the successful production of ischemia in experimental animals, especially in the rodent, became possible. Previously, several experimental studies have been reported on the morphological changes in the hippocampus following ischemia (Brierley et al., 1971; Brown and Brierley, 1972). The changes in affected neurons within the vulnerable hippocampal area in these experiments were reported to be identical to the well-defined, predictable pattern of ischemic cell change. The alteration in the selectively vulnerable hippocampal region was believed not to differ from the ischemic neuronal damage seen elsewhere in the brain.

Experimental cerebral ischemia in the gerbil

The Mongolian gerbil *(Meriones unguiculatus)* was introduced as an experimental animal for stroke by Levine and Payan (1966), who noticed that unilateral ligation of the carotid artery at the neck produces cerebral infarction. Later works have revealed that ischemia in the gerbil is due to a lack of the interconnection in the circle of Willis at the base of the skull (Levine and Sohn, 1969; Tamura et al., 1981). Almost all gerbils have no connection between the carotid and the vertebrobasilar circulation. In addition, about 30–60% of gerbils lack the communication between left and right carotid systems. At the beginning, the gerbil was used as a focal ischemia model by occluding the unilateral carotid artery (Kahn, 1972; Ito et al., 1975; Levy et al., 1975). Later, it has come to be realized that bilateral occlusion of the carotid arteries brings about uniform forebrain ischemia, during which the value of blood flow is close to zero (Crockard et al., 1980; Suzuki et al., 1983a).

Although the gerbil model for cerebral ischemia has several beneficial features, the model has a disadvantage. The animal develops "seizure-like" abnormalities, especially during and after relatively prolonged ischemia (Levy et al., 1975), which are sometimes so severe that they may jeopardize experimental data (Pulsinelli and Brierley, 1979). Ischemia of longer than 7 min frequently precipitates "seizure-like" abnormal behavior (Kirino and Sano, 1984a) and the severity and duration of this abnormality differ from animal to animal, especially when the ischemic insult becomes more protracted. One should therefore be careful in interpreting experimental data when ischemia lasts longer than 20–30 min in the gerbil. Brief ischemia, however, usually does not cause overt "epileptic" movement during ischemia and after recirculation. Moreover, the gerbil brain is known to be electrically silent during ischemia and consequently "epileptic" movement, if any, does not arise from the ischemic brain itself during ischemia (Cohn, 1979).

Materials and methods

Adult Mongolian gerbils (60–80 g) were subjected to transient ischemia by occluding the bilateral carotid arteries at the neck using aneurysm clips. Five groups of animals were prepared according to the duration of carotid occlusion, i.e., 3 min, 5 min, 10 min, 20 min, and 30 min. The gerbils were allowed to survive for 3 h, 6 h, 12 h, 1 day, 2 days, 4 days, and 7 days after ischemia, and they were perfusion fixed. The fixative contained 2.5% glutaraldehyde and 2% paraformaldehyde in 0.1 M cacodylate buffer (pH = 7.3). Specimens containing the dorsal hippocampus were obtained and processed for light and electron microscopy. Selected specimens were examined immunocytochemically using an antibody raised against neuron-specific enolase (NSE) which specifically exists in neurons (Pickel et al., 1975). Further details have been given elsewhere (Kirino and Sano, 1984a; Kirino et al., 1983).

Brief ischemia (5–10 min)

After 3 min of occlusion, one out of five animals developed scattered destruction of the CA1 pyramidal cells, whereas the brains of the other gerbils looked normal. After ischemia of longer than 5 min, most of the brains showed damage in the hippocampus. The extent of cell injury in the hippocampus was clearly demonstrated by immunocytochemistry using the anti-NSE antibody (Fig. 3). The frequency of brain damage following an ischemic insult of longer than 5 min was 93.9%.

In serial sections of gerbil brains fixed 7 days following 5 min of ischemia no neuronal damage was observed outside the hippocampus. Specimens cut coronally or obliquely (perpendicularly to the 2.0 mm long axis of the dorsal hippocampus) demonstrated that hippocampal damage was present throughout the dorsal hippocampus. At the most posterior pole of the hippocampus where it bends ventrally, as examined by horizontal sections, tissue damage was slight or non-existent. The changes in

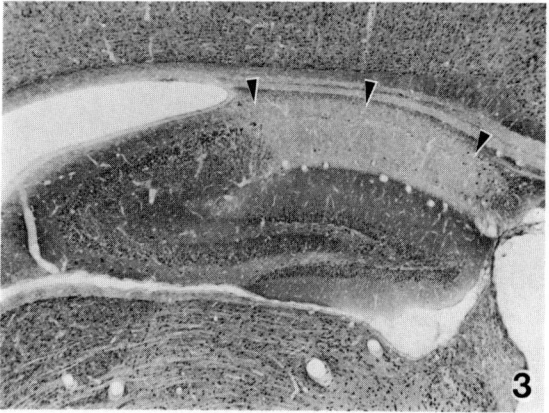

Fig. 3. The hippocampal region of the gerbil stained immunocytochemically using an antibody raised against neuron-specific enolase (NSE). Six months following ischemia, the CA1 subfield (arrowheads) is devoid of staining, indicating that neuronal elements in the CA1 have been eliminated for the most part, × 22.

each sector of the hippocampus following brief ischemia were as follows.

The *CA4* pyramidal cells showed a fast change (Fig. 4). They became darkly stained with shrunken cell bodies and empty spaces surrounding them. This change became obvious within 3–6 h following ischemia. Occasionally, injured cells contained numerous vacuoles. These darkly stained cells were scattered in the CA4 subfield among seemingly unaffected pyramidal cells.

Alteration in the *CA2* and *CA3* subfields took place within a day (Fig. 5). Following brief ischemia, pyramidal cells in the CA2 sector became swollen. Numerous dark granules were seen in the enlarged cytoplasm and the cell nuclei were displaced to the periphery and had a crescent shape. This cell alteration culminated on days 1 and 2; then it resulted in cell death for the most part.

The change in the *CA1* (Sommer's sector) developed slowly (Figs. 6, 7). On day 1 following brief ischemia, no definite alteration was seen except that the cell nucleus occasionally looked more inhomogeneous than normal. On day 2 (Fig. 6), the pyramidal cells showed a slight clumping of the nuclear chromatin and slits developed in the basal side of the cytoplasm. These initial signs of alteration were followed by extensive destruction of most of the pyramidal cells when observed on the 4th day (Fig. 7). In the later stage of the CA1 cell change, some pyramidal cells were darkly stained whereas others were swollen and stained only slightly. No uniform type of cell decomposition was detected at this stage.

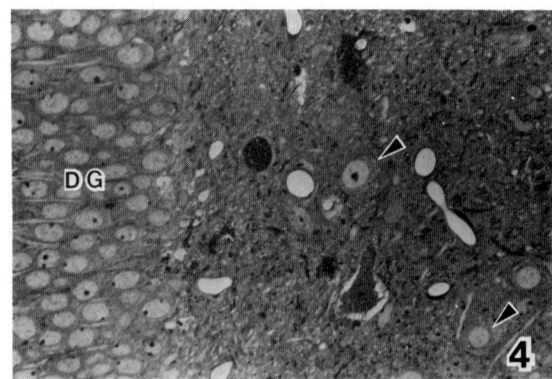

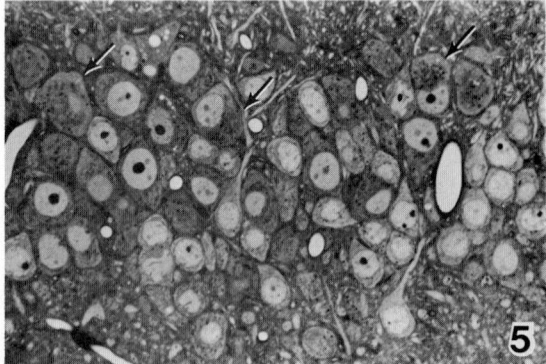

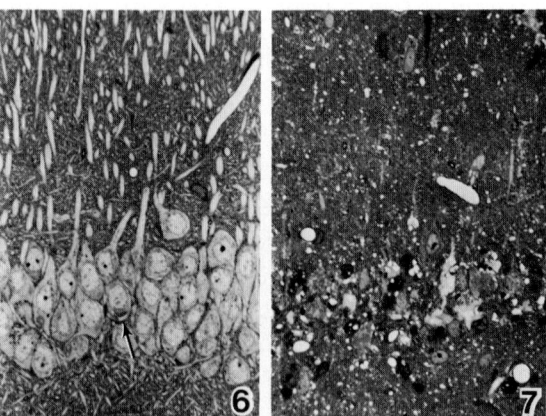

Fig. 4. Gerbil. One day following 5 min of ischemia. Scattered CA4 neurons are affected, darkly stained, and shrunken. Other pyramidal cells (arrowheads) look unchanged. The dentate granule cells (DG) appear similar to normal. Plastic section, toluidine blue, × 352.

Fig. 5. Gerbil. One day following 5 min of ischemia. In the CA2 subfield, there are few swollen pyramidal cells with increased intracytoplasmic granules (arrows). The cell nuclei are displaced to the periphery. Plastic section, toluidine blue, × 344.

Fig. 6–7. Gerbil hippocampal CA1 subfield. Plastic section, toluidine blue, × 290.

Fig. 6. Two days following 5 min of ischemia, the pyramidal cells appear almost normal, but a slit-like change is seen (arrow) on the basal side of the perikarya.

Fig. 7. Four days following 5 min of ischemia, most of the pyramidal cells in this field have been destroyed. The neuropil above and below the pyramidal cell layer is spongy.

Relatively longer ischemia (20–30 min)

In gerbils subjected to transient forebrain ischemia of longer than 20 min, cell damage extended to the CA3 subfield, and the whole hippocampus was lost, while the dentate gyrus usually looked intact.

In the *CA1* subfield, the changes appeared faster than in the case of brief ischemia. One day after 20 min of ischemia, the tendency for slit formation in the cytoplasm was accentuated, and cell nuclei were more inhomogeneous than after brief ischemia. On day 2 (Fig. 8), the majority of the pyramidal cells showed increased staining with toluidine blue. Twelve hours following 30 min of occlusion (Fig. 9), some CA1 pyramidal cells were at the stage of overt cell disintegration. They had darkly stained, shrunken cell bodies with surrounding empty spaces. These findings in the CA1 pyramidal cells following the longer ischemia resembled the classical ischemic cell change of neurons in their light-microscopic appearance.

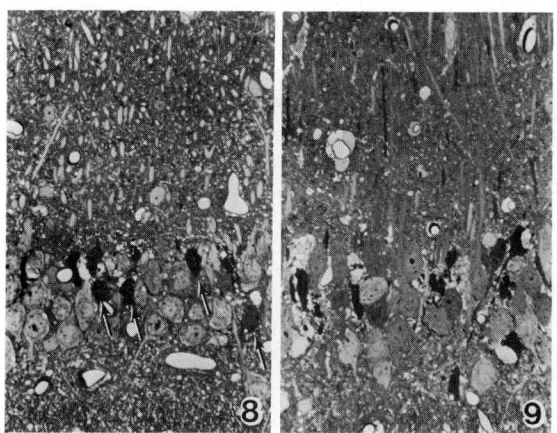

Fig. 8–9. Gerbil hippocampal CA1 subfield. The change appears faster following recirculation when the ischemic period lasts longer. Plastic section, toluidine blue, × 297.

Fig. 8. Twenty-minute ischemia causes faster neuronal changes in the CA1 subfield. Some pyramidal cells are darkly stained and look shrunken (arrows). There are small vacuoles in the cytoplasm.

Fig. 9. Twelve hours following 30 min of ischemia, the change appears much faster. Some neurons are intensely dark and shrunken. They are surrounded by empty spaces.

The changes in the *CA2* and the *CA3* appeared faster and in more severe form. Giant pyramidal cells in the CA3 showed widespread reactive change. This was most conspicuous in the CA3 area which is contiguous to the CA2. This cell alteration resulted in almost total loss of the pyramidal cells in the hippocampus.

The number of cells injured in the *CA4* increased as ischemic insult was prolonged. However, the morphological characteristics of the change in the CA4 neurons was not different from those following brief ischemia.

Summary of the gerbil experiment

Following ischemia, three different types of change were observed in the CA4, CA2, and CA1 subfields. In the CA4, the change was rapid and corresponded to the previously known ischemic cell change. Affected neurons became dark and shrunken within a few hours after ischemia. When the ischemia was longer, the number of injured CA4 neurons increased but the structural change was similar. The change in the CA4 seems to represent an irreversible type of ischemic neuronal injury.

The alteration in the CA2 was relatively slow and identical to what has been known as reactive change. This alteration was seen in gerbils which did not develop overt "epileptiform" abnormalities.

The CA1 pyramidal cells developed a strikingly slow cell death process. It became apparent by light microscopy 2 days following brief ischemia (5–10 min). Four days after the ischemic insult, most of the CA1 neurons were destroyed. All of these findings suggest that the delayed neuronal death in the CA1 is a novel type of cell change resulting from ischemia. Following longer ischemia (20–30 min), the change in the CA1 pyramidal cells took place faster and resembled the well-defined ischemic cell change. This problem of transition in morphology from the "delayed neuronal death" type to the "ischemic cell change" type prompted us to further study using electron microscopy (see below).

Experimental cerebral ischemia in the rat

A rat forebrain ischemia model was described by Pulsinelli and Brierley (1979). They electrocoagulated bilateral vertebral arteries in the rat at the point just beneath the alar foramina of the 1st cervical vertebra. The animal showed no abnormalities in behavior or morphological findings following this procedure alone. On the day following the vertebral artery coagulation, bilateral carotid arteries were obliterated by clasps. This produced profound ischemia in the rat forebrain.

Using their model, Pulsinelli et al. (1982b) reported a temporal profile of neuronal alterations in rats. They demonstrated a remarkably slow development of cell death in the cerebral cortex and the hippocampus. To compare the morphological characteristics of the slow neuronal death in the rat hippocampus with that seen in the gerbil, an experiment was performed using the rat forebrain ischemia model.

Adult Osborne-Mendel rats were subjected to four-vessel occlusion as described by Pulsinelli and Brierley (1979). On the day following the vertebral artery coagulation, the bilateral carotid arteries were clipped for 20 to 40 min. The animals which showed positive ischemic symptoms (Pulsinelli and Brierley, 1979) were fixed by perfusion 1, 2, or 4 days after the ischemia. Fixed brains were processed for light and electron microscopy as described above. Further details have been given elsewhere (Kirino et al., 1984).

Selective vulnerability in the rat hippocampus

Four days following 20 min of ischemia, all the specimens obtained from seven symptom-positive rats showed similar changes. There was an extensive loss of the CA1 pyramidal cells and scattered neuronal deaths in the CA4 subfield. The dentate gyrus and the CA3 sector of the hippocampus remained unchanged.

In the *CA1,* most of the pyramidal cells did not show overt morphological changes 1 day following 20 min of ischemia, but a slight increase in stainability by toluidine blue was noticed in some of the CA1 neurons. Two days after 20 min of ischemia (Fig. 10), the CA1 pyramidal cells were intensely stained and shrunken. At the same time, some CA1 neurons displayed slightly swollen, pale cytoplasm. Four days after the ischemia (Fig. 11) the pathologic process in the CA1 subfield resulted in an extensive destruction of the pyramidal cells. Neurons appeared dark and shrunken with tiny vacuoles in the cytoplasm. Some of the CA1 pyramidal cells were empty and slightly swollen. The neuropil was spongy containing vacuoles and darkly stained granules. After ischemia lasting for 40 min, the changes seen 1 day following the ischemic insult were roughly comparable to those observed 2 days after ischemia of 20 min.

The change was faster in the *CA4* subfield than in the CA1. One day after ischemia, scattered CA4 neurons, more than ten in a section, suffered cell death. The cell bodies were stained dark, shrunken, and surrounded by empty spaces.

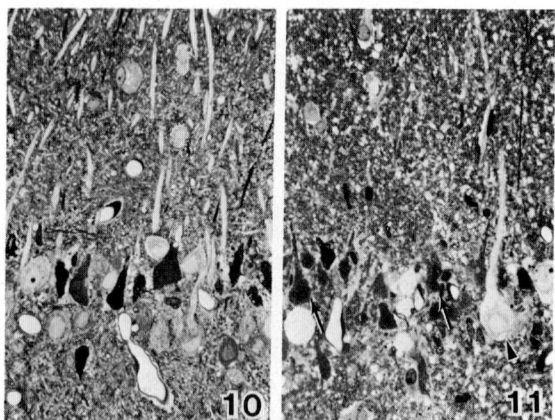

Fig. 10–11. Rat. The CA1 subfield following 20 min of ischemia. Plastic section, toluidine blue, × 340.

Fig. 10. Two days following ischemia, some pyramidal cells are stained intensely dark (arrows) and others pale with slightly swollen cytoplasm.

Fig. 11. Four days following ischemia, most of the neurons have been damaged. Some neurons are dark and shrunken with tiny vacuoles in the cytoplasm (arrows), others (arrowhead) are swollen and look empty.

Summary of the rat experiment

In the rat hippocampus, a similar pattern of ischemic neuronal damage developed. Following 20 min of ischemia, rapid cell disintegration was seen in the CA4, whereas the alteration in the CA1 was strikingly slow. These results suggest that the hippocampal selective vulnerability to ischemia is caused by an identical mechanism both in the gerbil and the rat. The light microscopic findings, however, differed between the two species. The change in the rat CA1 had more morphological similarity to the ischemic cell change which Brierley and his colleagues had defined (Brierley, 1976). To clarify this difference, further study using electron microscopy was done.

Electron microscopic observation of CA1 neurons

The unusually slow cell death in the hippocampus following ischemia posed several questions. First, does the change evolve gradually and steadily from the very beginning of the post-ischemic period? Or, does the alteration take place after the initial latent period during which neurons remain intact? Secondly, when ischemia lasts longer, the change develops more rapidly and resembles the well-defined ischemic cell change. In this case, is there any transitional form between the "delayed neuronal death" type to the "ischemic cell change" type, or is there a sudden shift from the former to the latter when the ischemia is prolonged? Thirdly, are there fundamental differences between the gerbil and the rat in the structural characteristics of the hippocampal neurons after ischemia.

Observations in the gerbil

Although definite structural change was hardly noticed by light microscopy in the CA1 pyramidal cell 1 day following brief ischemia (5–10 min), several fine structural alterations were already present. One was an increase in the cisterns of the endoplasmic reticulum (ER). At the periphery of the perikarya, parallel arrays of ER were formed. Ribosomes were usually disaggregated to form monoribosomes. Clusters of dense material were observed near, but not bound to, the cell surface membrane in the perikarya or in the dendrites. Two days following a brief ischemic insult (Fig. 12) an increased number of ER cisterns became apparent. Around the cell nucleus, fragmentary ER membranes had accumulated and, among them, lysosomes and clusters of dense material not limited by a membrane were seen. On the basal side of the CA1 pyramidal cell parallel stacks of ER cisterns were observed. Ribosomes, only as monoribosomes, were attached to these cisterns or located between them. The nuclear chromatin looked slightly clumped. Mitochondria appeared unchanged; between the 2nd and the 4th day after brief ischemia, most of the CA1 pyramidal cells were destroyed. They showed a condensed, shrunken cytoplasm or, conversely, they had a swollen, watery appearance. No definite uniform pattern of cell destruction was found at this stage.

After 20 min of ischemia (Fig. 13), the CA1 pyramidal cells contained massively proliferated ER cisterns and ribosomes in disaggregated form. Clusters of dark substance were seen scattered in the cytoplasm and in the dendrites. Although the fundamental pathologic changes thus did not differ from that after brief ischemia, they appeared faster. After this stage, the CA1 neurons were rapidly destroyed. Again, no uniform course of cell disintegration seemed to take place. Some neurons had swollen and empty cell bodies, whereas others looked dark and shrunken.

Twelve hours after 30 min of ischemia (Fig. 14), severe cell alteration was observed in some specimens, although the extent of cell changes differed from animal to animal. Some CA1 pyramidal cells displayed a change identical to what occurred after brief ischemia — their cytoplasm was filled with stacks of ER cisterns and clusters of darkly stained substances. Some CA1 neurons showed an advanced stage of cell destruction. Cell nuclei and perikarya were stained dark. Although some of these darkly stained cells showed proliferated ER cisterns in localized areas in their cytoplasm, they resembled the well-defined ischemic cell change on

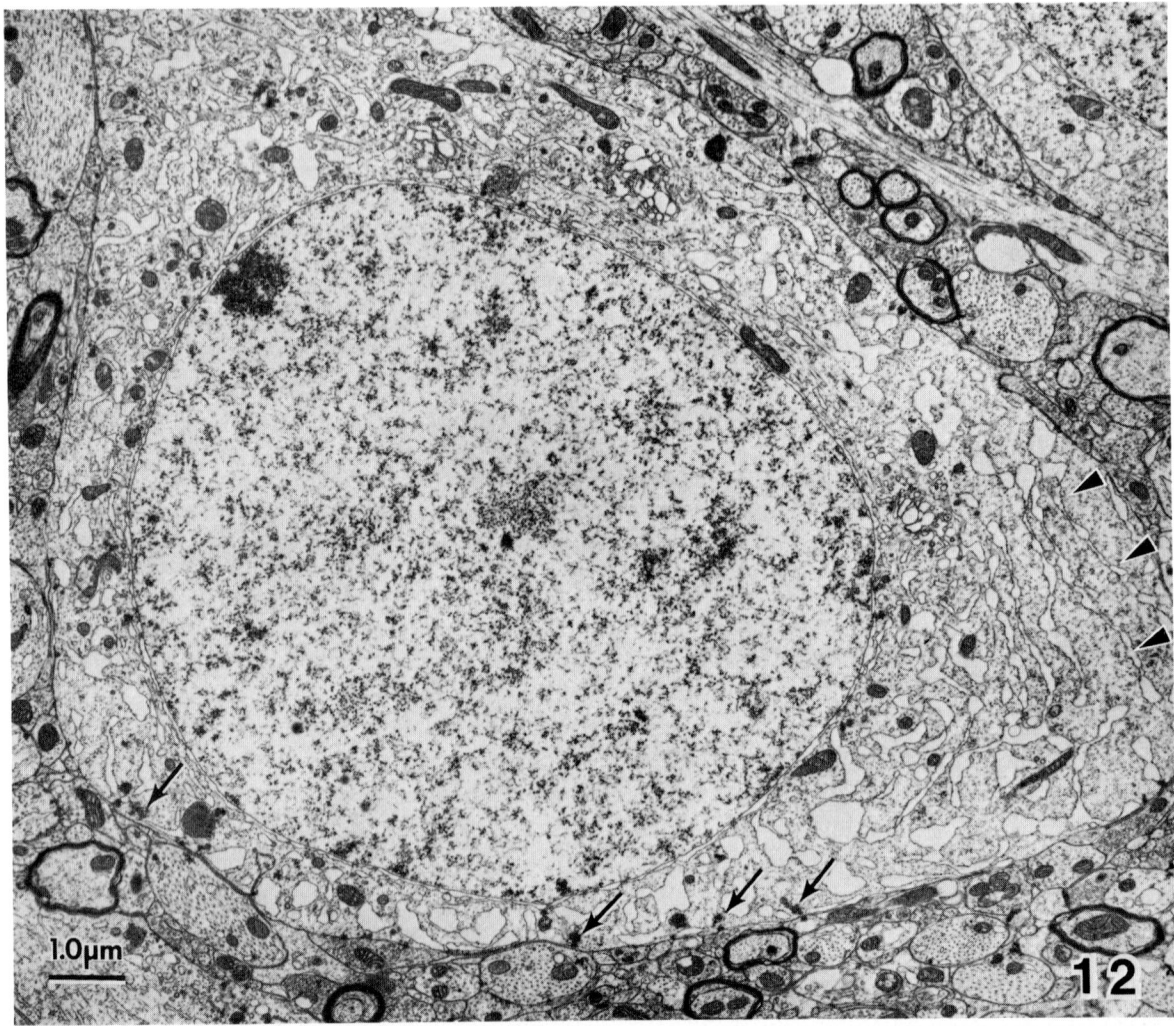

Fig. 12. Gerbil. Electron micrograph showing a CA1 pyramidal cell. Fragmentary membranous organelles fill the perikarya. They frequently form parallel stacks (arrowheads). Accumulation of dense substances in the cytoplasm is seen (arrows). Ribosomes are disaggregated into monoribosomes.

the other hand — their mitochondria frequently demonstrated empty swelling, and their cytoplasm was densely packed with dark ribosome-like granules.

Observations in the rat

One day following 20 min of ischemia (Fig. 15), although abnormalities by light microscopy were slight, the pyramidal cells presented overt ultrastructural alterations. There were increased numbers of membranous organelles scattered randomly as fragmentary cisterns in the cytoplasm. Occasionally they formed parallel arrays at the basal part of the cell body. Ribosomes, mainly monoribosomes, were attached to these membranous arrays or dispersed between the cisterns. Darkly stained substances in the cytoplasm, which were not limited by a membrane, were scattered throughout the perikarya and in the dendrites. Other organelles, such as the cell nucleus, mitochondria, and lysosomes looked unchanged. Two days following 20 min of

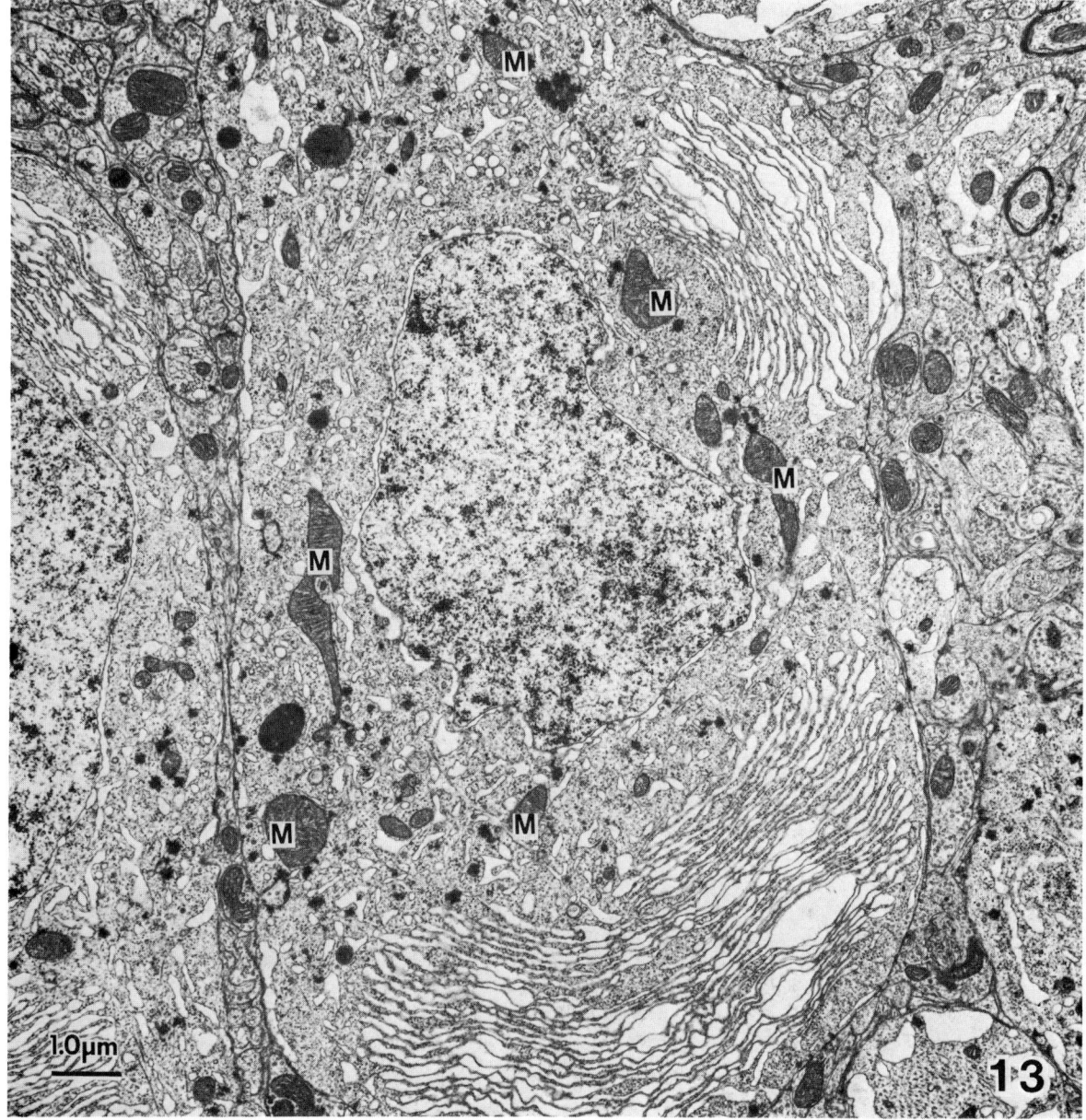

Fig. 13. Gerbil. One day following 20 min of ischemia, the change is more accentuated. All the neurons in this illustration show a similar change. ER cisterns have massively increased. Clusters of dark substances are scattered in the cytoplasm. Mitochondria (M) do not show empty swelling, but some of them are enlarged.

ischemia (Fig. 16), accumulation of dark granules and ribosomes made the nerve cells appear dark. The dark bodies and mitochondria tended to cluster around the central nucleus while multiple stacks of membranes lay at the periphery of the cell. At this stage, the astrocytic processes around neurons were swollen and empty. Four days after the ischemia, the CA1 region showed a glio-mesodermal reaction and an extensive destruction of neurons.

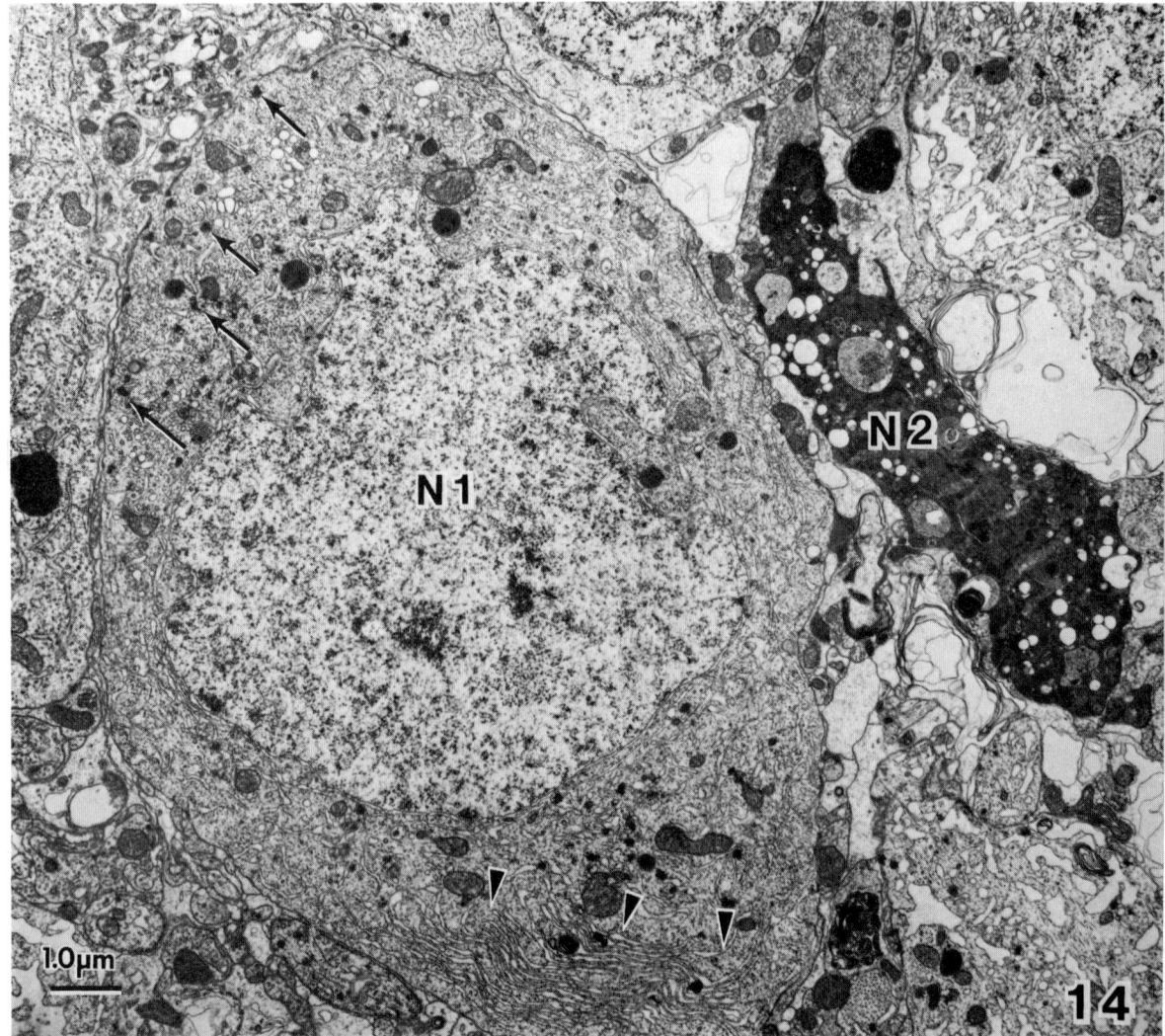

Fig. 14. Gerbil. Twelve hours following 30 min of ischemia. Some CA1 pyramical cells (N1) display similar change as is seen after brief ischemia. The cytoplasm is filled with stacks of ER cisterns (arrowheads) and clusters of dark substances (arrows). Other CA1 neurons (N2) show an advanced stage of cell destruction. The cell is shrunken and intensely dark.

Summary of the electron microscopic observation

The change in the majority of the CA1 neurons is slow but progressive. The full-blown pathologic state is only seen after the 2nd day by light microscopy, but an insidious process starts to take place by 24 h following brief ischemia. This slow change is clearly detected by electron microscopy. The main findings are an accumulation of increased ER cisterns, an increase of dark granules unbound by a membrane, and a disaggregation of polyribosomes into monoribosomes. These changes are never seen in the normal CA1 neurons. The delayed neuronal death in the hipoocampal CA1 subfield is a novel type of cell change after ischemia.

The cell alteration becomes, however, more similar to the previously known ischemic cell change as the intensity of the ischemic insult increases. Most of the neurons are darkly stained and shrunken, whereas some are watery and swollen. This

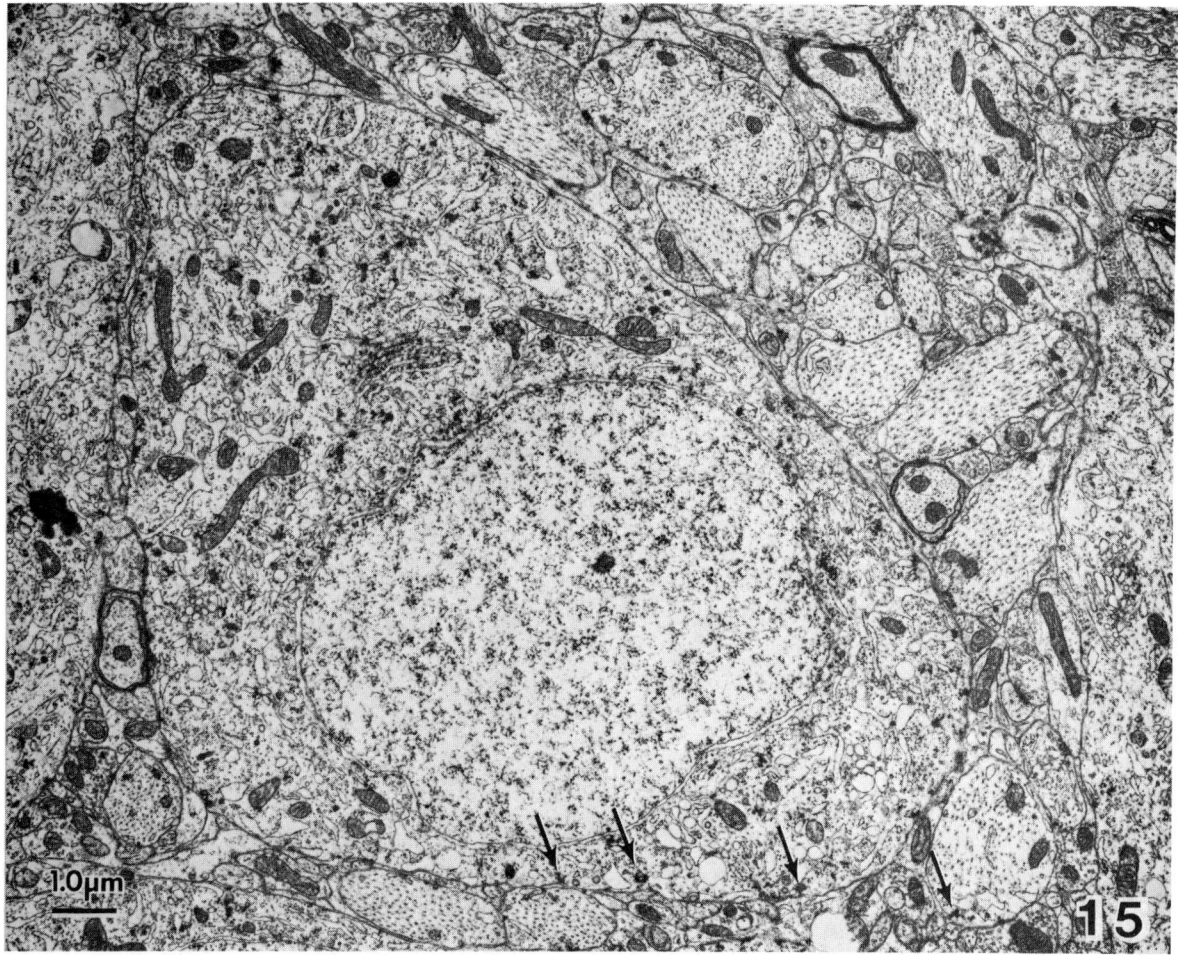

Fig. 15. Rat. One day following 20 min of ischemia. In the CA1 area cells contain fragmentary membranous organelles and scattered dark substances which are not limited by a membrane in the cytoplasm and dendrites (arrows).

full-blown state of ischemic neuronal damage, presumably, does not represent any specific pathological mechanism. The well-known ischemic cell change looks similar to other types of neuronal death. Following deafferentation, Johnson (1975) found dark neurons in the lateral vestibular nucleus in the rat, which are comparable to the ischemic cell change. During a period of development, "naturally occurring cell death" of spinal motoneurons is observed in the chick, with pathologic findings also close to the ischemic cell change (Chu-Wang and Oppenheim, 1978). It is unlikely that these changes are caused primarily by anoxia and/or ischemia.

Therefore the ischemic cell change, probably, is a type of cell change included within a wider category of acute neuronal injury and may not be exclusively specific to ischemia. As the cell change becomes more advanced and irreversible, the specific components of morphological changes seem to be lost gradually and a discussion on the pathogenesis of the cell change may, if done on a morphological basis only, become less practical. In the structural investigation of ischemia, it seems rather meaningful to study the boundary state between reversible and irreversible states.

Following prolonged, severe ischemia many CA1

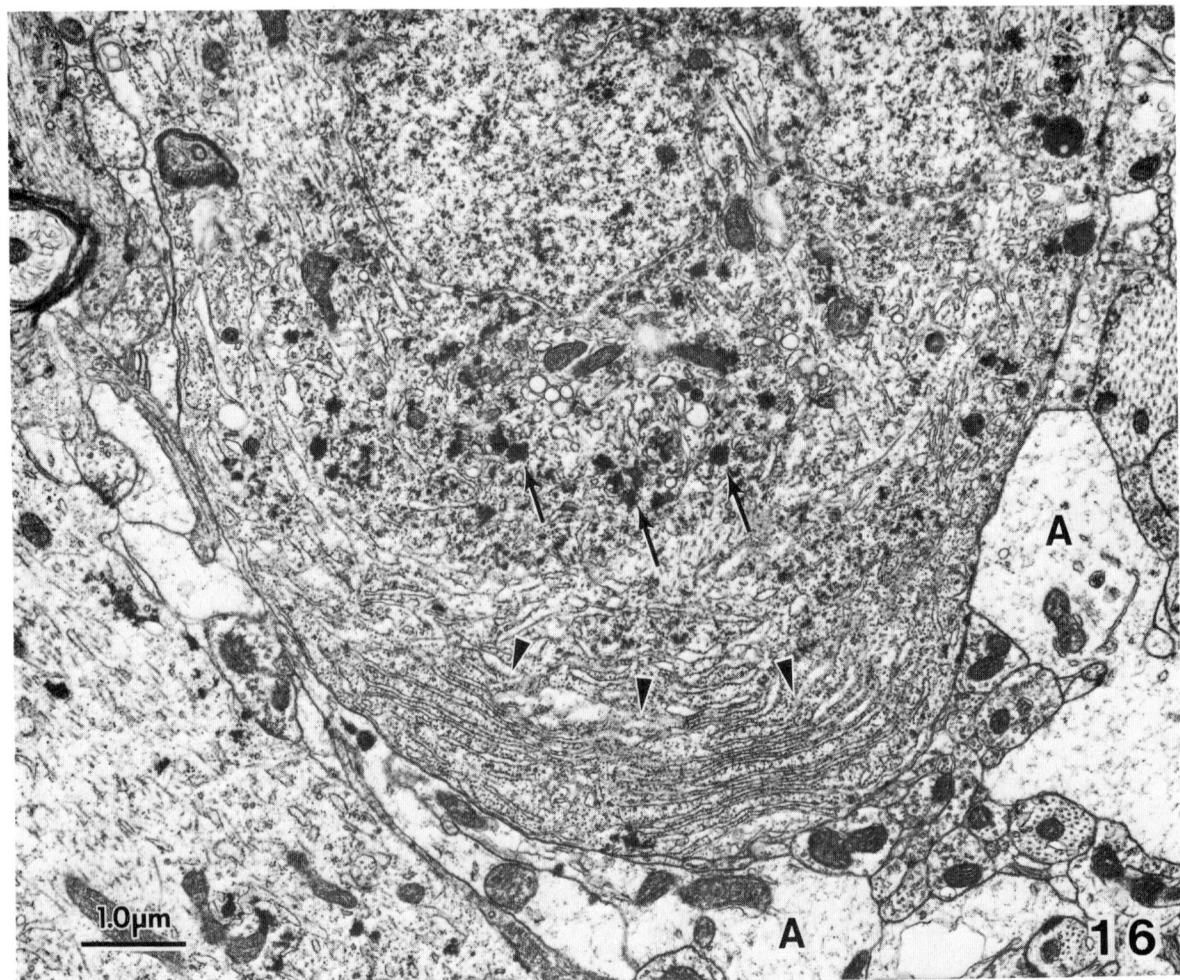

Fig. 16. Rat. One day following 20 min of ischemia. In some CA1 neurons increased membranous structures form parallel arrays (arrowheads) at the basal side of the cytoplasm. Accumulation of dark substances around the cell nucleus (arrowheads) is evident. Astrocytic processes (A) around the surface membrane look empty and swollen.

neurons bear a morphological resemblance, partially to the "ischemic cell change" type, and partially to the "delayed neuronal death" type. There is a transitional form of these two types. Therefore, the two forms of neuronal injury, in all likelihood, are not due to qualitative differences. When ischemia is too intense, neurons may lose their ability to counter the insult and may be destroyed quickly.

The changes in the CA1 following ischemia are very similar in both gerbils and rats in many respects. (1) The time course of the change in the CA1 is slow in both. It takes almost 2 days before the alteration in the CA1 can be observed by light microscopy. (2) The spatial distribution of the lesion is similar in both species. There are scattered cell deaths, which appear faster, in the CA4. Then an extensive neuronal destruction develops in the CA1. (3) Affected pyramidal neurons show similar fine structural changes in the rat and in the gerbil. In view of the resemblances mentioned above and the structural similarity of the normal hippocampus among various species, the alteration in the hippocampus following ischemia exhibited by various species including man may be fundamentally identical to the changes seen in the rodent.

Delayed neuronal death in the hippocampus

For the purpose of understanding the basic mechanism of ischemic neuronal damage, the hippocampus has proven to be one of the most suitable systems for experimental study. We have ample time to examine the CA1 neurons before these cells totally lose their viability. Most of the population of nerve cells in the particular location in the hippocampus behave almost synchronously and therefore it is easier to focus our attention than in a system where the neuronal change is scattered more sparsely. The hippocampus is an area where anatomical, physiological, and biochemical information has been copiously accumulated. This is another advantageous feature of the hippocampus model. In addition, as we will discuss later, the slow neuronal change in the hippocampal CA1 sector following brief ischemia is a potentially reversible alteration. We wish now to emphasize not only the basic but also clinical significance of the research on this hippocampal ischemic damage.

Mechanism of the delay of neuronal damage

The exact mechanism of delayed neuronal death is not known. The events following the reestablishment of recirculation after ischemia are thought to be primarily important in the process of an ischemic neuronal injury (Jenkins et al., 1981). Since a state of hypermetabolism has been reported to occur following recirculation (Diemer and Siemkowicz, 1980), an imbalance in the energy metabolism between supply and demand (Levy et al., 1979) may be the cause of the delayed neuronal death. The fact that the blood flow decreases for a certain period of time after recirculation — a phenomenon called postischemic hypoperfusion — is also known in the gerbil brain (Suzuki et al., 1983a). However, Arai et al. (1982) examined the CA1 subfield in the same gerbil ischemia model biochemically and they confirmed that there is no decrease of ATP that can account for cell deterioration. Pulsinelli et al. (1982a) also noticed a similar change in the energy metabolism in their rat ischemia model. They found that the imbalance of regional blood flow and glucose metabolism did not correlate with the pattern of neuronal injury. Although the phenomenon of metabolic uncoupling, i.e. an imbalance of supply and demand, may play some role, this is unsatisfactory to explain the highly specific cell loss in the hippocampus following brief ischemia.

Each subdivision of the hippocampus showed discrete forms of cell change after brief ischemia. It is better understood that the phenomenon of selective vulnerability depends on the position and interconnection of neurons in the total circuitry within the hippocampus. Since, in the cerebral cortex, inhibitory GABAergic neurons are believed to be highly susceptible to ischemic damage (Sloper et al., 1980), one possible explanation for the selective cell damage in the CA1 sector has been the following: inhibitory GABAergic neurons in the CA1 may be also highly vulnerable to ischemia. First, brief ischemia may cause cell damage in these neurons, then it may in turn precipitate excessive, detrimental firing of the CA1 neurons because of the loss of inhibitory synapses. This hypothesis, however, is not likely since Francis and Pulsinelli (1982) did not detect any selective decrease in the activity of glutamic acid decarboxylase (GAD), an enzyme related to GABA, in the CA1 sector following ischemia. On the contrary, a certain type of interneuron, presumably GABAergic, in the CA1 sector is not vulnerable to ischemia (Johansen et al., 1983).

The neurotoxicity of an amino acid, glutamate, has long been recognized. Olney and his colleagues have tested the toxicity of monosodium glutamate and considered that the excitatory activity of this amino acid is a major cause of this toxicity (Olney et al., 1971). They called this effect "excitotoxicity" (Olney and de Gubareff, 1978). In the CA1 subfield it is well known that most of the neurons have abundant glutamate receptors. It is yet to be clarified that glutamate in this area actually reaches a concentration high enough to activate a sustained excitation of neurons to causes "excitotoxicity". Interestingly kainic acid, a potent glutamate agonist, given intraventricularly, causes selective neuronal destruction in the CA3 sector of the hippocampus

(Nadler et al., 1978). The pattern of injury is completely different from that observed following ischemia. This kainic acid lesion does not appear after the destruction of glutaminergic input into the CA3 subfield and is thus dependent on the presence of excitatory afferents (Nadler and Cuthbertson, 1980).

The specific biochemical mechanism of the delayed neuronal death in the CA1 neurons following brief ischemia is still controversial. In the CA1 sector, the apical dendrites have high Ca^{2+} conductance which gives rise to burst discharges in the neurons (Traub and Llinas, 1979). In view of this fact Siesjö (1981) proposed the hypothesis that an excessive influx of Ca^{2+} into the cell following ischemia causes cell damage. Since an intracellular overload of Ca^{2+} is widely known to be detrimental, the working hypothesis that this ion is the common denominator of ischemic cell damage has attracted attention. Along this line, the events before and after Ca^{2+} entry are now being studied.

Rothman (1983) cultured the rat hippocampal neurons obtained from an embryo and tested their vulnerability to anoxia. He found that, before the establishment of synapses between cultured neurons, they are less susceptible to anoxia. However, as soon as neurons start to communicate by synapses, they became vulnerable to oxygen deprivation. At this stage, he added $MgCl_2$ to block synaptic activity and noticed that neurons can survive an anoxic insult. This result seems to suggest that synaptic activity is inevitably related to the neuronal vulnerability to anoxia or ischemia.

Although the CA1 neurons maintain their structural integrity for longer than 24 hours after brief ischemia, the fine structural changes are already seen at this stage. This change is an unusual form of neuronal alteration which follows ischemia. Such pathologic alteration is, however, not uncommon in the scope of general cell pathology. The increase of ER cisterns has been known especially in the pancreatic acinar cell and the hepatocyte (Suzuki and Zagoren, 1973, for refs.). In most cases the growth of ER cisterns is related to toxic substances. There may be two ways of interpreting the ER growth (Suzuki and Zagoren, 1973): the increase of the ER membrane may be due to a degenerative alteration of the endoplasmic reticulum or to a regenerative, repairing process of the membranous organelle. Disaggregation of polyribosomes into monoribosomes has been reported to occur following ischemia (Kleihues and Hossmann, 1971). Nevertheless, it may not be specific to an ischemic neuronal injury since various disease processes are known to show this phenomenon (Kleihues and Hossmann, 1971, for ref.).

Petito and Pulsinelli (1984) considered that the delayed neuronal death in the rat hippocampus has many morphological characteristics common with central chromatolysis which is usually seen as a result of axon reaction. Therefore, they proposed a hypothesis that the slow neuronal death in the CA1 neurons is caused by primary damage to neuronal processes. Some ultrastructural findings in the delayed neuronal death are indeed similar to those seen following axotomy. The changes which mimic central chromatolysis are, however, seen in various disease processes, including the change following excessive electrical stimulation (Peters et al., 1976, p. 12). Although the consequence of axon reaction on the survival of neurons is usually more severe in the brain of young animals (Lieberman, 1971), the effect of brief ischemia on the hippocampal CA1 neurons was less severe in young gerbils (Martinez et al., 1984). These facts, however, are not decisive enough to exclude the possibility of Petito's hypothesis.

Suzuki et al. (1983b) studied the gerbil CA1 neurons electrophysiologically following brief ischemia. They found that the CA1 neurons are electrically active for 1 day after ischemia. This means, at least electrophysiologically, that the neurons in the CA1 sector are alive for a certain period following brief ischemia. If this hypothesis is valid, neurons, following ischemia, are left in an unstable state between death and survival. As a consequence, there is the possibility of salvaging dying neurons following ischemia. To examine this hypothesis further, an experiment of drug effect on the change in the gerbil hippocampus following ischemia was performed.

Drug treatment of ischemic neuronal damage in the hippocampus

Mongolian gerbils weighing 60–80 g were subjected to bilateral carotid occlusion for 5 min. Immediately following clip removal a certain amount of pentobarbital was injected intraperitoneally. The dosages of pentobarbital were 10 mg/kg, 20 mg/kg, or 40 mg/kg. Each dosage group had its controls, which received the same volume of saline injection. Each group consisted of about 10 gerbils, and a total of 64 gerbils including 8 normal unoperated animals was used in this experiment. The animals were perfusion fixed 1 week following the ischemia and paraffin sections were prepared. Then the length of the CA1 subfield was measured, and the number of the CA1 neurons counted, without knowing the details of the preceding treatment. Based on these data, the neuronal density, i.e. the number of neurons per 1 mm length of the CA1 subfield, was calculated. Statistical analysis was done using Wilcoxon's rank sum test.

In all the hippocampi obtained from unoperated, normal gerbils ($n = 8$) the neuronal density was 212 ± 4.3/mm (mean ± standard error), the lowest density being 178/mm. The hippocampus with a neuronal density below 80/mm, a density less than a half of the lowest value in the normal gerbils, was considered to be severely affected by ischemia. The density above 160/mm was thought to be within normal limit or within a minimal range of neuronal damage.

When all the control animals ($n = 27$) which were subjected to ischemia and had not been treated by pentobarbital were counted as one group, 79.6% of 54 hippocampi were severely affected, and 9.3% were near normal. The overall average of neuronal density for the control group was 47 ± 8.4/mm.

In the gerbils ($n = 9$) injected with 10 mg/kg of pentobarbital the average neuronal density was 106 ± 16.4/mm. There was a tendency of favorable drug effect but this was not statistically significant. The corresponding controls ($n = 8$) had an average neuronal density of 64 ± 17.0/mm. Pentobarbital treatment with a dosage of 20 mg/kg ($n = 10$) showed a definite effect, with 75% of 20 hippocampi being almost normal or minimally damaged. The average density was 168 ± 13.0/mm, whereas the average density in the corresponding controls ($n = 9$) was 53 ± 13.8/mm. This difference was statistically significant ($p < 0.01$). Pentobarbital, 40 mg/kg ($n = 10$), showed a similar effect. The average density was 181 ± 16.1/mm, and the density of the controls ($n = 10$) was 29 ± 12.2/mm. This was statistically significant as well ($p < 0.01$).

Neurons which are to succumb without treatment survive when pentobarbital is given. Therefore, this result obtained by using pentobarbital indicates that the CA1 neurons, which are destined to die in a few days for the most part, are still alive immediately following brief ischemia. This means that drug treatment of ischemic stroke is effective at least in a restricted situation.

A number of drugs have known protective effects against ischemic neuronal injury, but pentobarbital is one of the best known and the most used. The precise pharmacological mechanism in cerebral ischemia is, however, yet to be clarified. Following the drug treatment, even if it is effective, one may not be able to tell the exact location of neurons which react to the drug administration, especially when such neurons are scattered sparsely. One advantage of the gerbil model in this regard is that the location of the neuronal population which will enjoy favorable drug effects is predictable.

The clinical usefulness of pentobarbital is still somewhat limited. In this experiment as well we don't know up to what degree of ischemia the drug is effective. Practically, how long the treatment can be delayed is still another important question. Our preliminary data concerning this latter problem is so far pessimistic since pentobarbital, which is effective if given immediately after brief ischemia in the gerbil, has no effect of protecting neurons when injected 1 h following ischemia. This result reminds us of the fact that protein synthesis in the CA1 neurons is already suppressed 2 h following brief ischemia (Bodsch et al., 1985). The metabolic state of the CA1 neurons seems to be greatly disturbed far earlier than we can detect any morphological changes.

Clinical significance of the delayed neuronal death in the hippocampus

The active function of the central nervous system depends, roughly speaking, on the number of working neurons. Since neurons in the brain do not regenerate, preservation of neurons is of primary importance in clinical neurology and neurosurgery. We would like to emphasize the importance of, if it actually exists, reversible ischemic injury.

In clinical cases of ischemic stroke, a rapid, irreversible type of ischemic neuronal injury is the major problem. The slow, potentially reversible type of change as seen in the gerbil hippocampus may play only a minor role in stroke patients. In addition, we have no evidence whether this slow type of ischemic neuronal damage is encountered in other areas of the brain or if it is only seen in the hippocampus.

The practical significance of this slowly progressing neuronal damage, however, should not be underestimated. Not only in the hippocampus but in other areas of the brain, as well as in the periphery of focal ischemia, there is a possibility of finding a less destructive type of ischemic neuronal damage. This type of neuronal injury may not progress rapidly and could be reversible. We hope that future experiments will make it clear that delayed neuronal death is one of the examples in which successful treatment of sick neurons becomes possible following ischemia.

References

Arai, H., Lust, W.D. and Passonneau, J.V. (1982) Delayed metabolic changes induced by 5 min of ischemia in gerbil brain. *Trans. Am. Soc. Neurochem.*, 13: 177.

Bliss, T.V.P. and Dolphin, A.C. (1982) What is the mechanism of long-term potentiation in the hippocampus. *Trend Neurosci.*, 289–290.

Bodsch, W., Takahashi, K., Barbier, A., Grosse Ophoff, B. and Hossmann, K.-A. (1985) Cerebral protein synthesis and ischemia. *This volume*, pp. 197–210.

Bouchet and Cazauvieilh (1825) De l'épilepsie considérée dans ses rapports avec l'aliénation mentale. Paris, cited by Spielmeyer (1927).

Bratz, E. (1899) Ammonshornbefunde der Epileptischen. *Arch. Psychiat.*, 31: 820–836.

Brierley, J.B. (1976) Cerebral hypoxia. In: W. Blackwood and J.A.N. Corsellis (Eds.), *Greenfield's Neuropathology. 3rd edn.*, Edward Arnold, London, pp. 41–85.

Brierley, J.B., Brown, A.W. and Meldrum, B.S. (1971) The nature and time course of the neuronal alterations resulting from oligaemia and hypoglycaemia in the brain of *Macaca mulatta*. *Brain Res.*, 25: 483–499.

Brown, A.W. and Brierley, J.B. (1972) Anoxic-ischemic cell change in rat brain. Light microscopic and fine-structural observations. *J. Neurol. Sci.*, 16: 59–84.

Brown, A.W., Levy, D.E., Kublik, M., Harrow, J. and Plum, F. (1979) Selective chromatolysis of neurons in the gerbil brain: a possible consequence of "epileptic" activity produced by common carotid artery occlusion. *Ann. Neurol.*, 5: 127–138.

Bubis, J.J., Fujimoto, T., Ito, U., Mrsulja, B.J., Spatz, M. and Klatzo, I. (1976) Experimental cerebral ischemia in Mongolian gerbils. V. Ultrastructural changes in H3 sector of the hippocampus. *Acta Neuropathol. (Berl.)*, 36: 285–294.

Chu-Wang, I. and Oppenheim, R.W. (1978) Cell death of motoneurons in the chick embryo spinal cord. I. A light and electron microscopic study of naturally occurring and induced cell loss during development. *J. Comp. Neurol.*, 177: 33–58.

Coceani, F. and Gloor, P. (1966) The distribution of the internal carotid circulation in the brain of the Macaque monkey (*Macaca mulatta*). *J. Comp. Neurol.*, 128: 419–428.

Cohn, R. (1979) Convulsive activity in gerbils subjected to cerebral ischemia. *Exp. Neurol.*, 65: 391–397.

Crockard, A., Iannotti, F., Hunstock, A.T., Smith, R.D., Harris, R.J. and Symon, L. (1980) Cerebral blood flow and edema following carotid occlusion in the gerbil. *Stroke*, 11: 494–498.

Diemer, N.H. and Siemkowicz, E. (1980) Increased 2-deoxyglucose uptake in hippocampus, globus pallidus, and substantia nigra after cerebral ischemia. *Acta Neurol. Scand.*, 61: 56–63.

Francis, A. and Pulsinelli, W. (1982) The response of GABAergic and cholinergic neurons to transient cerebral ischemia. *Brain Res.*, 243: 271–278.

Isaacson, R.L. (1982) *The limbic system*, 2nd edn. Plenum Press, New York, London.

Isaacson, R.L. and Pribram, K.H. (Eds.) (1975) *The hippocampus, a comprehensive treatise* (2 vols.) Plenum Press, New York.

Ito, U., Spatz, M., Walker, J.T. and Klatzo, I. (1975) Experimental cerebral ischemia in Mongolian gerbils. I. Light microscopic observations. *Acta Neuropathol. (Berl.)*, 32: 209–223.

Jenkins, L.W., Povlishock, J.T., Lewelt, W., Miller, J.D. and Becker, D.P. (1981) The role of postischemic recirculation in the development of ischemic neuronal injury following complete cerebral ischemia. *Acta Neuropathol. (Berl.)*, 55: 205–220.

Johansen, F.F., Jørgensen, M.B. and Diemer, N.H. (1983) Resistance of hippocampal CA-1 interneurons to 20 min of transient cerebral ischemia in the rat. *Acta Neuropathol. (Berl.)*, 61: 135–140.

Johnson, J.E. Jr. (1975) The occurrence of dark neurons in the normal and deafferentated lateral vestibular nucleus in the rat. Observations by light and electron microscopy. *Acta Neuropath. (Berl.)*, 31: 117–127.

Kahn, K. (1972) The natural course of experimental cerebral infarction in the gerbil. *Neurology (Minneap.)*, 22: 510–515.

Kalimo, H., Rehncrona, S., Soderfeldt, B., Olsson, Y. and Siesjö, B.K. (1981) Brain lactic acidosis and ischemic cell damage. 2. Histopathology. *J. Cereb. Blood Flow Metabol.*, 1: 313–327.

Kirino, T. (1982) Delayed neuronal death in the gerbil hippocampus following ischemia. *Brain Res.*, 239: 57–69.

Kirino, T. and Sano, K. (1984a) Selective vulnerability in the gerbil hippocampus following transient ischemia. *Acta Neuropathol. (Berl.)*, 62: 201–208.

Kirino, T. and Sano, K. (1984b) Fine structural nature of delayed neuronal death following ischemia in the gerbil hippocampus. *Acta Neuropathol. (Berl.)*, 62: 209–218.

Kirino, T., Brightman, M.W., Oertel, W.H., Schmechel, D.E. and Marangos, P.J. (1983) Neuron-specific enolase as an index of neuronal regeneration and reinnervation. *J. Neurosci.*, 3: 915–923.

Kirino, T., Tamura, A. and Sano, K. (1984) Delayed neuronal death in the rat hippocampus following transient forebrain ischemia. *Acta Neuropathol. (Berl.)*, 64: 139–147.

Kleihues, P. and Hossmann, K.-A. (1971) Protein synthesis in the cat brain after prolonged cerebral ischemia. *Brain Res.*, 35: 409–418.

Levine, S. and Payan, H. (1966) Effects of ischemia and other procedures on the brain and retina of the gerbil *(Meriones unguiculatus)*. *Exp. Neurol.*, 16: 255–262.

Levine, S. and Sohn, D. (1969) Cerebral ischemia in infant and adult gerbils. Relation to incomplete circle of Willis. *Arch. Pathol.*, 87: 315–317.

Levy, D.E., Brierley, J.B. and Plum, F. (1975) Ischaemic brain damage in the gerbil in the absence of "no-reflow". *J. Neurol. Neurosurg. Psychiat.*, 38: 1197–1205.

Levy, D.E., Van Uitert, R.L. and Pike, C.L. (1979) Delayed postischemic hypoperfusion: a potentially damaging consequence of stroke. *Neurology*, 29: 1245–1252.

Lieberman, A.R. (1971) The axon reaction: A review of the principal features of perikaryal responses to axon injury. In: *International Review of Neurobiology*, Vol. 14. Academic Press, New York, London, pp. 49–124.

Lorente de Nó, R. (1934) Studies on the structure of the cerebral cortex. II. Continuation of the study of the ammonic system. *J. Psychol. Neurol.*, 46: 113–117.

Martinez, H., Cahn, R., Mrsulja, B.B. and Klatzo, I. (1984) Reactivity of young gerbil brain to cerebral ischemia. *J. Neuropathol. Exp. Neurol.*, 43: 352.

McGee-Russel, S.M., Brown, A.W. and Brierley, J.B. (1970) A combined light and electron microscope study of early anoxic-ischaemic cell change in rat brain. *Brain Res.*, 20: 193–200.

Nadler, J.V. and Cuthbertson, G.J. (1980) Kainic acid neurotoxicity toward hippocampal formation: dependence on specific excitatory pathways. *Brain Res.*, 195: 47–56.

Nadler, J.V., Perry, B.W. and Cotman, C.W. (1978) Intraventricular kainic acid preferentially destroys hippocampal pyramidal cells. *Nature*, 271: 676–677.

O'Keefe, J. and Nadel, L. (1978) *The Hippocampus as a Cognitive Map*. Oxford University Press, Oxford.

Olney, J.W. and de Gubareff, T. (1978) Extreme sensitivity of olfactory cortical neurons to kainic acid toxicity. In: E.G. McGeer, J.W. Olney and P.L. McNeer (Eds.), *Kainic Acid as a Tool in Neurobiology*. Raven Press, New York, pp. 201–217.

Olney, J.W., Ho, O.L. and Rhee, V. (1971) Cytotoxic effects of acidic and sulphur containing amino acids on the infant mouse central nervous system. *Exp. Brain Res.*, 14: 61–76.

Peters, A., Palay, S.L. and Webster, H de F. (1976) *The Fine Structure of the Nervous System. The Neurons and Supporting Cells*. W.B. Saunders, Philadelphia, London, Toronto.

Petito, C.K. and Pulsinelli, W.A. (1984) Delayed neuronal recovery and neuronal death in rat hippocampus following severe cerebral ischemia: possible relationship to abnormalities in neuronal processes. *J. Cereb. Blood Flow Metabol.*, 4: 194–205.

Pfleger, L. (1880) Beobachtung über Schrumpfung und Sclerose des Ammonshornes bei Epilepsie. *Allg. Z. Psychiat.*, 36: 359–365.

Pickel, V.M., Reis, D.J., Marangos, P.J. and Zomzely-Neurath, C. (1975) Immunocytochemical localization of nervous system specific protein (NSR-P) in rat brain. *Brain Res.*, 105: 184–187.

Pulsinelli, W.A. and Brierley, J.B. (1979) A new model of bilateral hemispheric ischemia in the unanesthetized rat. *Stroke*, 10: 267–272.

Pulsinelli, W.A. and Duffy, T.E. (1983) Regional energy balance in rat brain after transient forebrain ischemia. *J. Neurochem.*, 40: 1500–1503.

Pulsinelli, W.A., Levy, D.E. and Duffy, T.E. (1982a) Regional cerebral blood flow and glucose metabolism following transient forebrain ischemia. *Ann. Neurol.*, 11: 499–509.

Pulsinelli, W.A., Brierley, J.B. and Plum, F. (1982b) Temporal profile of neuronal damage in a model of transient forebrain ischemia. *Ann. Neurol.*, 11: 491–498.

Rothman, S.M. (1983) Synaptic activity mediates death of hypoxic neurons. *Science*, 220: 536–537.

Salford, L.G., Plum, F. and Brierley, J.B. (1973) Graded hypoxia-oligemia in rat brain. II. Neuropathological alterations and their implications. *Arch. Neurol.*, 29: 234–238.

Sano, K. and Malamud, N. (1953) Clinical significance of sclerosis of the cornu ammonis: ictal "psychic phenomena". *Arch. Neurol. Psychiat.*, 70: 40–53.

Scharrer, E. (1940) Vacularization and vulnerability of the cornu ammonis in the opossum. *Neurol. Psychiat. (Chic.)*, 44: 483–506.

Shepherd, G.M. (1979) *The synaptic organization of the brain*, 2nd edn. Oxford University Press, New York, Oxford.

Siesjö, B.K. (1981) Cell damage in the brain: a speculative synthesis. *J. Cereb. Blood Flow Metabol.,* 1: 155–185.

Sloper, J.J., Johnson, P. and Powell, T.P.S. (1980) Selective degeneration of interneurons in the motor cortex of infant monkeys following controlled hypoxia: a possible cause of epilepsy. *Brain Res.,* 198: 204–209.

Sommer, W. (1880) Erkrankung des Ammonshorns als ätiologisches Moment der Epilepsie. *Arch. Psychiatry,* 10: 631–675.

Spielmeyer, W. (1925) Zur Pathogenese der örtlich elektiver Gehirnveränderungen. *Z. Ges. Neurol. Psychiat.,* 99: 756–776.

Spielmeyer, W. (1927) Die Pathogenese des epileptischen Krampfes. *Z. Neurol. Psychiat.,* 109: 501–520.

Spielmeyer, W. (1929) Über örtliche Vulnerabilität. *Z. Ges. Neurol. Psychiat.,* 118: 1–16.

Suzuki, K. and Zagoren, J.C. (1973) Effect of the hypocholesterolemic drug AY-9944 on developing central nervous system of rats: alteration of endoplasmic reticulum in oligodendroglia. *J. Neurocytol.,* 2: 216–222.

Suzuki, R., Yamaguchi, T., Kirino, T., Orzi, F. and Klatzo, I. (1983a) The effects of 5-minute ischemia in Mongolian gerbils: I. Blood-brain barrier, cerebral blood flow, and local cerebral glucose utilization changes. *Acta Neuropathol. (Berl.),* 60: 207–216.

Suzuki, R., Yamaguchi, T., Li, C.L. and Klatzo, I. (1983b) The effects 5-minute ischemia in Mongolian gerbils. II. Changes of spontaneous neuronal activity in cerebral cortex and CA1 sector of hippocampus. *Acta Neuropathol. (Berl.),* 60: 217–222.

Tamura, A., Horizoe, H. and Fukuda, T. (1981) Relationship of cerebral vasculature to infarcted areas following unilateral common carotid artery ligation in the Mongolian gerbil. *J. Cereb. Blood Flow Metabol.,* 1, Suppl. 1: S194–195.

Traub, R.D. and Llinas, R. (1979) Hippocampal pyramidal cells: significance of dentritic ionic conductances for neuronal function and epileptogenesis. *J. Neurophysiol.,* 42: 476–498.

Uchimura, J. (1928) Über die Gefäßversorgung des Ammonshornes. *Z. Ges. Neurol. Psychiat.,* 112: 1–19.

Van Harreveld, A., Crowell, J. and Malhotra, S.K. (1965) A study of extracellular space in central nervous tissue by freeze-substitution. *J. Cell Biol.,* 25: 117–137.

Vogt, C. and Vogt, O. (1922) Erkrankungen der Großhirnrinde im Lichte der topistik Pathoklise und Pathoarchitektonik. *J. Psychol. Neurol.,* 28: 1–171.

Microphysiology of selectively vulnerable neurons

Ryuta Suzuki[a], Takekane Yamaguchi[a], Yutaka Inaba[a] and Henry G. Wagner[b]

[a]Department of Neurosurgery, Tokyo Medical and Dental University, Tokyo Medical and Dental University, 1-5-45 Yushima Bunkyo-ku, Tokyo 113, Japan, and [b]Laboratory of Neuropathology and Neuroanatomical Sciences, NINCDS, National Institutes of Health, USA

Introduction

The consequences of ischemic insult to neurons are quite heterogeneous topographically and also chronologically. The topographical heterogeneity is known as "selective vulnerability", and the chronological heterogeneity is known as "maturation phenomenon" (Ito et al., 1975). These phenomena are responsible for the complexity of the sequential changes of neurons following ischemic insult but, on the other hand, they provide the opportunity for the study of the mechanisms of ischemic cell death. Kirino (1982) observed that a brief ischemic insult produced selective neuronal damage in the neurons of the hippocampal CA1 subfield (CA1N), with high chronological and topographical reproducibility, in Mongolian gerbils. According to his work, CA1N showed slowly progressing destruction which became dramatically pronounced at 3–4 days following 5 min of bilateral common carotid artery (CCA) occlusion. The phenomenon was termed "delayed neuronal death" (DND) because of the characteristic time course. DND provides the opportunity to observe the development of morphological, electrophysiological and pathophysiological changes in selectively vulnerable neurons following ischemic insult. With these data it may be possible to come close to the understanding of the mechanisms of "ischemic cell death", and to find a treatment for cerebral ischemia.

In the present paper changes of neuronal function and other physiological parameters following brief CCA occlusion in Mongolian gerbils as well as regional differences of these parameters, are described.

Material and methods

1. Animal preparation

The limbs of Mongolian gerbils (3–4 months old) were loosely fixed with adhesive tapes, and the animals were anesthetized with a mixture of 20–30% oxygen, 70–80% nitrous oxide, and 1–2% halothane. CCA were exposed bilaterally through a midline cervical incision and Heifetz clips were applied on both CCA, as the anesthesia was discontinued. After 5 min, the clips were removed for recirculation of the brain.

2. Morphological observations

Five minutes forebrain ischemia were produced by bilateral CCA occlusion in 89 animals. The animals were perfused transcardially with paraformaldehyde at 3, 6, 12 hours, 1, 2, 3, 4, 5, 6 days, and 1, 2 weeks after the insult. Brains were removed 2 h later, kept in the same fixative overnight and embedded in paraffin. Brain sections were stained with HE and cresyl violet, and studied by light microscopy.

3. Quantitative measurement of regional cerebral blood flow (rCBF)

The method of rCBF measurement using ^{3}H-nicotine described by Ohno et al. (1979) was modified for our experiments (Suzuki et al., 1983a, 1984). Ten μCi of ^{3}H-nicotine (Amersham, specific activity 1.27 Ci/mmol) was infused in 45 animals at various times after the onset of ischemia, while arterial blood was sampled at a constant rate using a withdrawal pump. The animals were decapitated 35 seconds after the start of ^{3}H-nicotine infusion. Each brain was rapidly dissected into its cerebellum, hippocampus, frontal and occipital cortex sections, and weighed. rCBF (ml/100 g per min) was calculated as: rCBF = $100 \times Qb \times Fs/Qs \times Mb$, where Qb represents quantity of indicator in brain mass, Fs is the known withdrawal rate of arterial blood sample (ml/min), Qs represents quantity of indicator in the blood sample and Mb is brain mass in grams.

4. Qualitative assay of rCBF

In 25 gerbils rCBF was studied qualitatively before, during and at various times after ischemia, using ^{14}C-iodoantipyrine autoradiography. The animals received 10 μCi of ^{14}C-iodoantipyrine (New England Nuclear Co., specific activity 58.9 mCi/mmol) by constant infusion into the femoral vein over 40 seconds; at the end of this period they were decapitated. Brains were immersed into liquid nitrogen, cut coronally into 20-μm sections, and prepared for autoradiography (Sakurada et al., 1978).

5. Qualitative assay of local cerebral glucose utilization (lCGU)

In 34 gerbils lCGU was evaluated qualitatively before and at various times after ischemia using ^{14}C-2-deoxyglucose. The animals received 10 μCi of ^{14}C-2-deoxyglucose (New England Nuclear Co., specific activity 52.2 mCi/mmol) by bolus injection into the femoral vein, and were decapitated 20 or 45 min later. The brains were immersed into liquid nitrogen, and processed for autoradiography.

To assess cerebral glucose transport 10 μCi of 3-O-methyl-^{14}C-D-glucose (New England Nuclear Co., specific activity 53.5 mCi/mmol) was injected into 12 gerbils, and the brains were processed for autoradiography.

6. Recordings of spontaneous neuronal activity (SNA)

Procedures in acute experiments: 35 animals were anesthetized as before, surgical exposure of CCA was performed, and 4–0 silk loops were placed around the CCA. During the following procedure the animals were anesthetized with a mixture of 20–30% oxygen, 70–80% nitrous oxide, and 0.7–1.0% halothane. The animals were placed on a warm blanket, and their heads were fixed in a stereotaxic instrument. A small opening in the cranium was made at 2.0–2.5 mm posterior and 1.8–2.0 mm lateral to the bregma, and the dura was incised. A glass microelectrode with a tip of 1–2 μm, filled with 2 M NaCl, was advanced to a predetermined depth, either into the cortex or into the hippocampal CA1 subfield. According to the frozen sections from 20 gerbil brains, the thickness of the cortex was 1.055 ± 0.059 mm and the depth of CA1 sector from the cortical surface was 1.355 ± 0.053 mm (mean ± SD). For recording of SNA from the cerebral cortex the electrodes were placed at 0.8 ± 0.1 mm depth from the surface. The placement in CA1 subfield was ascertained by recording SNA in the cortex and, after passing a "silent zone" of white matter, by reappearance of SNA at a depth of about 1.355 mm below cortical surface. After obtaining stable action potential recordings, the silk loops around CCA were pulled by a weight to occlude the circulation. Five minutes later the silk loops were cut and removed to restore blood flow. SNA recordings were continued for 40–70 min after beginning of recirculation. During the procedure, a bipolar electroencephalogram (EEG) was also recorded from the epidural surface of the frontal and temporal cortex. To confirm the placement of the microelectrodes fast green or neutral red were in-

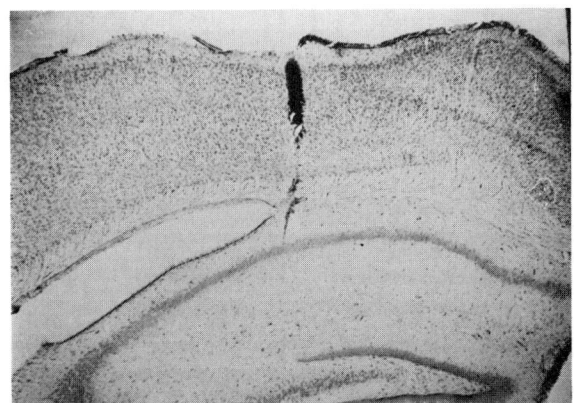

Fig. 1. Track of microelectrode, stained iontophoretically with neutral red, showing the tip located in the CA1 subfield of the hippocampus. Cresyl violet staining of Vibratome section. (With permission from Suzuki et al., 1983b.)

jected by iontophoretic method at the end of the experiment. After the experiment the brains were taken out from the animals and Vibratome brain sections were examined with cresyl violet staining (Fig. 1).

Procedures in chronic experiments: 26 animals, each being previously submitted to 5 min of forebrain ischemia, were prepared for the experiments. At 7–10 h, 1 and 2 days after the ischemic insult, the animals were reanesthetized with a mixture of oxygen, nitrous oxide and halothane, and fixed in the stereotaxic apparatus. SNA recordings were obtained from neurons of the cortex (CorN) and CA1N. The frequencies of action potentials were determined with a signal analyser, operating in the histogram mode. A more detailed description has been published elsewhere (Suzuki et al., 1983b).

7. Measurement of extracellular potassium ($[K^+]e$) and calcium ($[Ca^{2+}]e$) activity

Ten animals were prepared by the same procedure as used for SNA recordings, except for the anesthesia which was induced by pentobarbital (40 mg/kg i.p.). A multibarrelled glass pipette with a tip diameter of 10–20 μ was used. One barrel was filled with a potassium ion-selective resin (Corning 477317), another was filled with a calcium ion-selective resin (WPI IE-202). The third barrel was filled with 154 mM NaCl and used as the reference electrode, and for recording of local EEG. Calibration of each ion-selective electrode was performed before and after each experiment, using calibration fluids of known concentrations of KCl and $CaCl_2$. The electrode tips were positioned by a micromanipulator in the extracellular space of cerebral cortex or hippocampal CA1 subfield. After allowing 20–30 min for stabilization of electrodes, CCA were occluded bilaterally for 5 min, then CCA were recirculated. Recordings were discontinued 25–30 min after the beginning of recirculation.

Results

1. Morphological observations

The morphological changes in the brains after 5 min of ischemia were restricted to the hippocampus, thus confirming earlier observations of Kirino (1982). With respect to CA1N, notable changes were observed first at 2 days following ischemia, at which time neurons showed some loss of Nissl substance, a more accentuated staining of dendrites, and appearance of clear clefts in the cytoplasm. After 3 days most of CA1N showed severe ischemic injury, followed by neuronal disintegration at 4 days (Fig. 2). The cortex showed no pathological changes during the whole observation period.

2. Quantitative measurements of rCBF

The results are presented in the Table 1. Bilateral CCA occlusion produced severe ischemia in both cortex and hippocampus. In contrast, cerebellum showed increased flow as a consequence of high blood pressure during occlusion. The release of occlusion resulted in reactive hyperemia in the previously ischemic territories. Reactive hyperemia was followed by post-ischemic hypoperfusion after 10 min recirculation. Within 2 days rCBF returned to normal except in the cerebellum, which showed significant low perfusion at 1 day after recirculation.

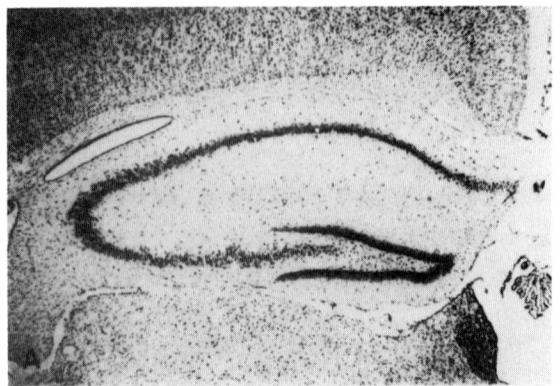

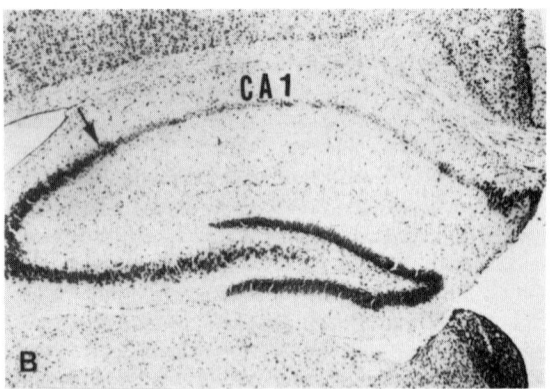

Fig. 2. Hippocampus of sham-operated gerbil (A) and of gerbil after 4 days recirculation following 5 min of forebrain ischemia (B). There is widespread neuronal destruction in the CA1 subfield, the border of which is indicated by the arrow. Cresyl violet staining.

3. Qualitative assay of rCBF

The autoradiographic observations of rCBF are described elsewhere (Suzuki et al., 1983a) and corroborate the quantitative rCBF measurements. During CCA occlusion the forebrain revealed severe ischemia followed by heterogeneous hyperemia after the occlusion was released. In animals killed after 10 min recirculation, hypoperfusion affecting diffusely both hemispheres was present. In gerbils killed later than 6 h of recirculation significant differences from the normal rCBF pattern were absent.

4. Qualitative assay of lCGU

As described in detail elsewhere (Suzuki et al., 1983a), 2 out of 6 animals killed 1 day after recirculation showed high lCGU in CA1 subfield of hippocampus; the others showed spotty increase of lCGU in the mesial part of CA1 subfield and in the border zone between CA1 and CA2 subfields. At 2 days a strikingly low lCGU was noticed in the CA1 subfield of hippocampus.

The brains of gerbils injected with 3-O-methyl-^{14}C-D-glucose showed a homogeneous pattern of isotope distribution, and there was no difference between autoradiograms of sham-operated controls and of animals killed in the post-ischemic period.

TABLE 1

rCBF before, during and after 5 min bilateral CCA occlusion in gerbils

	Numbers of animals	Frontal cortex	Occipital cortex	Hippocampus	Cerebellum
1. Sham-operated	7	131 ± 6.0	143 ± 8.0	93 ± 5.3	137 ± 6.4
2. During occlusion	5	5 ± 1.3[b]	7 ± 2.2[b]	8 ± 2.7[b]	169 ± 42.9
3. Immediately after recirculation	6	207 ± 45.7	190 ± 55.9	202 ± 25.3[b]	160 ± 15.9
4. 2 min after recirculation	5	221 ± 33.4[a]	178 ± 36.3	173 ± 38.4	165 ± 19.4
5. 10 min after recirculation	5	70 ± 4.9[b]	81 ± 5.3[b]	72 ± 2.2[b]	149 ± 13.0
6. 6 h after recirculation	6	122 ± 8.2	121 ± 8.2	93 ± 8.2	124 ± 6.5
7. 1 day after recirculation	5	117 ± 10.7	120 ± 19.7	93 ± 9.4	107 ± 8.0[a]
8. 2 days after recirculation	6	126 ± 8.6	129 ± 10.6	99 ± 5.3	123 ± 9.0

Values and means ± SEM, ml/100 g per min.
[a] $p < 0.05$ significance as compared with sham-operated controls ([b] $p < 0.01$).
(With permission from Suzuki et al., 1983a.)

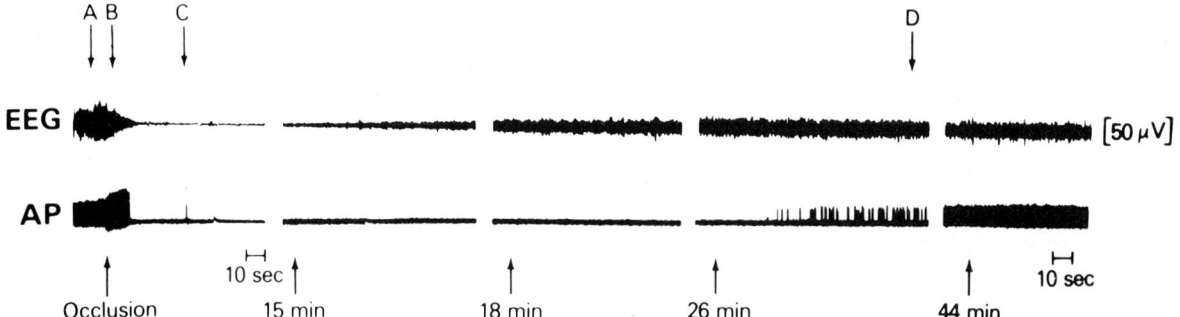

Fig. 3. EEG and action potential recordings from a CA1 neuron (AP) during and after 5 min of forebrain ischemia in gerbils. The letters A–D indicate the time of hippocampal unit recordings shown in Fig. 4. (With permission from Suzuki et al., 1983b.)

5. Recordings of SNA

In the acute experiments single unit recordings of 13 CorN and 15 CA1N were analyzed. The average frequency of spontaneous action potentials under anesthesia was 7.4 ± 2.5/s in CorN and 9.2 ± 4.7/s (mean ± SD) in CA1N and never exceeded 20/s. Immediately after the occlusion, there was an abrupt increase in the frequency of spike discharges. This rapid firing persisted for 1–5 seconds, then gradually became less rapid, and finally ceased within 20–30 seconds after the occlusion, when the EEG became isoelectric (Figs. 3 and 4). Several neurons exhibited groups of few spikes after the EEG flattened. The average time of disappearance of action potentials after onset of ischemia was 20.9 ± 11.1 s for the CorN and 21.8 ± 16.6 s for the CA1N. Recovery occurred at 18.4 ± 10.2 min in CorN and 14.8 ± 7.4 min in CA1N after the onset of ischemia. Spike frequency of CorN and CA1N after reestablishment of continuous firing was 4.3 ± 1.0/s, 5.6 ± 3.3/s, respectively (Fig. 5).

In the chronic experiments, action potentials from 64 neurons could be recorded long enough for analysis. A considerable number of CA1N revealed high frequency spike discharges up to 90/s, when recorded at 7–10 h or at 1 day after recirculation, whereas at the same time most of CorN showed normal activity (Fig. 6). At 2 days after recirculation single unit activities of CorN were easily detectable, and their discharge frequencies were within a control range. On the other hand, recording of electrical activity from the CA1 subfield were not obtained in any of nine tested hemispheres with the exception of some weak activity from one neuron. The recordings of SNA in CorN and CA1N are summarized graphically in Fig. 7.

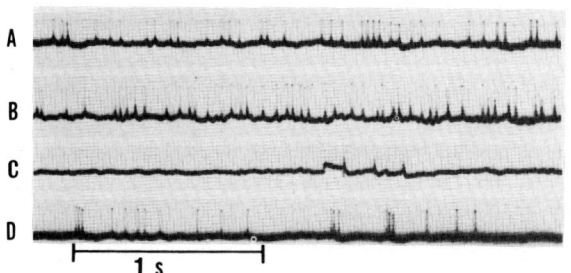

Fig. 4. Action potentials recorded from hippocampal CA1 neuron before, during and after 5 min of forebrain ischemia in gerbils. Time of recording is indicated by letters A–D in Fig. 3. (With permission from Suzuki et al., 1983b.)

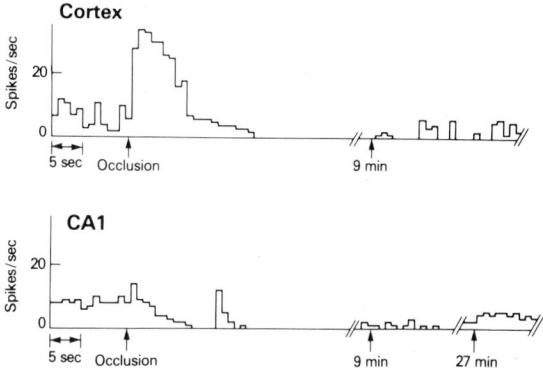

Fig. 5. Spike frequency histograms of action potentials from single cortical and single CA1 neurons. Note immediate changes in frequency following occlusion. (With permission from Suzuki et al., 1983b.)

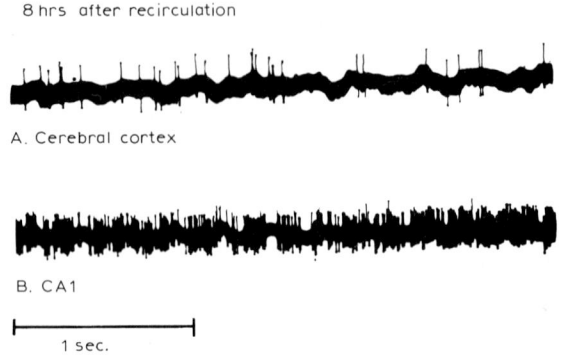

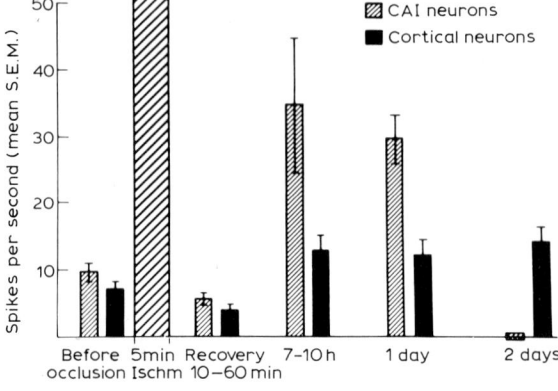

Fig. 6. Spontaneous neuronal activity recorded after 8 h recirculation from single cortical and CA1 neurons. The latter shows markedly increased frequency of action potentials. (With permission from Suzuki et al., 1983b.)

Fig. 7. Histogram of frequency of action potentials in cortical and CA1 neurons at various periods after 5 min of forebrain ischemia. (With permission from Suzuki et al., 1983b.)

6. Measurement of $[K^+]e$ and $[Ca^{2+}]e$

The extracellular ion activities in the cortex and CA1 subfield showed basically similar profiles after ischemia, though exact values of ion activities and the durations of each phase were slightly different (Figs. 8 and 9). Initially, $[K^+]e$ and $[Ca^{2+}]e$ increased slowly for about 49 seconds after the onset of CCA occlusion both in the cortex and CA1. Then suddenly $[K^+]e$ rapidly increased to about 54 mM in the cortex and to 41 mM in the CA1 subfield (in the following, values from the cortex appear in the text, and those from the CA1 subfield in parentheses, respectively). Thereafter $[K^+]e$ gradually increased to 75 mM (78 mM). In contrast, $[Ca^{2+}]e$ abruptly fell during ischemia, synchronously with the sharp rise in $[K^+]e$, and decreased to a value of less than 50% of control. At the moment of recirculation $[K^+]e$ started to decrease promptly, while $[Ca^{2+}]e$ further declined for several minutes. $[K^+]e$ returned to the base line in 10 min (8 min), while recovery of $[Ca^{2+}]e$ required 23 min (20 min) of recirculation.

Discussion

The morphological observations revealed that 5 min of forebrain ischemia in gerbils lead to highly

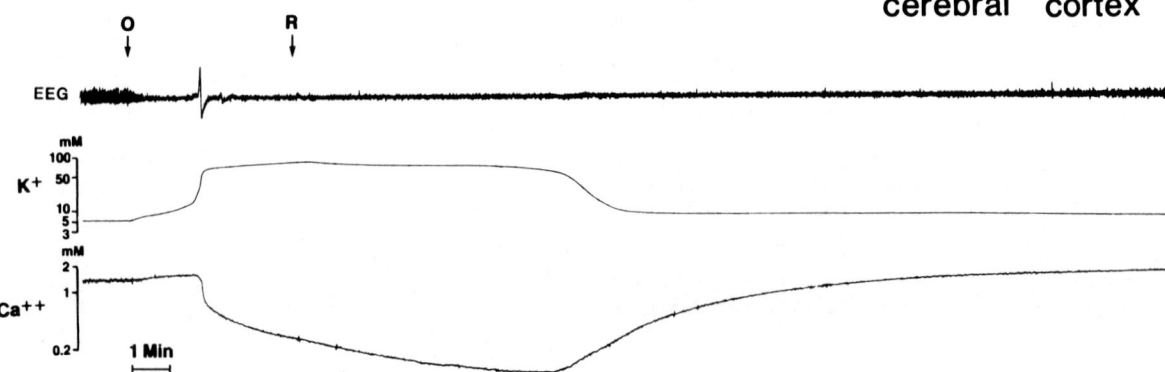

Fig. 8. Time course of changes in extracellular potassium and calcium concentrations in cerebral cortex before, during and after 5 min of forebrain ischemia. (O) indicates moment of occlusion, (R) time of release of the occlusion. (With permission from Yamaguchi et al., 1985.)

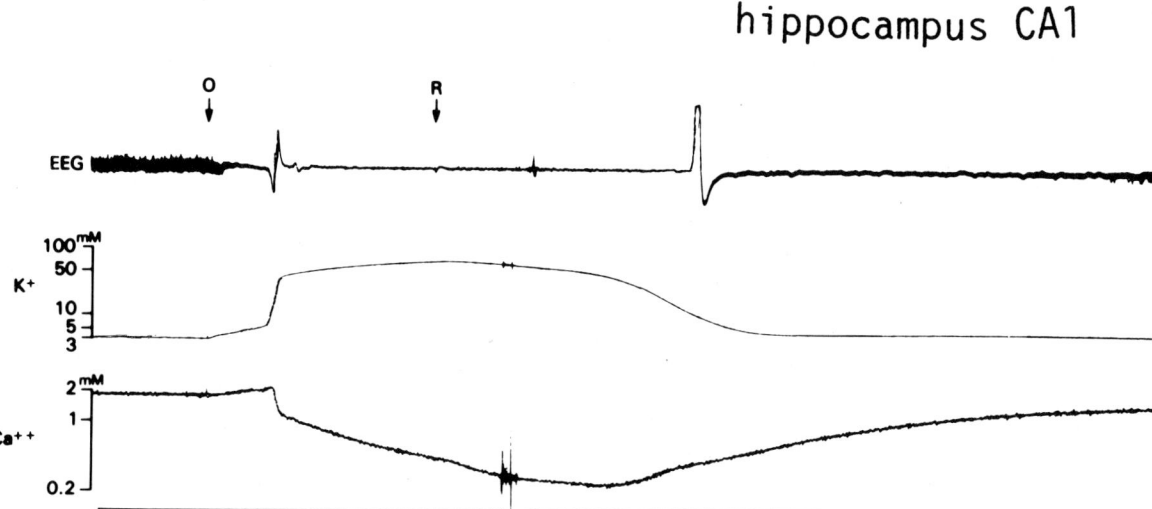

Fig. 9. Time course of changes in extracellular potassium and calcium concentrations in the hippocampus before, during and after 5 min of forebrain ischemia. (With permission from Yamaguchi et al., 1985.)

reproducible delayed destruction of neurons in the hippocampal CA1 subfield. We believe that the model has great advantages for further research of ischemic brain damage because of its simplicity, high reproducibility and little invasiveness into the animals. Brown et al. (1979) suggested that ischemic cell changes in gerbils were possibly caused in part by their epileptic activity, which was thought to be a characteristic of gerbils. However, this is unlikely because Pulsinelli et al. (1982a) reported slowly progressive neuronal damage in the hippocampal CA1 sector following 30-min four-vessel occlusion in rats. Recent electronmicroscopical observations confirmed that there are no apparent differences of the lesions in either gerbils or rats (Kirino et al., 1984). According to these studies, we conclude that the phenomenon of slowly progressive damage in selectively vulnerable neurons occurs in various species.

Our observations of rCBF changes corroborate other reports (Levy et al., 1979; Pulsinelli et al., 1982b), i.e. during vascular occlusion both the CorN and the CA1N suffered from the same degree of severe ischemia. Immediately after recirculation, a heterogenous type of hyperemia was noticed. The cause of this short-lasting reactive hyperemia is still unknown; however, lactic acid and extracellular potassium ions released from intracellular pools may play an important role due to their vasodilating effect (Kuschinski et al., 1972). This is supported by our observation that changes in $[K^+]e$ normalized within 10 min after recirculation when post-ischemic hypoperfusion was noticed. The mechanisms of post-ischemic hypoperfusion have been explained by several hypotheses, including mechanical compression of microvasculature by edema and vasoconstriction due to increased vascular smooth muscle tone. The latter hypothesis was preferred by several authors (Miller et al., 1980; Pulsinelli et al., 1982b), Suzuki et al. (1983a) reported that an early opening of the blood-brain barrier occurs during initial hyperemia. It is, therefore, conceivable that a vasoconstricting agent enters the brain at this time. Since post-ischemic hypoperfusion occurred simultaneously in all cerebral regions which were affected by the ischemic insult, hypoperfusion itself may not be responsible for neuronal death in CA1N. On the other hand, our observations of lCGU showed significant heterogeneity during the post-ischemic period. This was most evident in hippocampus, in which lCGU was increased after up to 24 h of recirculation, and in which pronounced discrepancies between rCBF and lCGU were noticed after 10 min recirculation. A similar dissociation was observed by other authors (Diemer et al., 1980; Pulsinelli et al., 1982b; Choki et al., 1983), and uncoupling of rCBF and lCGU may be a potential cause of the neuronal damage. However, as long as the mechanism and the significance of high lCGU are unclear, the observed phenomena are insufficient to explain why neuronal death occurs following ischemia. It may only be a secondary change reflecting other sequential events occurring after the ischemic insult.

The recordings of action potentials from neurons suffering from ischemia give us more direct and detailed information on neuronal function. Disappearances of SNA after the onset of ischemia correlated well with the flattening of the EEG. Recovery started at 10 min after restoration of cerebral circulation, first with intermittent and later with continuous discharges of both CorN and CA1N. CA1N — but not CorN — showed pronounced hyperactivity after 7–24 h recirculation (Fig. 7). These findings are in agreement with our observations on lCGU: during the phase of hyperactivity lCGU was increased in the hippocampus, but it became subnormal when neurons proved to be functionally dead 2 days after recirculation.

We were able to demonstrate hyperactivity of CA1N by direct recordings of action potentials. However, the possible cause of excitation is unclear. Siesjö (1981) pointed out that the selectively vulnerable neurons of hippocampus exhibit high conductance for Ca^{2+} ions, and according to Meldrum (1981) abnormal influx of Ca^{2+} into CA1N may be related to hyperactivity and bursting activity of these cells. This theory was supported by the histochemical demonstration at the ultrastructural level of excessive entry of Ca^{2+} into CA1 and CA3 neurons in status epilepticus (Griffiths et al., 1982). Based on those findings, we measured $[K^+]e$ and $[Ca^{2+}]e$ simultaneously in both the cortex and the hippocampus. Our findings confirmed other reports (Harris et al., 1981; Hansen, 1981; Harris and Symon, 1984) on changes of extracellular ions during and after ischemia, but significant differences between the cortex and the hippocampus were absent during the observation period. This is in agreement with recent observations of Simon et al. (1984), who found that Ca^{2+} deposits could be seen not only in the selectively vulnerable neurons but also in other neurons. Although pentobarbital anesthesia was used in our study of extracellular ion activity, these observations suggest that high Ca^{2+} conductivity in CA1N was not a significant factor for hyperactivity of CA1N during the early phase of recirculation. On the other hand, recent neurochemical findings revealed that γ-aminobutyric acid (GABA) was significantly reduced after 12 h of recirculation following 5 min of forebrain ischemia in gerbils (Arai and Yasumoto, personal communication, 1984). Since GABA plays an important role for neuronal inhibition, hyperactivity of CA1N may be due to depletion of GABA.

Kirino and Sano (1984a, 1984b) recently described pathological changes of neurons in gerbils following various durations of ischemia. They confirmed that DND of CA1N was an expression of the maturation phenomenon. They observed that 3 min of ischemia was not sufficient to produce neuronal damage, but 20–30 min of ischemia produced more rapid and intense neuronal damage of hippocampal neurons than 5-min ischemia, although the fundamental pathological changes did not differ except for mitochondrial alterations. The mitochondria did not show any significant pathological changes until 2 days after 5-min ischemia, whereas they enlarged and occasionally exhibited bizarre forms on day 2 following 20–30 min ischemia (Kirino et al., 1984b). Petito and Pulsinelli (1984) investigated the electronmicroscopic changes in CA1N in rats following 30 min of forebrain ischemia. During the early post-ischemic period mitochondrial swelling was noted in CA1N but mitochondria appeared normal at 24 h after ischemia. Subsequently, neuronal cell death occurred after 48–72 h. They concluded that the morphological appearance indicated the possibility of neuronal recovery. Recently, Simon et al. (1984) reported massive

Ca^{2+} deposits in the mitochondria of selectively vulnerable neurons during the late observation period by using the oxalate/pyroantimonate procedure following 30 min of ischemic insult in rats. Considering these observations, including our SNA recordings, it can be concluded that reversibility of neuronal function, i.e. reversibility of neuronal unit activity, is well correlated with the reversibility of morphological changes of mitochondria. It is also noteworthy to mention that the major degradative enzyme for GABA is a mitochondrial enzyme which is not associated with neuronal membranes (Hammerschlag et al., 1976).

Recovery of neurons following various insults has been estimated by recording electrical activity, such as EEG or evoked potentials. Hossmann and Kleihues (1973) reported EEG recovery in cats and monkeys after up to 60 min global cerebral ischemia. Heiss and Rosner (1983) recorded SNA in cats following transient middle cerebral artery occlusion, and observed that neuronal function recovered after severe ischemia with regional blood flow of less than 0.09 ml/g per min when the ischemic insult lasted less than 20 min. However, these observations were not correlated with the morphological changes after the insult. Our observations of SNA of CA1N also showed initial recovery although these neurons are destined to die, indicating that the neurons need support to survive during the recovery phase. In other words, the neurons are accessible to treatment during the recirculation phase as well as during the ischemic phase.

The described changes of various parameters resulting from 5 min ischemia in gerbils demonstrate

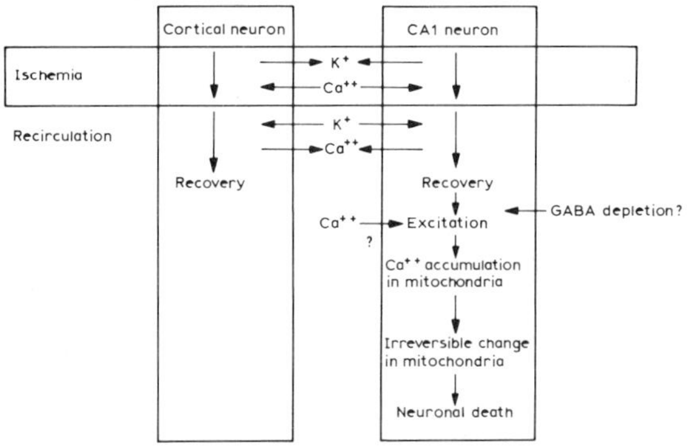

Fig. 10. Hypothetical representation of pathophysiological events following brief ischemia of cortical and CA1 neurons.

that ischemic death of CA1N takes place during the recirculation period. Other reports mentioned here also provide strong support for this assumption. Fig. 10 represents a hypothetical scheme of mechanisms responsible for DND. We propose that during initial recovery the selectively vulnerable neurons behave similar as other neurons. After a latent period, however, Ca^{2+} enters secondarily into CA1N because of high conductivity for Ca^{2+} following GABA depletion. This causes excitation of neurons and excessive accumulation of Ca^{2+} in mitochondria, resulting in destruction of the mitochondria followed by neuronal disintegration. The actual sequence of pathophysiological changes following ischemic insult may not be as simple as the proposed hypothesis, and other factors such as calmodulin, pH, glutamate, etc., may also play important roles in neuronal death. However, we are able to come close to the truth only by a stepwise accumulation of evidence.

References

Brown, A.W., Levy, D.E., Kublik, M., Harrow, J., Plum, F. and Brierley, J.B. (1979) Selective chromatolysis of neurons in the gerbil brain: a possible consequence of "epileptic" activity produced by common carotid artery occlusion. *Ann. Neurol.*, 5: 127–138.

Choki, J., Greenberg, J. and Reivich, M. (1983) Regional cerebral glucose metabolism following transient forebrain ischemia. *Ann. Neurol.*, 11: 568–574.

Diemer, N.H. and Siemkowicz, E. (1980) Increased 2-deoxyglucose uptake in hippocampus, globus pallidus and substantia nigra after cerebral ischemia. *Neurol. Scand.*, 61: 56–63.

Griffiths, T., Evans, M.C. and Meldrum, B.S. (1982) Intracellular sites of early calcium accumulation in the rat hippocampus during status epilepticus. *Neurosci. Lett.*, 30: 329–334.

Hammerschlag, R. and Roberts, E. (1976) Overview of chemical transmission. In: G.J. Siegel, R.W. Albers, R. Katzman and B.W. Agranoff (Eds.), *Basic Neurochemistry*. Little, Brown Comp., Boston, pp. 167–179.

Hansen, A.J. (1981) Extracellular ion concentrations in cerebral ischemia. In: T. Zeuthen (Ed.), *The Application of Ion-selec-*

tive Microelectrodes. Elsevier/North-Holland Biomedical Press, Amsterdam, pp. 239–254.

Harris, R.J., Symon, L., Branston, N.M. and Bayhan, M. (1981) Changes in extracellular calcium activity in cerebral ischemia. *J. Cereb. Blood Flow Metabol.,* 1: 203–209.

Harris, R.J. and Symon, L. (1984) Extracellular pH, potassium, and calcium activities in progressive ischemia of rat cortex. *J. Cereb. Blood Flow Metabol.,* 4: 178–186.

Heiss, W.D. and Rosner, G. (1983) Functional recovery of cortical neurons as related to degree and duration of ischemia. *Ann. Neurol.,* 14: 294–301.

Hossmann, K.-A. and Kleihues, P. (1973) Reversibility of ischemic brain damage. *Arch. Neurol.,* 29: 375–384.

Ito, U., Spatz, M., Walker, J.T. and Klatz, I. (1975) Experimental cerebral ischemia in Mongolian gerbils. *Acta Neuropathol. (Berl.),* 32: 209–223.

Kirino, T. (1982) Delayed neuronal death in the gerbil hippocampus following ischemia. *Brain Res.,* 239: 57–69.

Kirino, T. and Sano, K. (1984a) Selective vulnerability in the gerbil hippocampus following transient ischemia. *Acta Neuropathol. (Berl.),* 62: 201–208.

Kirino, T. and Sano, K. (1984b) Fine structural nature of delayed neuronal death in rat hippocampus following ischemia in the gerbil hippocampus. *Acta Neuropathol. (Berl.),* 62: 209–218.

Kirino, T., Tamura, A. and Sano, K. (1984) Delayed neuronal death in the rat hippocampus following transient forebrain ischemia. *Acta Neuropathol. (Berl.),* 64: 139–147.

Kuschinski, W., Wahl, M., Bosse, O. and Thuran, K. (1972) Perivascular potassium and pH as determinants of local pial artery diameter in cats. *Circ. Res.,* 31: 240–247.

Levy, D., Van Uitert, R. and Pike, C. (1979) Delayed post-ischemic hypoperfusion: a potentially damaging consequence of stroke. *Neurology,* 29: 1245–1252.

Meldrum, B.S. (1981) Metabolic effects of prolonged epileptic seizures and the causation of epileptic brain damage. In: F.C. Rose (Ed.), *Metabolic Disorders of the Nervous System.* Pitman, London, pp. 175–187.

Miller, C., Lampard, D., Alexander, K. and Brown, W. (1980) Local cerebral blood flow following transient cerebral ischemia. *Stroke,* 11: 534–541.

Ohno, K., Pettigrew, K.D. and Rapoport, S.I. (1979) Local cerebral blood flow in the conscious rat as measured with ^{14}C-antipyrine, ^{14}C-iodo-antipyrine and ^{3}H-nicotine. *Stroke,* 10: 62–67.

Petito, C.K. and Pulsinelli, W.A. (1984) Delayed neuronal recovery and neuronal death in rat hippocampus following severe cerebral ischemia: possible relationship to abnormalities in neuronal processes. *J. Cereb. Blood Flow Metabol.,* 4: 194–205.

Pulsinelli, W.A., Brierley, J.B. and Plum, F. (1982a) Temporal profile of neuronal damage in a model of transient forebrain ischemia. *Ann. Neurol.,* 11: 491–498.

Pulsinelli, W.A., Levy, D.E. and Duffy, T.E. (1982b) Regional cerebral blood flow and glucose metabolism following transient forebrain ischemia. *Ann. Neurol.,* 11: 499–509.

Sakurada, O., Kennedy, C., Jehle, J.W., Brown, J.D., Carbin, G.L. and Sokoloff, L. (1978) Measurement of local cerebral blood flow with iodo ^{14}C antipyrine. *Am. J. Physiol.,* 234: H59–H66.

Siesjö, B.K. (1981) Cell damage in the brain: a speculative synthesis. *J. Cereb. Blood Flow Metabol.,* 1: 155–184.

Simon, R.P., Griffiths, T., Evans, M.C., Swan, J.H. and Meldrum, B.S. (1984) Calcium overload in selectively vulnerable neurons of the hippocampus during and after ischemia: an electron microscopy study in the rat. *J. Cereb. Blood Flow Metabol.,* 4: 350–361.

Suzuki, R., Yamaguchi, T., Kirino, T., Orzi, F. and Klatzo, I. (1983a) The effect of 5-minute ischemia in Mongolian gerbils. I. Blood-brain barrier, cerebral blood flow, and local cerebral glucose utilization changes. *Acta Neuropathol. (Berl.),* 60: 207–216.

Suzuki, R., Yamaguchi, T., Li, C.L. and Klatzo, I. (1983b) The effects of 5-minute ischemia in Mongolian gerbils. II. Changes of spontaneous neuronal activity in cerebral cortex and CA1 sector of hippocampus. *Acta Neuropathol. (Berl.),* 60: 217–222.

Suzuki, R., Nitsch, C., Fujiwara, K. and Klatzo, I. (1984) Regional changes in cerebral blood flow and blood-brain barrier permeability during epileptiform seizures and in acute hypertension in rabbits. *J. Cereb. Blood Flow Metabol.,* 4: 96–102.

Yamaguchi, T., Wagner, H.G. and Klatzo, I. (1985) Observations on the post-ischemic pathophysiology in the gerbil brain including K^+ and Ca^{2+} changes. In: *Proceedings of NATO Advised Research Workshop on Mechanisms of Secondary Brain Damage.* Plenum Press, New York, in press.

Neurochemical correlates to selective neuronal vulnerability

Tadeusz Wieloch

Laboratory for Experimental Brain Research, University of Lund, S-221 85 Lund, Sweden

Introduction

With the development of small animal models allowing long-term recovery following ischemic (Ito et al., 1975; Diemer and Siemkowicz, 1981; Pulsinelli and Brierley, 1979; Smith et al., 1984a; Blomqvist and Wieloch, 1985) and hypoglycemic (Auer et al., 1984a) insults, it is possible to challenge the concept of selective neuronal vulnerability with histological and biochemical approaches.

Two major histopathological findings obtained from these investigations are of importance when mechanisms of selective neuronal necrosis are discussed. First, in a brain area suffering a homogeneous ischemic insult some neurons will be irreversibly damaged and disintegrate during the recovery phase, while others, initially showing acute morphological changes, will recover and survive (Ito et al., 1975; Kirino, 1982). Secondly, in some brain areas an interval of several days, when brain damage is minimal, is required before neuronal necrosis commences (Ito et al., 1975; Kirino, 1982; Pulsinelli et al., 1982). Consequently, earlier neurochemical investigations of the molecular mechanisms of ischemic and hypoglycemic brain damage, conducted on relatively large samples, suffered a loss of sensitivity due to dilution effects. More important, though, is the fact that many studies of the cell damage following the insults have been, and still are, conducted in the acute phase of the insult, with no or only few hours of recovery, thus not taking into consideration the phenomenon of delayed neuronal necrosis. As no correlation has been demonstrated between regional cerebral blood flows during the ischemic (Suzuki et al., 1983a) and hypoglycemic insult (Abdul-Rahman et al., 1980) and regional neuronal necrosis, the vulnerable neurons must be subjected to local external stress, or possess particular properties making them prone to these insults.

This chapter describes some of the special neurochemical features of the areas of the brain selectively vulnerable to ischemic and hypoglycemic insults. The discussion will focus on the neuronal connections to the vulnerable brain areas, on the distribution of receptors and transmitter content in the vulnerable areas, and on some current hypothesis of neuronal damage. Emphasis will be placed on a possible imbalance between excitation and inhibition of neurons as a factor in the development of neuronal necrosis, in particular the importance of excitatory transmitters, recently suggested to mediate ischemic (Jørgensen and Diemer, 1982; Rothman, 1984a; Simon et al., 1984a; Wieloch et al., 1985) and hypoglycemic (Auer et al., 1984b; Wieloch et al., 1985) brain damage.

Selective neuronal vulnerability and afferent input

Neuronal circuits

Transient complete or incomplete cerebral ischemia in rats (Jørgensen and Diemer, 1982; Pulsinelli et al., 1982; Smith et al., 1984b; Blomqvist and Wie-

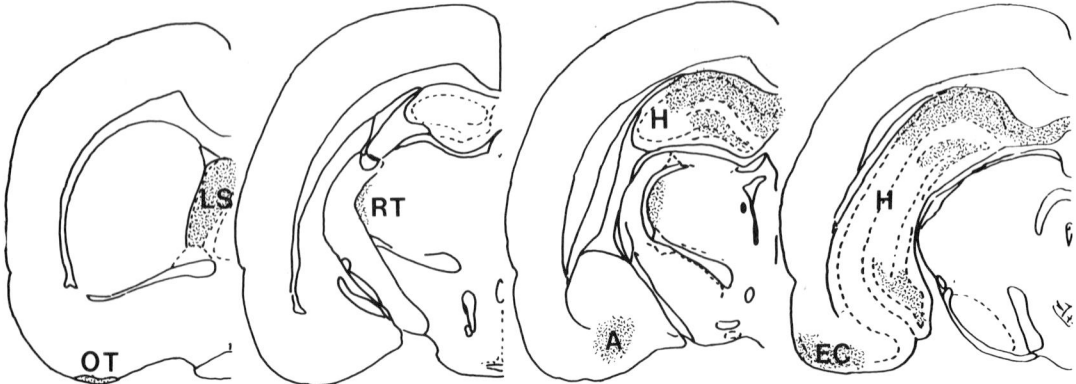

Fig. 1. The distribution of neuronal necrosis in the rat brain following short periods of cerebral ischemia (2–5 min) with 1 week of survival. A, amygdala; EC, entorhinal cortex; H, hippocampus; LS, lateral septum; OT, olfactory tubercle; RT, reticular nucleus of the thalamus. (Data from Smith et al., 1984b; Blomquist and Wieloch, 1985.)

loch, 1985) leads to selective neuronal necrosis in discrete brain areas. Following ischemia of 2–5 min duration and 1 week recovery, neuronal necrosis is confined to the CA1 and subicular regions of the hippocampus, the hilus of the dentate gyrus, the reticular nucleus of the thalamus, the lateral septum, the olfactory tubercle, the primary olfactory cortex, the amygdaloid nuclei and the entorhinal cortex (Fig. 1). It is evident from the distribution pattern of the neuronal necrosis that limbic brain areas are mainly affected. This suggests that neuronal activation in the limbic system, as in limbic seizures (Collins et al., 1983a), may act as an important mediator and amplifier of the deleterious reactions leading to neuronal damage following short periods of cerebral ischemia.

This is further substantiated in studies on sustained stimulation of the perforant path (Sloviter and Damiano, 1981; Sloviter, 1983; Olney et al., 1982) and amygdala kindling epilepsy (McIntyre et al., 1982). Morphological changes were observed in the CA1 region, hilus of the dentate gyrus, the lateral septum, the amygdala and thalamic nuclei, i.e. regions also showing neuronal necrosis following short periods of ischemia.

Prolonged periods of ischemia of 6–30 min with 1 week of recovery recruit neuronal damage in the middle layers of cerebral cortex, the caudate nucleus, the substania nigra pars reticulata, and ventral thalamic nuclei of the rat brain (Fig. 2) (Jørgensen and Diemer, 1982; Pulsinelli et al., 1982; Smith et al., 1984b). Metabolic activation and neu-

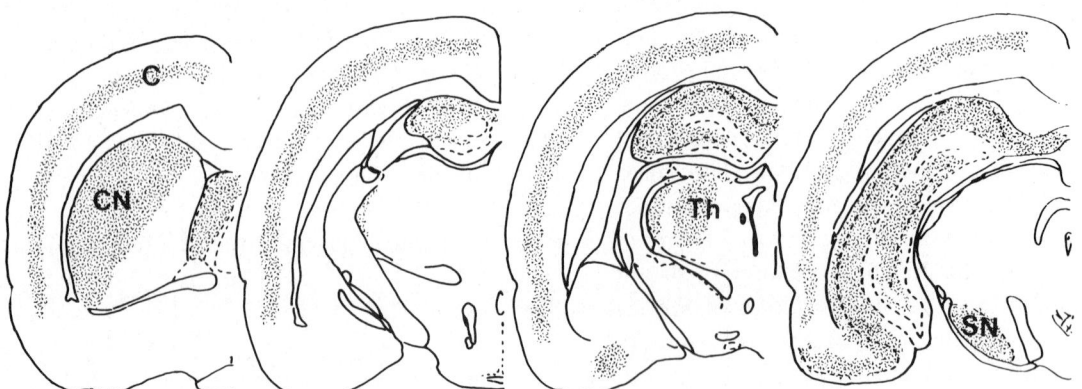

Fig. 2. Selective neuronal necrosis in the rat brain following extended periods of ischemia (5–10 min) and 1 week survival. C, cortex (layers III–V); CN, caudate nucleus; SN, substantia nigra; Th, thalamic nuclei (Data from Smith et al., 1984b).

ronal damage in some of these brain areas have been reported when focal seizures were elicited in the cerebral cortex (Collins and Olney, 1982; Collins et al., 1983b). Increased 2-deoxyglucose uptake in areas of selective vulnerability have been reported in the early recovery phase following an ischemic insult (Diemer and Siemkowicz, 1980; Suzuki et al., 1983b; Choki et al., 1983), though the relevance of these observations is still obscure.

The correlation between selective neuronal necrosis and activation of certain neuronal circuits thus provides indirect evidence of a possible transsynaptic mediation of neuronal necrosis following cerebral ischemia. However, it has to be stressed that the distribution of the damage is different from that observed following 2 hours of status epilepticus. In a model of status epilepticus allowing long-term survival, neuronal necrosis was not observed in the septal nucleus, the reticular nucleus of the thalamus or in the caudate nucleus (Nevander et al., 1984, 1985). Thus, other mechanisms apart from neuronal hyperactivity must also prevail in the pathogenesis of ischemic brain damage.

In hypoglycemia, the distribution of neuronal necrosis is different. Following 30 min of hypoglycemic coma and 1 week recovery, necrotic neurons are mainly confined to the surface layers of the cerebral cortex, the outer blade of the dentate gyrus, areas facing the subarachnoid spaces, and cerebellar Purkinje cells at the foramen of Luschka (Auer et al., 1984b). The distribution of the damage suggests a deleterious action of a neurotoxin transported via the route of the cerebro spinal fluid (Auer et al., 1984b). After the onset of recovery following a hypoglycemic insult, damage is recruited in the dorsolateral caudoputamen, affecting small and medium-sized neurons (Kalimo et al., 1985). As the major afferents to the striatum are the cortico-striatal fibres, suggested to be glutamatergic (Spencer, 1976; Divac et al., 1977; McGeer et al., 1977), neuronal necrosis could be envisaged to be caused by a transsynaptic mechanism in the post-hypoglycemic period.

Although there are major differences between the distribution of neuronal necrosis following ischemia and hypoglycemia, the release of a toxic substance, be it an excitatory transmitter or related compound, could be a common pathogenic factor. The next section will thus focus on the distribution of excitatory and inhibitory transmitters and their receptors in relation to the areas of neuronal necrosis, and some properties which may be important for brain pathology.

Excitatory transmitters

Excitatory amino acids (EAA)

The amino acids glutamate and aspartate are major excitatory transmitters in the central neurons system (Cotman et al., 1981; Watkins and Evans, 1981; Fonnum, 1984). When present in high concentration they are neurotoxic (Lucas and Newhouse, 1957; Olney, 1978; Nadler et al., 1981; Köhler and Schwarcz, 1981) and could play a role in the pathogenesis of several neurological diseases such as temporal lobe epilepsy, Huntington's disease (see Coyle et al., 1981), and olivopontocerebellar dystrophy (Plaitakis et al., 1982).

In the present context the distribution of afferents containing acidic amino acids are of particular interest (Storm-Mathisen, 1977; Fagg and Foster, 1983) (Fig. 3). A striking feature of this distribution is that all brain areas selectively vulnerable to an ischemic insult receive a dense excitatory aminoacidergic innervation. For example, the vulnerable hippocampal CA1 neurons receive an excitatory

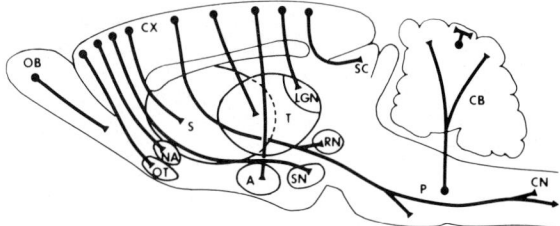

Fig. 3. Some neuronal pathways, proposed to use acidic amino acid transmitters in the mammalian brain. A, amygdala; CB, cerebellum; CN, caudate nucleus; CX, cerebral cortex; LGN, lateral geniculate nucleus; NA, nucleus accumbens; OB, olfactory bulb; OT, olfactory tubercle; P, pons; RN, red nucleus; S, striatum; SC, superior colliculus; SN, substantia nigra; T, thalamus. (From Fagg and Foster 1983, with permission.)

(Glu/Asp) input from the CA3 zone (Schaffer collaterals), the contralateral hippocampus (commissural fibres), and the entorhinal cortex (perforant path) (Steward, 1976; Wyss, 1981; Doller and Weight, 1982) (Fig. 4). The lateral septum receives an excitatory input (Glu/Asp) (Malthe-Sørenssen et al., 1979; Storm-Mathisen and Opsahl, 1978) from another branch of the CA3 pyramidal cell axons (Swanson and Cowan, 1979). The perforant path is considered to be the main excitatory pathway to the hippocampus. An increased transmitter release in the CA1 area could be envisaged by stimulation of the direct pathway or through the multisynaptic pathway via the dentate gyrus granule cells and the CA3 pyramidal neurons.

Several recent investigations have provided indirect evidence suggesting EAA's as mediators of neuronal necrosis following anoxia/ischemia. During ischemia excessive amounts of glutamate are released into the extracellular space in the hippocampus (Benveniste et al., 1984), and striatum (Wieloch and Tossman, unpublished). The glutamate levels were still elevated after 5 min of recirculation (Fig. 5). In an in vitro study glutamate toxicity was demonstrated in cultures of hippocampal neurons under anoxic conditions (Rothman, 1983, 1984a). In a recent study, unilateral transections of the perforant path were performed and the neuronal necrosis was assessed in the CA1 region following

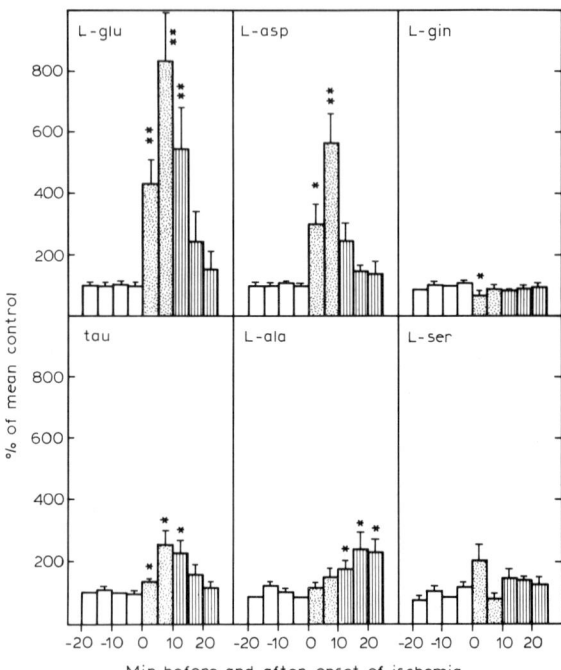

Fig. 5. Changes in the extracellular levels of some amino acids during and following 10 min of forebrain ischemia, as measured by a microdialysis technique. Note the significant increase in glutamate and aspartate levels following the onset of ischemia. The levels are still elevated following 5 min of recirculation. (From Benveniste et al., 1984, with permission.)

6 min of ischemia induced by cardiac arrest and 1 week recovery (Wieloch et al., 1985). There was a significant decrease in the number of necrotic neurons ipsilateral to the lesion (Fig. 6), demonstrating the important role of excitatory afferents in ischemic neuronal damage in the CA1 region. If the released glutamate or aspartate are important for the development of neuronal necrosis, it still remains to be determined whether the causal events are elevated transmitter levels during ischemia, in the early recovery period and/or during postischemic neuronal hyperactivity.

All neurons receiving a glutamatergic input are not equally sensitive to an ischemic insult. Thus the CA3 pyramidal neurons, innervated by afferents presumably using glutamate as transmitter (Storm-Mathisen, 1977), are more resistant to ischemia than the pyramidal neurons in the CA1 and subi-

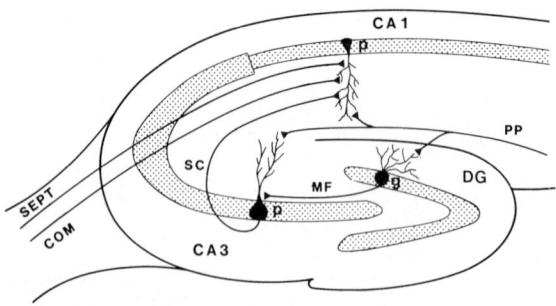

Fig. 4. The neuronal connections in the hippocampal formation proposed to use excitatory amino acids (PP, COM, SC, MF) or acetylcholine (SEPT) as transmitter. DG, dentate gyrus; COM, commissural fibres; g, granule cell layer of the dentate gyrus; MF, mossy fibres; p, pyramidal cell layer of CA1 or CA3; pp, perforant path; SC, Schaffer collaterals; SEPT, cholinergic fibres from the medial septal nucleus.

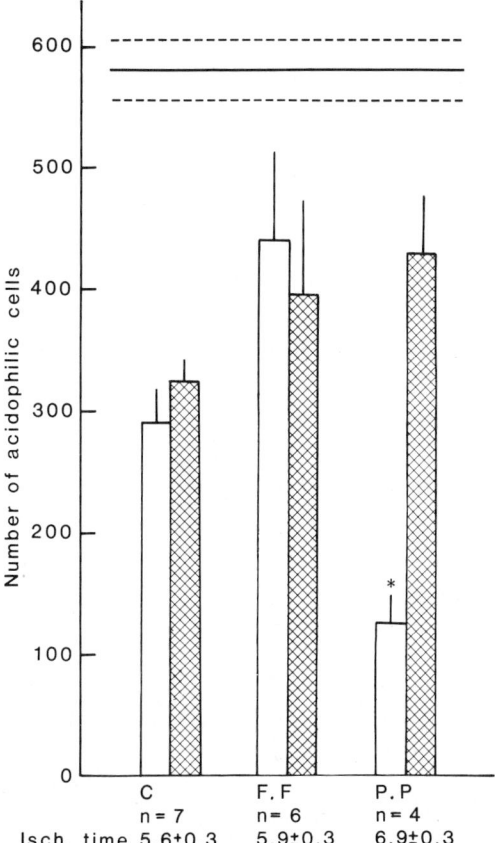

Fig. 6. The extent of neuronal necrosis in the CA1 region of the hippocampus measured as the number of acidophilic neurophagic neurons following 5–6 min of cerebral ischemia induced by cardiac arrest. The dashed lines indicate the number of pyramidal cells in the area studied, in control animals not subjected to ischemia. C, animals without lesions; FF, lesions of the septal input to the hippocampus by ablation of the fimbria-fornix; PP, lesions of the perforant path. A significant decrease ($p < 0.01$, Newman Kuhl's test) of neuronal necrosis was observed in the CA1 region of the hippocampus ipsilateral to the PP lesion. (From Wieloch et al., 1985, with permission.)

cular neurons (Smith et al., 1984b). This difference in susceptibility could partly be explained by the differences in excitatory amino acid receptors at the postsynaptic loci in different brain regions.

Receptors for EAA's have been defined in terms of agonist/antagonist binding and by their electrophysiological properties (Foster and Fagg, 1984). At least three different types of receptors have been characterized (Watkins and Evans, 1981). Two of these, the N-methyl-D-aspartate (NMDA) and the quisqualate (QA) receptors are confined to the areas of selective vulnerability. A particularly high concentration of NMDA receptors was found in the outer layers of cerebral cortex, the stratum oriens and radiatum in the CA1 and subicular regions, and stratum moleculare in the CA3 region of the hippocampus (Fig. 7). (Monaghan et al., 1983; 1985a,b.) The QA receptor measured as α-amino-3-hydroxy-5-methyl-4-isoazolepropionic acid (AMPA) binding sites were distributed in high concentration in the subiculum, cerebral cortex (layers I–III), anterior striatum, dorsolateral septum, and hippocampus (Monaghan et al., 1985b).

The NMDA receptor has several biophysical

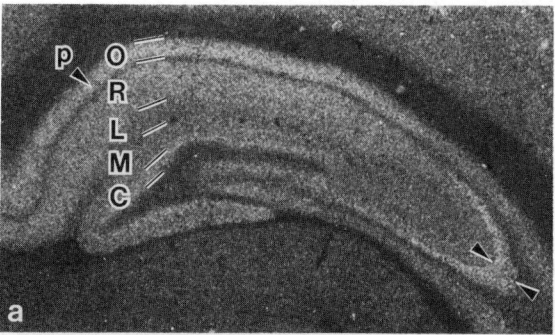

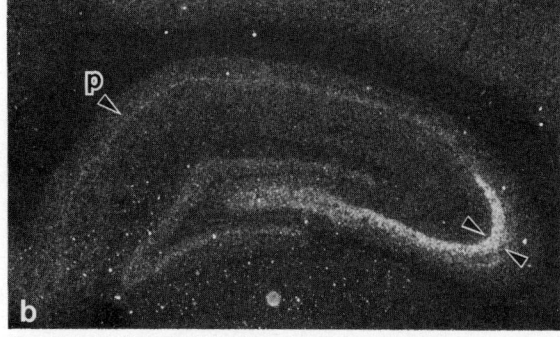

Fig. 7. The distribution of ³H-glutamate binding in the dorsal hippocampus in the absence (a) and presence (b) of 100 μM N-methyl-D-aspartate (NMDA). Note the high density of ³H-glutamate in the CA1 region and subiculum (a), which is abolished in the presence of NMDA (b). O, stratum oriens; P, stratum pyramidale; R, stratum radiatum; L, stratum lacunosum-moleculare; M, outer two third of the molecular layer of the dentate gyrus; C, commissural/associational layer of the dentate gyrus. For details see Monaghan et al., 1983. (From Monaghan et al., 1983, with permission.)

properties, which might have important pathophysiological implications. When stimulated with agonist it induces neuronal burst firing (Flatman et al., 1983; Herrling et al., 1983). Furthermore, when the membrane potential is decreased an increased inward current is observed when neurons are stimulated by agonists (Flatman et al., 1983; Nowak et al., 1984). Moreover glutamate stimulation of the NMDA receptor is potentiated when magnesium concentrations are reduced (Nowak et al., 1984). This implies that the cellular response to glutamate or aspartate binding to the NMDA receptor may be enhanced in the postischemic period, when total cortical magnesium concentrations are decreased (Hillered et al., 1984), and if the plasma membrane potential is unstable due to leakage (see Siesjö and Wieloch, 1985).

Selective antagonists to EAA receptors have been developed (Davies et al., 1983), and proved efficient against EAA neurotoxicity (Schwarcz et al., 1982; Olney, 1983) and epileptic convulsions (Croucher et al., 1982). Selective and efficient antagonists of the NMDA receptors are the 2-amino phosphonic acid derivatives, in particular 2-amino-5-phosphono-pentanoic acid (APP) and 2-amino-7-phosphono-heptanoic acid (APH) (Evans et al., 1982; Davies et al., 1983). In a recent investigation APH was reported to be protective against cerebral ischemia of 30-min duration (Simon et al., 1984a). However, a short recovery period following ischemia was employed, and the effects of the drug on cerebral circulation during ischemia were not investigated.

The caudate nucleus receives a dense innervation from the anterior neocortex of presumably glutamatergic afferents (see Fagg and Foster, 1983; Fonnum, 1984). Neocortical ablations ameliorate the neuronal damage in the subjacent caudate nucleus induced by 30 min of severe hypoglycemic coma

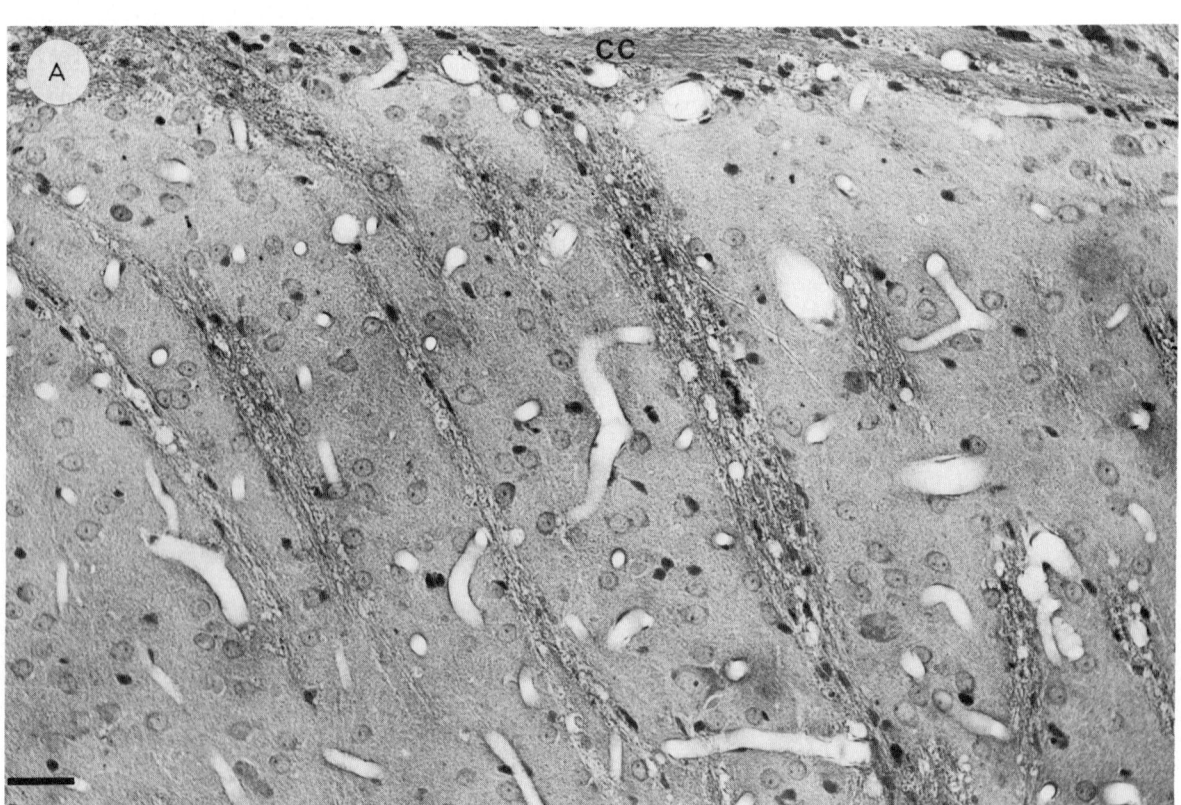

Fig. 8A.

while the contralateral caudate nucleus displays 70–90% neuronal necrosis (Fig. 8A and B) (Wieloch et al., 1985). Similarly, unilateral injections of the glutamate antagonist APH into the striatum ameliorated neuronal necrosis following hypoglycemic coma in the injected hemisphere (Fig. 9A and B). Hypoglycemic brain damage may thus also involve the action of an excitotoxin presumably an excitatory amino acid or related compound.

Other toxic compounds

Apart from the EAA's several other endogenous excitants have been shown to have neurotoxic properties (Roberts and Foster, 1983; Schwarcz et al., 1984). Two of these are pertinent in the present discussion. Quinolinic acid is a tryptophan metabolite recently found in the brain (Wolfensberger et al., 1983; Moroni et al., 1984) and has documented neurotoxic properties (Schwarcz et al., 1983a). Although the levels of quinolinic acid have not been determined in ischemic, postischemic or hypoglycemic brains, the compound merits consideration, particularly in the hypoglycemic situation when the brain utilizes endogenous compounds for energy production (Agardh et al., 1981). Furthermore the neurotoxic properties of quinolinic acid have been shown to be mediated via the NMDA receptors and its neurotoxicity was inhibited by NMDA receptor antagonists such as APH (Schwarcz et al., 1983b).

Cholinomimetics have demonstrated cytotoxic effects. Carbachol and anticholinesterases induce myopathy at the neuromuscular junction, which

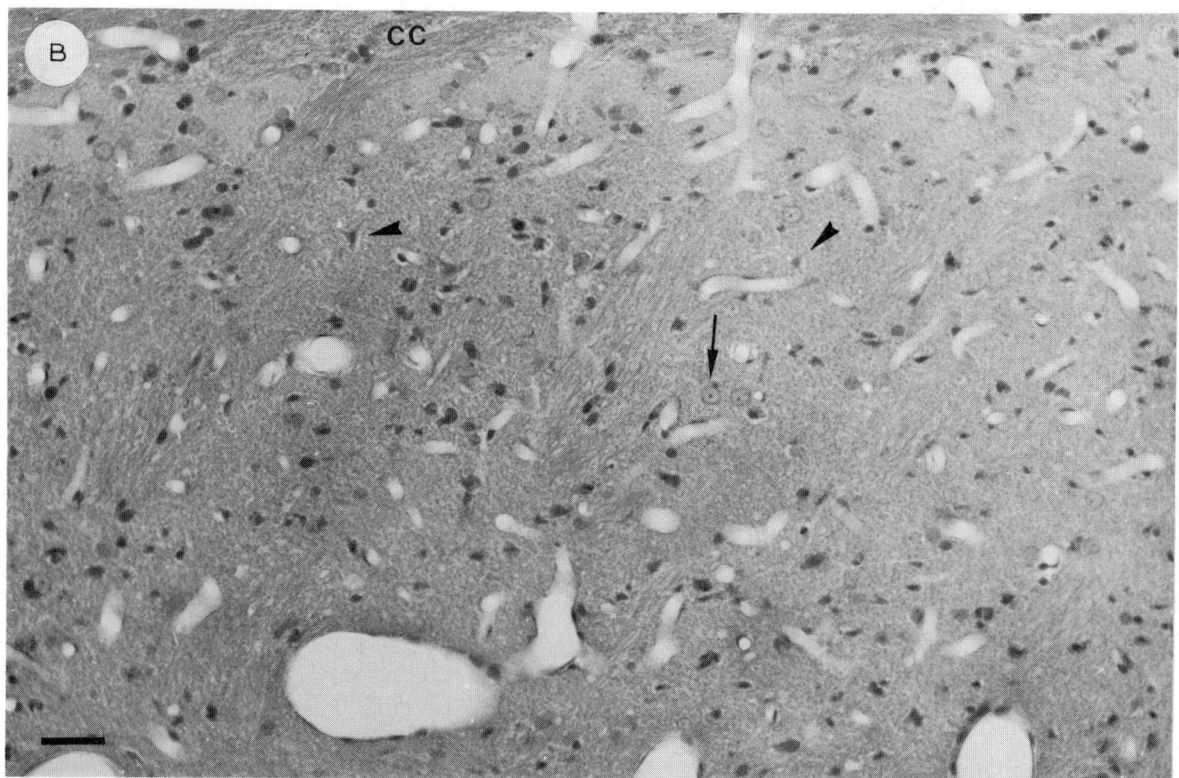

Fig. 8 (A and B). Transection of the cortico-striatal fibres ameliorate hypoglycemic brain damage in the ipsilateral caudate nucleus (CN). Unilateral removal of the motorcortex was performed 2–3 weeks prior to induction of 30 min of insulin-induced hypoglycemia, and the neuronal necrosis was assessed after 1 week recovery. (A) Ipsilateral to the lesion no degeneration of cell bodies could be observed in the CN subjacent to the lesion. (B) Contralateral to the lesion 80% of neuronal necrosis (arrowhead) is seen, mainly affecting the small and medium-seized neurons. Arrow indicates a normal neuronal body. CC, corpus callosum. Bar = 100 μm. (Wieloch, Engelsen, Westerberg and Auer, unpublished; see also Wieloch et al., 1985.)

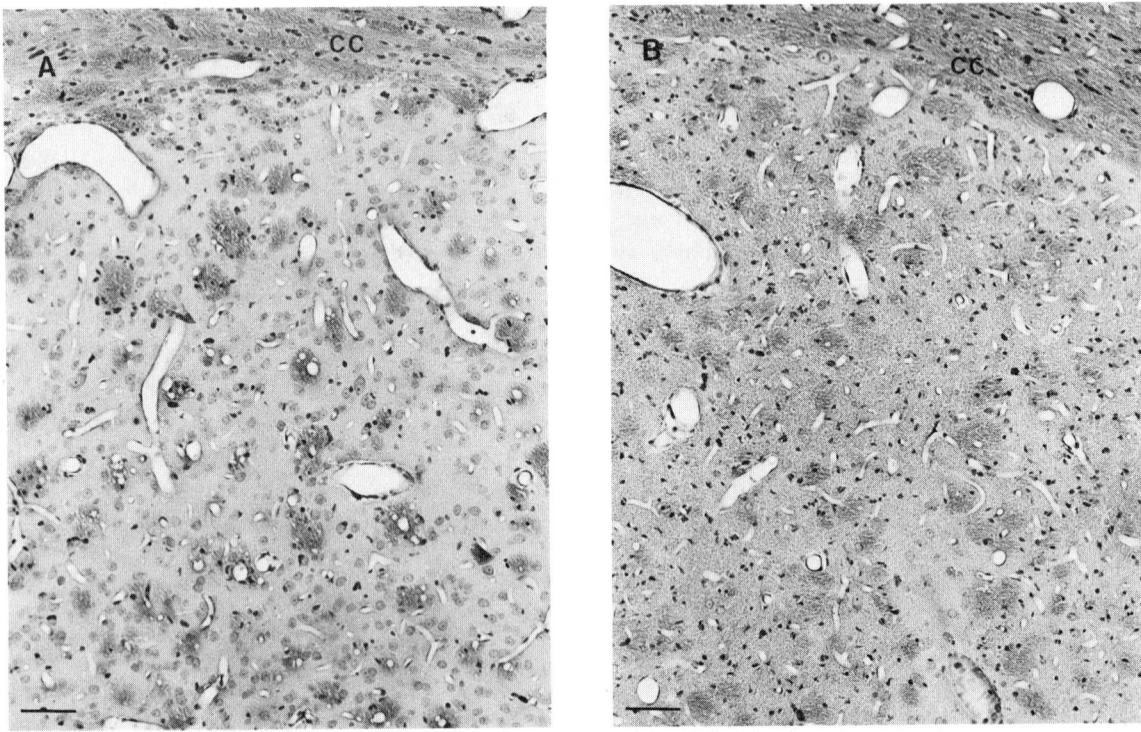

Fig. 9. 2-Amino-7-phosphonoheptanoic acid (APH) ameliorates neuronal necrosis in the caudate nucleus, following 30 min of insulin-induced hypoglycemia. (A) Fourty μg APH in 2 μl solution was injected unilaterally into the caudate nucleus. No damage is seen in the area surrounding the injection site. (B) Two μl of NaCl (9 mg/ml) was injected unilaterally into the caudate nucleus. Extensive necrosis (approximately 80%) of small and medium-seized neurons is seen. Bar = 200 μm. (Wieloch, unpublished.)

could be prevented by bungarotoxin and abolishment of calcium from the extracellular fluid (Leonard and Salpeter, 1979). Several cholinomimetics and acetylcholinesterase inhibitors induced a seizure-related neurotoxicity (Olney et al., 1982). The hippocampus also receives a cholinergic innervation. The medial septum projects excitatory cholinergic fibres to the hippocampus (Storm-Mathisen, 1977) (Fig. 4). However, transection of the fibres did not affect the density of neuronal necrosis in the CA1 region following cerebral ischemia (Wieloch et al., 1985) (Fig. 6).

Inhibitory transmitters

GABA

The neuronal necrosis following short periods of cerebral ischemia affects a part from the pyramidal cells in CA1 and subiculum, also neurons that are most probably GABA-ergic. Thus the damaged neurons in the hilar region of the dentate gyrus have been shown to be GABA-ergic (Amaral, 1978; Ribak and Andersson, 1980). Similarly the damaged cells in the dorsolateral septum (Fig. 10) are probably GABA-ergic (Panula et al., 1984), as are the neurons of the reticular nucleus of the thalamus (Houser et al., 1980).

A potential damage to the GABA-ergic neurons, occurring after short periods of ischemia (Smith et al., 1984b), could further aggravate the brain damage by, for example, decreasing the feedback or feedforward inhibitory input (Collins et al., 1983b; Buszaki, 1984), as in the case of epileptic neuronal damage (Ribak and Reffenstein, 1982). In hypoglycemia, selective loss of presumed GABA-ergic neurons in the caudate nucleus has been reported (Kalimo et al., 1985).

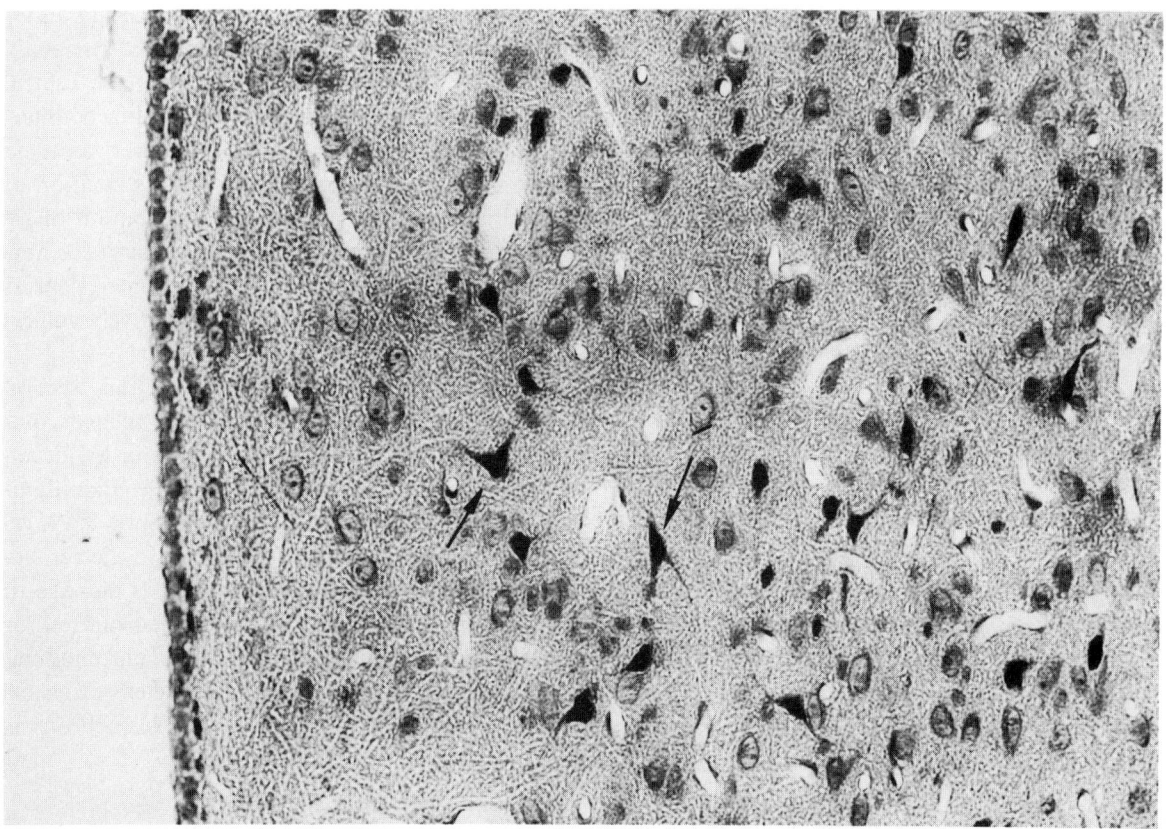

Fig. 10. Ischemic neuronal damage in the dorsolateral septum following 6 min of ischemia induced by cardiac arrest and 1 week recovery. Several pyknotic neurons are seen (arrows). Acid fuchsin-cresyl violet stain. Bar = 100 μm.

Adenosine

Adenosine is a neuromodulator in the central nervous system thoroughly investigated both in slice preparation and in vivo (see Phillis and Wu, 1981; Williams, 1984). In the present context the inhibitory action of adenosine on neuronal firing (Dunwiddie and Hoffer, 1980; Okada and Kuroda, 1975), by its action on pre- and postsynaptic A1 and A2 receptors, is of particular interest. The A1 receptors show a heterogenous distribution in the brain. They are mainly confined to the lateral septal nucleus (Lewis et al., 1981) and the CA1 region of the hippocampus (Lee et al., 1985a,b) (Fig. 11), with a higher receptor density in the dorsal portion than in the ventral portion of the hippocampus (Lee et al., 1983). The density and distribution of the A1 receptors correlates with the higher density of neuronal necrosis in the dorsal hippocampus as compared to the ventral (Smith et al., 1984b; Blomqvist and Wieloch, 1985). Electrophysiological and lesion experiments have demonstrated that the A1 receptors are confined to the postsynaptic membrane of the CA1 region (Lee et al., 1984, 1985a). A most interesting result from these experiments is that adenosine ameliorates the spontaneous after discharges following antidromic stimulation of slices in low calcium media. This is particularly important in view of the increased postischemic firing rate of the CA1 pyramidal cells (Suzuki et al., 1983b). Following 5 min of ischemia the tissue levels of adenosine increase from approximately 1 μmol $\cdot$ kg^{-1} to 400 μmol $\cdot$ kg^{-1} (Rehncrona et al., 1978). In the recirculation period following short periods of cerebral ischemia the levels of the total

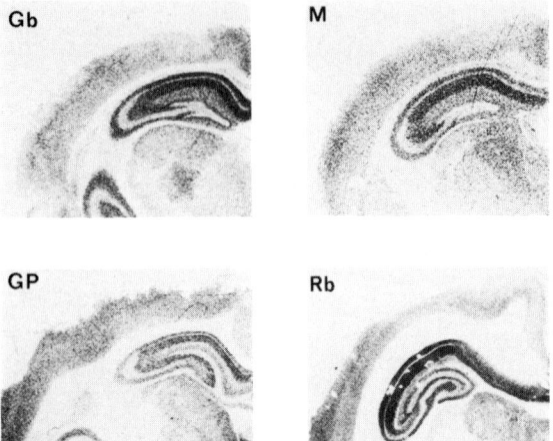

Fig. 11. Autoradiographic visualization of the distribution of adenosine A1 receptors in the hippocampus of gerbil (Gb), mouse (M), guinea pig (GP), and rabbit (Rb), as binding of ^{3}H-cyclohexyladenosine (CHA) to brain slices. Note the high density of ^{3}H-CHA in the CA1 region and subiculum in all animal species. (From Lee et al., 1985b, with permission.)

phosphorylated adenine compounds in the hippocampus are decreased by 22% while the energy charge of the tissue is normal (Blomqvist et al., 1985). The ATP levels are depressed up to 6 hours following reperfusion (Pulsinelli and Duffy, 1983). It can thus be envisaged that in a situation when the brain is recovering from a catabolic insult, the adenosine may preferentially be utilized for the formation of ATP rather than for use as modulator. Consequently the inhibitory action of adenosine would be decreased. Alternatively, the dramatic increase in the levels of adenosine during ischemia could change the cellular response to postischemic adenosine stimulation (P. Schubert, personal communication).

Noradrenaline

Noradrenaline is an inhibitory neurotransmitter (Phillis and Kostopoulos, 1977) widely distributed in the brain. Its depressant effect on neuronal epileptic acitivity is also well recognized (Mason and Corcoran, 1979; see Burley and Ferendelli, 1984). Following cerebral ischemia there is a rapid decrease in the levels of noradrenaline (Calderini et al., 1978; Blomqvist et al., 1985), indicating an increased turnover of the transmitter (Calderini et al., 1978). The postischemic activation of the central noradrenergic system can be envisaged to counteract neuronal hyperexcitability. However, as there is no clear correlation between the distribution of noradrenergic afferents and the distribution of selective neuronal necrosis, the activation of the noradrenaline system may not be sufficient to depress the neuronal hyperexcitability in selectively vulnerable areas.

In summary, data presented in this section strongly suggests that EAA's and/or related compounds are major pathogenic factors in the development of ischemic and hypoglycemic brain damage, preferentially acting on postsynaptic EAA receptor sites. A concomitant decrease in the activity of inhibitory neuronal systems such as damage to potentially inhibitory GABA-ergic neurons and/or an insufficient release of inhibitory neuromodulators might further aggravate the deleterious effects of an excitatory stress on the vulnerable neurons as well as of spontaneous firing activity.

Possible intracellular mediators of cell damage

Although the *extracellular* mediators of regional selective neuronal necrosis following ischemic and hypoglycemic insults are likely to be excitatotoxins, knowledge of the lethal *intracellular* mediators is still scant. This is mainly due to the limited knowledge of the molecular properties of these receptors. Postsynaptic densities can be isolated with retained specific binding of glutamate agonists such as NMDA and QA (Fagg and Matus, 1985). Further research on the properties of the receptors will be of great value in the evaluation of their importance in pathological situations. It is not fully clear what second messenger is used by the EAA receptors (Watkins and Evans, 1981; Roberts and Foster, 1983). However, the ionic movements over the plasma membrane induced by agonist-receptor interactions include influx of chloride, sodium and water (Watkins and Evans, 1981) and calcium ions (Schwartzkroin and Wyler, 1979; Berdichevsky et al., 1983). Two hypotheses regarding the mechanisms of ischemic neuronal death based on the deleterious effects of elevation of the intracellular concentrations of these ions have recently been proposed.

The calcium hypothesis

The deleterious effects of an excessive influx of calcium into cells were first proposed for hepatocytes by Schanne and coworkers (1979). In the central nervous system calcium ions were hypothesized to be responsible for the induction of neuronal necrosis following cerebral ischemia (Hass, 1981; Siesjö, 1981), in hypoglycemia and status epilepticus (Siesjö, 1981). The deleterious reactions activated by calcium ions have been recently reviewed (Siesjö and Wieloch, 1985).

The calcium toxicity on the cellular level has elegantly been discussed by Rasmussen and Waisman (1983) in terms of rate constants of calcium influx and efflux over cell membranes. Briefly, the theory predicts that, as a consequence of a known higher influx rate of calcium over the plasma membrane and into the mitochondria as compared to the efflux rates, the calcium ions will accumulate in the mitochondria with time. The predicted increase in cytosolic calcium concentrations (10^{-6} M) is sufficient to activate most cellular calcium-regulated physiological processes. An excessive mitochondrial calcium accumulation could inhibit ADP phosphorylation (see Fiskum, 1984). Although ATP depletion has not been observed in the recirculation period in the vulnerable areas of the hippocampus (Mies et al., 1983), local energy failure at sites of excessive calcium influx such as at postsynaptic densities in the dendrites of CA1, could be involved. The cytosolic concentrations of calcium could be further increased if the concentrations of cytosolic calcium binding proteins are decreased. The hippocampus has a peculiar distribution of a calcium buffering protein (CaBP), mainly confined to the CA1 and the granule cells of the dentate gyrus but less in the CA3 region (Baimbridge and Miller, 1982). The levels of this protein drastically decrease following amygdala kindling (Miller and Baimbridge, 1983). The possible decrease in the levels of CaBP in the postischemic period could further increase the cytosolic calcium concentrations.

What is the experimental evidence for a calcium toxicity following ischemia and hypoglycemia? At the onset of ischemia and hypoglycemic coma, calcium ions flow down its concentration gradient from the extracellular to the intracellular spaces (Hansen and Zeuthen, 1981; Harris et al., 1984). This takes place concomitantly with a series of deleterious reactions such as energy failure and lipolysis, leading to elevation of free fatty acids, in particular arachidonic acid (Bazan, 1976; Rehncrona et al., 1982; Wieloch et al., 1984). This elevation of arachidonic acid is marked in vulnerable brain structures such as the hippocampus (Blomqvist et al., 1985). In the recirculation phase the levels of extracellular calcium ion concentrations are rapidly restored and normal levels attained within 15 min (Hansen and Zeuthen, 1981). In a study using intravenously injected ^{45}Ca, an increased radioactivity in all regions of the hippocampus was observed within 24 hour following ischemia without an increase in the total levels of calcium; after 72 hours, when neuronal necrosis was evident by light microscopy, an increase in the total levels of calcium was noted (Dienel, 1984). The increase in radioactive calcium in the hippocampal formation without a concomitant increase in total calcium suggested an increased turnover of the ion over the plasma membrane. With the oxalate-pyroantimonate stain it has been demonstrated that calcium accumulates in neurons following anoxia/ischemia (Van Reempts and Borgers, 1982; Van Reempts et al., 1984; Simon et al., 1984b). Analogous findings have been reported in excitotoxin-induced damage to hypothalamic neurons (Olney et al., 1984) where intracellular calcium deposits were observed, and following kainic acid induced seizures (Korf and Postema, 1984). Recently, it was shown that treatment of animals with flunarizine, a "calcium entry blocker", decreased the hippocampal CA1 damage following 10 min of forebrain ischemia (Deshpande and Wieloch, 1984).

Although circumstantial evidence suggests that calcium ions might be responsible for the deleterious reactions leading to neuronal death, an important question still remaining is whether the observed increase in cytosolic calcium concentration precedes the neuronal death or is its consequence.

The chloride hypothesis

In two recent articles it was demonstrated that hippocampal neuronal cultures subjected to anoxia, induced by KCN poisoning, or by decreased oxygen tension, degenerated due to mechanisms related to synaptic activity (Rothman, 1983), and that this process was enhanced if glutamate was present in the medium (Rothman, 1984a). Glutamate did not enhance neuronal degeneration if chloride ions were substituted by the impermeable sulfate or isothionate ions, and sodium ions by benzoylcholine. Furthermore, the presence of calcium was not required for neurotoxicity of glutamate (Rothman, 1984b). Similar results were obtained in preparations of chick embryo retina (Olney et al., 1984). The authors concluded that glutamate exerts its neurotoxic effect on the neurons through osmolysis, by enhancing chloride influx concomitantly with sodium and water, and that calcium ions are not an obligatory factor.

Whether these mechanisms prevail in the ischemic, postischemic or hypoglycemic situation has not been substantiated. No dendritic swelling could be observed in the stratum radiatum of CA1 in the gerbil subjected to bilateral common carotid occlusion for 5 min and 3, 6 and 12 hours of recovery (Kirino, 1982). In an electron microscopic study of the dentrites in the CA1 region, Petito and Pulsinelli (1984) demonstrated dendritic *shrinkage* rather then swelling 24 hours following an ischemic insult. Pre- and postsynaptic membrane breaks were reported, 60 min following a 10-min ischemia period (Ekström von Lubitz and Diemer, 1982; Johansen et al., 1984) but they were not preceded by extensive cellular swelling. Thus no conclusive *in vivo* support for the chloride hypothesis is available at the moment. However, an extensive temporal study of the ultrastructural changes in the dendrites of the pyramidal cells following ischemia seems warranted.

Other intracellular mediators

In the immediate postischemic phase the levels of *cyclic nucleotides* such as cAMP and cGMP (Kobayashi et al., 1977; Blomqvist et al., 1985) are dramatically increased. Since neither noradrenaline, nor prostaglandins, nor adenosine seem to induce the elevation of cAMP (Blomqvist et al., 1985), the EAA's may be plausible candidates (see Roberts and Foster, 1983; Watkins and Evans, 1981). Excessive elevations of the levels of cAMP or cGMP could have a dramatic effect on plasma membrane properties (Delgado-Escueta and Horan, 1983) and protein synthesis (Benne et al., 1978).

Free radicals are another class of compounds with potential cytotoxic properties. The most sensitive targets in the cell for free radical attack are the DNA, the unsaturated fatty acid double bonds in the membranes, and sulfhydryl and amino groups on proteins (see Tappel, 1975; Pryor, 1978). The arachidonic acid, released during ischemia and hypoglycemic coma (see above), may serve as initiator of free radical formation and a postischemic hyperexcitability could be further aggravating (Siesjö et al., 1982). The relation between these potentially toxic compounds and cell death is still obscure, but if such compounds are formed they could have devastating effects on the integrity of the plasma membrane and protein synthesis mechanisms.

Acknowledgements

This study was supported by grants from the Swedish Medical Research Council (No. 14X-263), and from U.S. Public Health Service (NIH grant No. 2 RO1 NSO7838). The author wishes to thank Erna Björkengren for skilful secretarial help.

References

Abdul-Rahman, A., Agardh, C.-D. and Siesjö, B.K. (1980) Local cerebral blood flow in the rat during severe hypoglycemia and in the recovery period following glucose injection. *Acta Physiol. Scand.,* 109: 307–314.

Agardh, C.-D., Chapman, A.G., Nilsson, B. and Siesjö, B.K. (1981) Endogenous substrate utilized by rat brain in severe insulin-induced hypoglycemia. *J. Neurochem.,* 36: 490–500.

Amaral, D.G. (1978) A Golgi study of cell types in the hilar region of the hippocampus in the rat. *J. Comp. Neurol.,* 182: 851–914.

Auer, R.N., Olsson, Y. and Siesjö, B.K. (1984a) Hypoglycemic brain injury in the rat. *Diabetes,* 33: 1090–1098.

Auer, R.N., Wieloch, T., Olsson, Y. and Siesjö, B.K. (1984b) The distribution of hypoglycemic brain damage. *Acta Neuropathol. (Berl.),* 64: 177–191.

Baimbridge, K.G. and Miller, J.J. (1982) Immunohistochemical localization of calcium-binding protein in the cerebellum, hippocampal formation and olfactory bulb of the rat. *Brain Res.,* 245: 223–229.

Bazán, N.G. (1976) Free arachidonic acid and other lipids in the nervous system during early ischemia and after electroshock. *Adv. Exp. Med. Biol.,* 72: 317–335.

Benne, R., Edman, J., Traut, R.R. and Hershey, J.W.B. (1978) Phosphorylation of eukaryotic protein synthesis initiation factor. *Proc. Natl. Acad. Sci. USA,* 75: 108–112.

Benveniste, H., Drejer, J., Schousboe, A. and Diemer, N.H. (1984) Elevation of the extracellular concentrations of glutamate and aspartate in rat hippocampus during transient cerebral ischemia monitored by intracerebral microdialysis. *J. Neurochem.,* 43: 1369–1374.

Berdichevsky, E.N., Riveros, N., Sanchez-Armass, S. and Orrego, F. (1983) Kainate, N-methylaspartate and other excitatory amino acids increase calcium influx into rat brain cortex cells in vitro. *Neurosci. Lett.,* 36: 75–80.

Blomqvist, P. and Wieloch, T. (1985) Ischemic brain damage in the rat following cardiac arrest using a long term recovery model. *J. Cereb. Blood Flow Metab.,* in press.

Blomqvist, P., Lindvall, O. and Wieloch, T. (1985) Cyclic AMP concentrations in rat neocortex and hippocampus during and following incomplete ischemia: influence of central noradrenergic neurons, prostaglandins and adenosine. *J. Neurochem.,* 44: 1345–1353.

Burley, E.S. and Ferendelli, J.A. (1984) Regulatory effects of neurotransmitters on electroshock and pentylentetrazol seizures. *Fed. Proc.,* 43: 2521–2524.

Buzsáki, G. (1984) Feed-forward inhibition in the hippocampal formation. *Prog. Neurobiol.,* 22: 131–153.

Calderini, G., Carlsson, A. and Nordström, C.-H. (1978) Influence of transient ischemia on monoamine metabolism in the rat brain during nitrous oxide and phenobarbitone anesthesia. *Brain Res.,* 157: 303–310.

Choki, J., Greenberg, J. and Reivich, M. (1983) Regional cerebral glucose metabolism during and after bilateral cerebral ischemia in the gerbil. *Stroke,* 14: 568–579.

Collins, R.C. and Olney, J. (1982) Focal cortical seizures cause distant neuronal thalamic lesions. *Science,* 218: 177–179.

Collins, R.C., Lothman, E.W. and Olney, J.W. (1983a) Status epilepticus in the limbic system: biochemical and pathological changes. In: A.V. Delgado-Escueta, C.G. Wasterlein, D.M. Treiman and R.J. Porter (Eds.), *Advances in Neurology, Vol. 34, Status Epilepticus.* Raven Press, New York, pp. 277–288.

Collins, R.C., Olney, J.W. and Lothman, E.W. (1983b) Metabolic and pathological consequences of focal seizures. In: A.A. Ward, Jr., J.K. Penry and D. Purpura (Eds.), *Epilepsy.* Raven Press, New York, pp. 87–107.

Cotman, C.W., Foster, A. and Lanthorn, T. (1981) An overview of glutamate as a neurotransmitter. In: G. DiChiara and G.L. Gessa (Eds.), *Glutamate as neurotransmitter.* Raven Press, New York, pp. 1–27.

Coyle, J.T., Bird, S.J., Evans, R.H., Gulley, R.L., Nadler, J.V., Nicklas, W.J. and Olney, J.W. (1981) Excitatory amino acid neurotoxins: selectivity, specificity, and mechanism of action. *Neurosci. Res. Progr.,* 19: 330–427.

Croucher, M.J., Collins, J.F. and Meldrum, B.S. (1982) Anticonvulsant action of excitatory amino acid antagonists. *Science,* 216: 899–901.

Davies, J., Evans, R.H., Jones, A.W., Mewett, K.N., Smith, D.A.S. and Watkins, J.C. (1983) Recent advances in the pharmacology of excitatory amino acids in the mammalian central nervous system. In: K. Fuxe, P. Roberts and R. Schwarcz (Eds.), *Excitotoxins.* Macmillan Press, London, pp. 43–54.

Delgado-Escueta, A.V. and Horan, M. (1983) Effects of seizures on ion transport and membrane protein phosphorylation. In: A.V. Delgado-Escueta, C.G. Wasterlain, D.M. Treiman and R.J. Porter (Eds.), *Advances in Neurology, Vol. 34.* Raven Press, New York, pp. 311–323.

Deshpande, J. and Wieloch, T. (1985) Amelioration of ischemic brain damage by postischemic treatment with flunarizine. *Neurol. Res.,* 7: 27–29.

Diemer, N.H. and Siemkowicz, E. (1980) Increased 2-deoxyglucose uptake in hippocampus, globus pallidus and substantia nigra after cerebral ischemia. *Acta Neurol Scand.,* 61: 56–63.

Diemer, N.H. and Siemkowicz, E. (1981) Regional neuronal damage after cerebral ischemia in the normo- and hypoglycemic rat. *Neuropathol. Appl. Neurobiol.,* 7: 217–227.

Dienel, G.A. (1984) Regional accumulation of calcium in postischemic rat brain. *J. Neurochem.,* 43: 913–925.

Divac, I., Fonnum, F. and Storm-Mathisen, J. (1977) High affinity uptake of glutamate in terminals of corticostriatal axons. *Nature,* 266: 377–378.

Doller, H.J. and Weight, F.F. (1982) Perforant pathway activation of hippocampal CA1 stratum pyramidale neurons: electrophysiological evidence for a direct pathway. *Brain Res.,* 237: 1–13.

Dunwiddie, T.V. and Hoffer, B.J. (1980) Adenine nucleotides and synaptic transmission in the in vitro rat hippocampus.

Br. J. Pharmacol., 69: 59–68.

Ekström von Lubitz, D.K.J. and Diemer, N.H. (1982) Complete cerebral ischemia in the rat: an ultrastructural and stereological analysis of the distal stratum radiatum in the hippocampal CA1 region. Neuropathol. Appl. Neurol., 8: 197–215.

Evans, R.H., Francis, A.A., Jones, A.W., Smith, D.A.S. and Watkins, J.C. (1982) The effect of a series of ω-phosphonic-α-carboxylic amino acids on electrically evoked and excitant amino acid-induced responses in isolated spinal cord preparations. Br. J. Pharmacol., 75: 65–75.

Fagg, G.E. and Foster, A.C. (1983) Aminoacid neurotransmitter and their pathways in the mammalian central nervous system. Neuroscience, 9: 701–719.

Fagg, G.E. and Matus, A. (1985) Selective association of N-methyl-aspartate and quisqualate types of L-glutamate receptor with brain postsynaptic densities. Proc. Natl. Acad. Sci. U.S.A., in press.

Fiskum, G. (1984) Physiological aspects of mitochondrial calcium transport. In: H. Sigel (Ed.), Metal ions in biological systems, Vol. 17. Marcel Dekker, New York, pp. 187–214.

Flatman, J.A., Schwindt, P.C., Crill, W.E. and Stafstrom, C.E. (1983) Multiple actions of N-methyl-D-aspartate on cat neocortical neurons in vitro. Brain Res., 266: 169–173.

Fonnum, F. (1984) Glutamate: a neurotransmitter in mammalian brain. J. Neurochem., 1: 1–11.

Foster, A.C. and Fagg, G.E. (1984) Acidic amino acid binding sites in mammalian neuronal membranes: their characteristics and relationship to synaptic receptors. Brain Res. Rev., 1: 103–164.

Hansen, A.J. and Zeuthen, T. (1981) Extracellular ion concentrations during spreading depression and ischemia in the rat brain cortex. Acta Physiol. Scand., 113: 437–445.

Harris, R.J., Wieloch, T., Symon, L. and Siesjö, B.K. (1984) Cerebral extracellular calcium activity in severe hypoglycemia: relation to extracellular potassium and energy state. J. Cereb. Blood Flow Metab., 4: 187–193.

Hass, W.K. (1981) Beyond cerebral blood flow, metabolism and ischemic thresholds: examination of the role of calcium in the initiation of cerebral infarction. In: J.S. Meyer, H. Lechner, M. Reivich, E.O. Ott and A. Arabinar (Eds.), Cerebral Vascular Disease, Vol. 3, Proceedings of the 10th Salzburger Conference on Cerebral Vascular Disease. Excerpta Medica, Amsterdam, pp. 3–17.

Herrling, P., Morris, R. and Salt, T.E. (1983) Effects of excitatory amino acids and their antagonists on membrane and action potentials of cat caudate neurones. J. Physiol. (Lond.), 339: 207–222.

Hillered, L., Siesjö, B.K. and Arfors, K. (1984) Mitochondrial response to transient forebrain ischemia and recirculation in the rat. J. Cereb. Blood Flow Metab., 4: 438–446.

Houser, C.R., Vaugh, J.E., Barber, R.P. and Roberts, E. (1980) GABA neurons are the major cell type of the nucleus reticularis thalami. Brain Res., 200: 341–354.

Ito, U., Spatz, M., Walker, J.T. and Klatzo, I. (1975) Experimental cerebral ischemia in mongolian gerbils. Acta Neuropathol. (Berl.), 32: 209–223.

Johansen, F.F., Jørgensen, M.B., Ekström von Lubitz, D.K.J. and Diemer, N.H. (1984) Selective dendrite damage in hippocampal CA1 stratum radiatum with unchanged axon ultrastructure and glutamate uptake after transient cerebral ischemia in the rat. Brain Res., 291: 373–377.

Jones, A.W., Croucher, M.J., Meldrum, B.S. and Watkins, J.C. (1984) Suppression of audiogenic seizures in DBA/2 mice by two new dipeptide NMDA receptor antagonists. Neurosci. Lett., 45: 157–161.

Jørgensen, M.B. and Diemer, N.H. (1982) Selective neuron loss after cerebral ischemia in the rat: possible role of transmitter glutamate. Acta Neurol. Scand., 66: 536–546.

Kalimo, H., Auer, R.N. and Siesjö, B.K. (1985) The temporal evolution of hypoglycemic brain damage. III. Light- and electron-microscope findings in the rat caudoputamen. Acta Neuropathol. (Berl.), in press.

Kirino, T. (1982) Delayed neuronal death in the gerbil hippocampus following ischemia. Brain Res., 239: 57–69.

Kobayashi, M., Lust, W.D. and Passenneau, J.V. (1977) Concentrations of energy metabolites and cyclic nucleotides during and after bilateral ischemia in the gerbil cerebral cortex. J. Neurochem., 32: 463–468.

Korf, J. and Postema, F. (1984) Regional calcium accumulation and cation shifts in rat brain by kainate. J. Neurochem., 43: 1052–1060.

Köhler, C. and Schwarcz, R. (1981) Monosodium glutamate: increased toxicity after removal of neuronal re-uptake sites. Brain Res., 211: 485–491.

Lee, K.S., Reddington, M., Schubert, P. and Kreutzberg, G. (1983) Regulation of the strength of adenosine modulation in the hippocampus by a differential distribution of the density of A_1 receptors. Brain Res., 260: 156–159.

Lee, K.S., Schubert, P. and Heinemann, U. (1984) The anticonvulsive action of adenosine: a postsynaptic, dendritic action by a possible endogenous anticonvulsant. Brain Res., in press.

Lee, K.S., Schubert, P. and Reddington, M. (1985a) Adenosine as a neuromodulator. In: V. Stefenovich and G.I. Okyazuz-Bakbuti (Eds.), The Role of Adenosine in Cerebral Metabolism and Blood Flow. VNU Boekengroep, Utrecht, in press.

Lee, K.S., Schubert, P., Reddington, M. and Kreutzberg, G.W. (1985b) The distribution of 5'-nucleotidase and adenosine A1 receptors: evidence for diversification and conservation in the hippocampi of several commonly employed experimental animals. Acta Histochem., in press.

Leonard, J.P. and Salpeter, M. (1979) Agonist-induced myopathy at the neuromuscular junction is mediated by calcium. J. Cell. Biol., 82: 811–819.

Lewis, M.E., Patel, J., Moon Edley, S. and Marangos, P.J. (1981) Autoradiographic visualization of rat brain adenosine receptors using N-6-cyclohexyl-^{3}H adenosine. Eur. J. Pharmacol., 73: 109–110.

Lucas, D.R. and Newhouse, J.P. (1957) The toxic effect of L-glutamate on the inner layers of the retina. *Arch. Ophthalmol.*, 58: 193–201.

Malthe-Sørenssen, D., Skrede, K. and Fonnum, F. (1979) Calcium dependent release of D-^{3}H-aspartate from the dorsal septum after electrical stimulation of the fimbria in vitro. *Neuroscience*, 5: 127–133.

Mason, S.T. and Corcoran, M.E. (1979) Cathecolamines and convulsions. *Brain Res.*, 170: 497–507.

McGeer, P.L., McGeer, E.G., Scherer, U. and Singh, K. (1977) A glutamatergic corticostriatal path? *Brain Res.*, 128: 308–314.

McIntyre, D.C., Nathanson, D. and Edson, N. (1982) A new model of partial status epilepticus based on kindling. *Brain Res.*, 250: 53–63.

Mies, G., Paschen, W., Hossmann, K.-A. and Klatzo, I. (1983) Simultaneous measurement of regional blood flow and metabolism during maturation of hippocampal lesions following short-lasting cerebral ischemia in gerbils. *J. Cereb. Blood Flow Metabol.*, 3: S329–330.

Miller, J.J. and Baimbridge, K.G. (1983) Biochemical and immunohistochemical correlates of kindling-induced epilepsy: role of calcium binding protein. *Brain Res.*, 278: 322–326.

Monaghan, D.T., Holets, V.R., Toy, D.W. and Cotman, C.W. (1983) Anatomical distributions of four pharmacologically distinct ^{3}H-L-glutamate binding sites. *Nature*, 306: 176–179.

Monaghan, D.T., Yao, D. and Cotman, C.W. (1985a) Distribution of ^{3}H-AMPA binding sites in rat brain as determined by quantitative autoradiography. *Brain Res.*, in press.

Monaghan, D.T., Yao, D., Olverman, H.J., Watkins, J.C. and Cotman, C.W. (1985b) Autoradiography of ^{3}H-D-2-amino-5-phosphonopentanoate binding sites in rat brain. *Neurosci. Lett.*, in press.

Moroni, F., Lombardi, G., Carla, V. and Moneti, G. (1984) The excitotoxin quinolinic acid is present and unevenly distributed in the rat brain. *Brain Res.*, 295: 352–355.

Nadler, J.V., Evenson, D.A. and Cuthbertson, G.J.L. (1981) Comparative toxicity of kainic acid and other acidic amino acids toward rat hippocampal neurons. *Neurosci.*, 6: 2505–2517.

Nevander, G., Ingvar, M., Auer, R. and Siesjö, B.K. (1984) Irreversible neuronal damage after short periods of status epilepticus. *Acta Physiol. Scand.*, 120: 155–157.

Nevander, G., Ingvar, M., Auer, R. and Siesjö, B.K. (1985) Status epilepticus in well oxygenated causes neuronal necrosis. *Ann. Neurol.*, in press.

Nowak, L., Bregestovski, P. and Ascher, P. (1984) Magnesium gates glutamate-activated channels in mouse central neurons. *Nature*, 307: 462–465.

Okada, Y. and Kuroda, Y. (1975) Inhibitory action of adenosine and adenine nucleotides on the postsynaptic potential of olfactory slices of guinea pig. *Proc. Jap. Acad.*, 51: 491–494.

Olney, J. (1978) Neurotoxicity of excitatory amino acids. In: E.G. McGeer, J.W. Olney and P.L. McGeer (Eds.), *Kainic as a Tool in Neurobiology*. Raven Press, New york, pp. 95–121.

Olney, J.W. (1983) Excitotoxins: an overview. In: K. Fuxe, P. Roberts and R. Schwarcz (Eds.), *Excitotoxins*. Macmillan Press, London, pp. 82–96.

Olney, J.W., Gubareff, de T. and Labruyere, J. (1982) Seizure related brain damage induced by cholinergic agents. *Nature*, 301: 520–522.

Olney, J.W., Gubareff, de T. and Sloviter, R.S. (1983) "Epileptic" brain damage in rats induced by sustained electrical stimulation of the perforant path. II. Ultrastructural analysis of acute hippocampal pathology. *Brain Res. Bull.*, 10: 699–712.

Olney, J.W., Price, M.T., Samson, L. and Labruyere, J. (1984) The ionic basis of excitotoxin-induced neuronal necrosis. Abstract. American Neuroscience Meeting 1984, p. 24.

Panula, P., Revuelta, A.V., Cheney, D.L., Wu, J.-Y. and Costa, E. (1984) An immunohistochemical study on the location of GABA-ergic neurons in rat septum. *J. Comp. Neurol.*, 222: 69–80.

Petito, C.K. and Pulsinelli, W.A. (1984) Delayed neuronal recovery and neuronal death in rat hippocampus following severe cerebral ischemia: possible relationship to abnormalities in neuronal processes. *J. Cereb. Blood Flow Metabol.*, 4: 194–205.

Phillis, J.W. and Kostopoulos, G.P. (1977) Activation of a noradrenergic pathway from the brain stem to rat cerebral cortex. *Gen. Pharmacol.*, 8: 207–211.

Phillis, J.W. and Wu, P.H. (1981) The role of adenosine and its nucleotides in central synaptic transmission. *Prog. Neurobiol.*, 16: 187–239.

Plaitakis, A., Berl, S. and Yahr, R. (1982) Abnormal glutamate metabolism in an adult-onset degenerative neurological disorders. *Science*, 216: 193–196.

Pryor, W.A. (1978) The formation of free radicals and the consequences of their reactions in vivo. *Photochem. Photobiol.*, 28: 787–801.

Pulsinelli, W.A. and Brierly, J.B. (1979) A new model of bilateral hemispheric ischemia in the unanesthetized rat. *Stroke*, 10: 267–272.

Pulsinelli, W.A. and Duffy, T.E. (1983) Regional energy balance in rat brain after transient forebrain ischemia. *J. Neurochem.*, 40: 1500–1503.

Pulsinelli, W.A., Brierley, J.B. and Plum, F. (1982) Temporal profile of neuronal damage in a model of transient forebrain ischemia. *Ann. Neurol.*, 11: 491–499.

Rasmussen, H. and Waisman, D.M. (1983) Modulation of cell function in the calcium messenger system. *Rev. Physiol. Biochem. Pharmacol.*, 95: 111–148.

Rehncrona, S., Siesjö, B.K. and Westerberg, E. (1978) Adenosine and cAMP in cerebral cortex of rats in hypoxia, status epilepticus and hypercapnia. *Acta Physiol. Scand.*, 104: 453–463.

Rehncrona, S., Westerberg, E., Åkesson, B. and Siesjö, B.K. (1982) Brain cortical fatty acids and phospholipids during and following complete and severe incomplete ischemia. *J. Neu-*

rochem., 38: 84–93.
Ribak, C.E. and Anderson, L. (1980) Ultrastructure of the pyramidal basket cells in the dentate gyrus of the rat. *J. Comp. Neurol.*, 192: 903–916.
Ribak, C.E. and Reffenstein, R.J. (1982) Selective inhibitory synapse loss in chronic cortical slabs: a morphological basis for epileptic susceptibility. *Can. J. Physiol. Pharmacol.*, 60: 864–870.
Roberts, P.J. and Foster, G.A. (1983) Receptors for excitotoxins. In: K. Fuxe, P. Roberts and R. Schwarcz (Eds.), *Excitotoxins*. MacMillan Press, London, pp. 66–81.
Rothman, S.M. (1983) Synaptic activity mediates death of hypoxic neurons. *Science*, 220: 536–537.
Rothman, S. (1984a) Synaptic release of excitatory amino acid neurotransmitter mediates anoxic neuronal death. *J. Neurosci.*, 4: 1884–1891.
Rothman, S.M. (1984b) Excitatory amino acid neurotoxicity is produced by passive chloride influx. Abstract: American Neuroscience Meeting 1984, p. 24.
Schanne, F.A.X., Kane, A., Young, E.E. and Faber, J. (1979) Calcium dependence of toxic death: a final common pathway. *Science*, 206: 700–702.
Schwarcz, R., Collins, J.F. and Parks, D.A. (1982) Amino-ω-phosphono carboxylates block ibotenate but not kainate neurotoxicity in rat hippocampus. *Neurosci. Lett.*, 33: 85–90.
Schwarcz, R., Whetsell, Jr. W.O. and Mangano, R.M. (1983a) Quinolinic acid: an endogenous metabolite that produces axon-sparing lesions in rat brain. *Science*, 219: 316–318.
Schwarcz, R., Whetsell, Jr. W.O. and Foster, A.C. (1983b) The neurodegenerative properties of intracerebral quinolinic acid and its structural analog cis-2,3-piperidine dicarboxylic acid. In: K. Fuxe, P. Roberts and R. Schwarcz (Eds.), *Excitotoxins*. MacMillan Press, London, pp. 122–137.
Schwarcz, R., Foster, A.C., French, E.D., Whetsell, Jr. W.O. and Köhler, C. (1984) Excitotoxic models for neurodegenerative disorders. *Life Sci.*, 35: 19–32.
Schwartzkroin, P.A. and Wyler, A.R. (1979) Mechanisms underlying epileptiform burst discharges. *Ann. Neurol.*, 7: 95–107.
Siesjö, B.K. (1981) Cell damage in the brain: a speculative synthesis. *J. Cereb. Blood Flow Metabol.*, 1: 155–185.
Siesjö, B.K., Ingvar, M. and Westerberg, E. (1982) The influence of bicuculline-induced seizures on free fatty acid concentrations in cerebral cortex, hippocampus, and cerebellum. *J. Neurochem.*, 39: 796–802.
Siesjö, B.K. and Wieloch, T. (1985) Cerebral metabolism in ischaemia: Neurochemical basis for therapy. *Br. J. Anaesth.*, 57: 47–63.
Simon, R.P., Swan, J.H., Griffith, T. and Meldrum, B.S. (1984a) Blockade of N-methyl-D-aspartate receptors may protect against ischemic damage in the brain. *Science*, 226: 850–852.
Simon, R.P., Griffith, T., Evans, M.C., Swan, J.H. and Meldrum, B.S. (1984b) Calcium overload in selectively vulnerable neurons of the hippocampus during and after ischemia: an electron microscopy study in the rat. *J. Cereb. Blood Flow Metabol.*, 4: 350–361.
Sloviter, R. (1983) "Epileptic" brain damage in rats induced by sustained electrical stimulation of the perforant path. I. Acute electrophysiological and light microscopic studies. *Brain Res. bull.*, 10: 675–697.
Sloviter, R.S. and Damiano, B.P. (1981) Sustained electrical stimulation of the perforant path duplicates kainate-induced electrophysiological effects and hippocampal damage in rats. *Neurosci. Lett.*, 24: 279–284.
Smith, M.-L., Bendek, G., Dahlgren, N., Rosén, I., Wieloch, T. and Siesjö, B.K. (1984a) Models for studying long-term recovery following forebrain ischemia in the rat. 2. A 2-vessel occlusion model. *Acta Neurol. Scand.*, 69: 385–401.
Smith, M.-L., Auer, R.N. and Siesjö, B.K. (1984b) The density and distribution of ischemic brain injury in the rat following 2–10 min of forebrain ischemia. *Acta Neuropathol. (Berl.)*, 64: 319–332.
Spencer, H.J. (1976) Antagonism of cortical excitation of striatal neurons by glutamic acid diethylester: evidence for glutamic acid as an excitatory transmitter in rat striatum. *Brain Res.*, 113: 563–574.
Storm-Mathisen, J. (1977) Localization of transmitter candidates in the brain: the hippocampal formation as a model. *Prog. Neurobiol.*, 8: 119–181.
Storm-Mathisen, J. and Opsahl, M. (1978) Aspartate and/or glutamate may be transmitters in hippocampal efferents to septum and hypothalamus. *Neurosci. Lett.*, 9: 65–70.
Steward, O. (1976) Topographic organization of the projections from the entorhinal area to the hippocampal formation. *J. Comp. Neurol.*, 167: 285–314.
Suzuki, R., Yamaguchi, T., Kirino, T., Orzi, F. and Klatzo, I. (1983a) The effects of 5-min ischemia in mongolian gerbils: I. Blood-brain barrier, cerebral blood flow, and local cerebral glucose utilization changes. *Acta Neuropathol. (Berl.)*, 60: 207–216.
Suzuki, R., Yamaguchi, T., Li, C.-L. and Klatzo, I. (1983b) The effects of 5 min ischemia in mongolian gerbils: II. Changes of spontaneous neuronal activity in cerebral cortex and CA2 sector of hippocampus. *Acta Neuropathol. (Berl.)*, 60: 217–222.
Swanson, L.W. and Cowan, W.M. (1979) The connections of the septal region in the rat. *J. Comp. Neurol.*, 186: 621–656.
Tappel, A.L. (1975) Lipid peroxidation and fluorescent molecular damage to membranes. In: B.F. Trump and A.V. Arstila (Eds.), *Pathobiology of Cell Membranes, Vol. 1*. Academic Press, New York, pp. 145–170.
Van Reempts, J. and Borgers, M. (1982) Morphological assessment of pharmacological brain protection. In: A. Waquier, W.S. Amery, M. Borgers and A. Waquier (Eds.), *Protection of Tissues in Brain Hypoxia*. Elsevier, Amsterdam, pp. 263–274.
Van Reempts, J., Haseldonckx, M., van de Ven, M. and Borgers, M. (1984) Morphology and ultrastructural calcium distribution in the rat hippocampus after severe transient ischemia. In: A. Bes, P. Braquet, R. Paoletti and B.K. Siesjö (Eds.),

Cerebral Ischemia, ICS 654. Excerpta Medica, Amsterdam-New York-Oxford, pp. 113–118.

Watkins, J.C. and Evans, R.H. (1981) Excitatory amino acid transmitters. *Ann. Rev. Pharmacol. Toxicol.,* 21: 165–204.

Wieloch, T., Harris, R., Symon, L. and Siesjö, B.K. (1984) Influence of severe hypoglycemia on brain extracellular calcium and potassium activities, energy charge, and phospholipid metabolism. *J. Neurochem.,* 43: 160–168.

Wieloch, T., Lindvall, O., Blomqvist, P. and Gage, F. (1985) Evidence for amelioration of ischemic neuronal damage in the hippocampal formation by lesions of the perforant path. *Neurol. Res.,* 7: 24–26.

Wieloch, T., Engelsen, B., Westerberg, E. and Auer, R. Lesions of the glutamatergic cortico-striatal projections in the rat ameliorate hypoglycemic brain damage in the striatum. *Neurosci. Lett.,* in press.

Williams, M. (1984) Mammalian central adenosine receptors. In: A. Lajtha (Ed.), *Handbook of Neurochemistry.* Plenum Press, New York, pp. 1–26.

Wolfensberger, M.A., Amsler, U., Cuenod, M., Foster, A.C., Whetsell, W.O. and Schwarcz, R. (1983) Identification of quinolinic acid in rat and human brain tissue. *Neurosci. Lett.,* 41: 247–252.

Wyss, J.M. (1981) An autoradiographic study of the efferent connections of the entorhinal cortex in the rat. *J. Comp. Neurol.,* 199: 495–512.

… SECTION II

Cellular Ca^{2+} and H^+ Homeostasis

Calcium entry blockers: autoradiographic mapping of their binding sites in rat brain

Porntip Supavilai, Roser Cortés, José M. Palacios and Manfred Karobath

Preclinical Research, Sandoz Ltd., 386/216, CH-4002 Basle, Switzerland

Introduction

Investigations with radiolabelled organic calcium entry blockers have recently lead to a rapid progress in an understanding of the molecular pharmacology of voltage-dependent calcium channels (VDCC) in some tissues like striated or smooth muscle (Glossmann et al., 1982). There is now strong evidence that the VDCC in these tissues contain several different drug receptors. One of them is a high affinity binding site which recognizes 1,4-dihydropyridines with a rank order of affinity which correlates with that predicted from classical pharmacological experiments (Glossmann et al., 1982). The binding of 1,4-dihydropyridines to their drug receptor can also be inhibited by other chemical classes of calcium entry blockers like verapamil and its analogs. However, these drugs do not compete with the 1,4-dihydropyridines for the same recognition site but they inhibit the binding of the 1,4-dihydropyridines in a selective allosteric manner, namely by increasing the dissociation of the 1,4-dihydropyridines from their specific binding sites (Glossmann et al., 1982; Gould et al., 1982; Murphy et al., 1983). These observations led to the concept that verapamil and chemically related organic calcium entry blockers interact with a specific phenylalkylamine drug receptor of VDCC. This notion has recently been supported in studies with (−)-[^{3}H]desmethoxyverapamil ((−)-[^{3}H]D888) which is more than 10 times as potent as calcium antagonist than (−)-verapamil in functional tests, and which appears to be a suitable ligand for the characterization of the properties of the phenylalkylamine drug receptor of VDCC (Ferry et al., 1984). Thirdly, there is evidence that D-*cis*-diltiazem interacts with a third distinct drug receptor of VDCC, which communicates with the 1,4-dihydropyridine drug receptor and with the phenylalkylamine receptor by reciprocal allosterism (Glossmann et al., 1982). In striated and in smooth muscle tissue the binding affinities of the various chemical classes of organic calcium entry blockers for their respective drug receptors correlate with the rank order of pharmacological potency in classical pharmacological test systems (Janis and Triggle, 1984). This suggests that the three binding sites for organic calcium entry blockers mentioned above are constituents of functional VDCC in these tissues (Janis and Triggle, 1984).

In the central nervous system the findings are more complex and controversial (for review see Miller and Freedman, 1984). Thus, in membranes from brain tissues high densities of binding sites for radiolabelled 1,4-dihydropyridines, for (−)-D888 and for D-*cis*-diltiazem have been described in several species, including man (Ehlert et al., 1982; Glossmann et al., 1982; Gould et al., 1982; Peroutka and Allen, 1983; Supavilai and Karobath, 1984). All these observations suggest that, in brain membranes, the three drug recognition sites of VDCC form a similar supramolecular complex as has been demonstrated for striated and smooth muscle.

However, in neuronal tissue, it has been difficult

to demonstrate a functional effect of organic calcium entry blockers. Thus, in pharmacologically meaningful concentrations or dosages these drugs have no marked psychotropic actions in a number of psychopharmacological and biochemical pharmacological test systems (Hoffmeister et al., 1982; for review see Miller and Freedman, 1984). Furthermore, in electrophysiological as well as in biochemical investigations of calcium metabolism or of calcium-dependent mechanisms, organic calcium entry blockers have been largely inactive (Miller and Freedman, 1984). This apparent lack of effect of organic calcium entry blockers in the central nervous system has led to the question whether the 1,4-dihydropyridine binding sites in brain are drug acceptors without a function (Miller and Freedman, 1984). It should be pointed out that a lack of brain penetration of 1,4-dihydropyridines does not appear to be responsible for the apparent lack of effect of these drugs in the central nervous system, since brain penetration of several 1,4-dihydropyridines and in vivo binding to their recognition sites in brain has recently been demonstrated (Shoemaker et al., 1983; Supavilai and Karobath, 1984).

In order to elucidate a possible functional role of organic calcium entry blockers in brain, we have performed receptor autoradiographic studies in this tissue using $(+)$-[^{3}H]PN200-110, $(\pm)$-[^{3}H]D600 and $(-)$-[^{3}H]D888 as ligands. The results of such studies can point to brain areas which contain a high density of these sites which could then be used in investigations aimed at detecting a possible functional role of VDCC in brain.

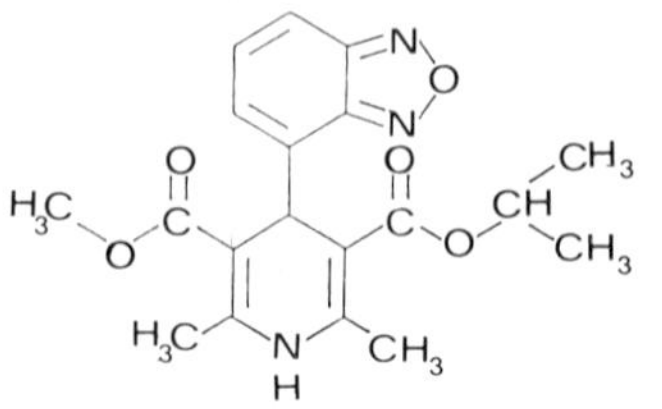

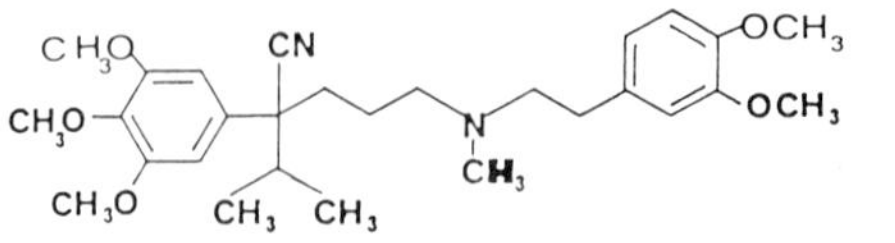

Materials and methods

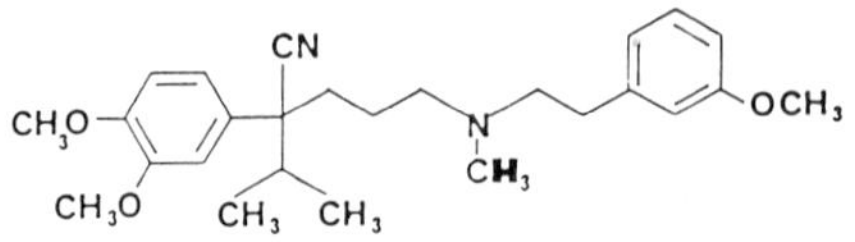

$(+)$-[^{3}H]PN200-110, (80 Ci/mmol) and $(-)$-[^{3}H]desmethoxyverapamil $(-)$-[^{3}H]D888 (83 Ci/mmol) were provided from Amersham Ltd., Buckinghamshire, UK, and $(\pm)$-[^{3}H]D600 (85 Ci/mmol) was provided by New England Nuclear, Boston, MA, USA. The structures of the ligands used in this investigation are shown in Fig. 1. PY108-068, PN200-110 and Bay K8644 were synthesized by P. Neuman and A. Vogel, Sandoz Ltd., Basle, Swit-

Fig. 1. Structure of PN 200-110, D 600 and D 888.

zerland. Other drugs and their sources were: verapamil and D600, Knoll, A.G., Ludwigshafen, FRG.

Autoradiography

These studies were performed with microtome-cryostat sections from the brains of adult male Wistar rats as previously described (Cortés et al., 1983, 1984). Rat brain slices (10 μm thick) were preincubated for 30 min in 50 mM Tris-HCl, pH 7.4, at room temperature. The slices were then incubated for 60 min in the presence of 0.1 nM $(+)$-[^{3}H]PN200-110 or of 1 nM $(\pm)$-[^{3}H]D600 or of 1 nM $(-)$-[^{3}H]D888. Values for non-specific binding were obtained by adding 1 μM unlabelled PY108-068 (when $(+)$-[^{3}H]PN200-110 was used as ligand) or 10 μM $(\pm)$-verapamil (when $(\pm)$-[^{3}H]D660 was used) or 10 μM $(\pm)$D600 (when $(-)$-[^{3}H]D888 was used). At the end of the incubation period, slices were transferred to ice cold buffer and washed for 20 min. Finally tissues were dried in a stream of cold air. Autoradiograms were obtained by apposing the labelled tissue sections to Ultrofilm (Cortés et al., 1984).

Results and discussions

Binding studies

It has already been demonstrated that the pattern of distribution of 1,4-dihydropyridine binding sites in brain is identical when [³H]PY108-068, [³H]-PN200-110 or [³H]nitrendipine are used as ligands (Cortés et al., 1984). These binding sites are distributed throughout the brain in a highly heterogenous manner with higher densities in gray matter, as compared to white matter tracts (Cortés et al., 1984). In the present study, the distribution of (+)-[³H]PN200-110 binding sites was compared with those of (±)-[³H]D600 and of (−)-[³H]D888 binding sites. The latter two compounds, both structural analogs of verapamil, have been proposed as ligands suitable for the characterization of the phenylalkylamine drug receptor of VDCC (Ferry et al., 1984; Reynolds et al., 1984). Fig. 2 shows autoradiograms obtained with (+)-[³H]PN200-110, (±)-[³H]D600 and with (−)-[³H]D888 in adjacent sagittal microtome-cryostat sections from rat brain. It can be seen that all three ligands bind to brain tissue in a very heterogenous mode. In the following the results obtained with these ligands are discussed separately.

(+)-[³H]PN200-110 binding

The results are in agreement with previous observations (Murphy et al., 1982; Cortés et al., 1983; Quirion, 1983) and a more detailed quantitative autoradiographic study (Cortés et al., 1984). The highest densities of (+)-[³H]PN200-110 binding sites are observed in the olfactory bulb, hippocampus and parts of the amygdala (Figs. 2 and 3, Table 1; Cortés et al., 1984). The neocortex also has high densities of (+)-[³H]PN200-110 binding sites, whereas in the basal ganglia, thalamus and hypothalamus intermediate levels are found (Figs. 2 and 3). The cerebellum, pons-medulla and white matter tracts contain low densities of (+)-[³H]PN200-110

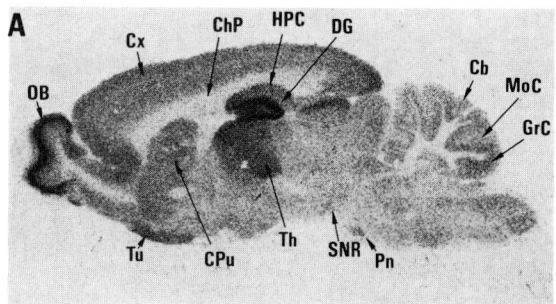
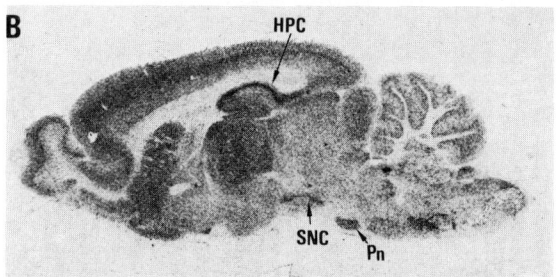
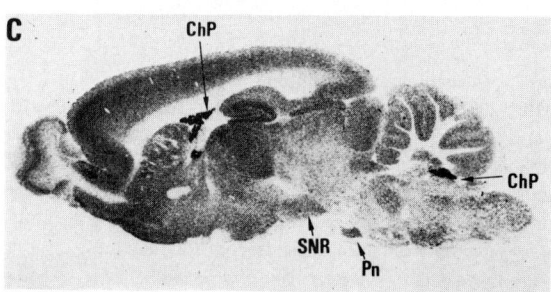

Fig. 2. Autoradiographic mapping of the distribution of (A) (+)-[³H]PN200-110; (B) (±)-[³H]D600; and (C) (−)-[³H]D888 binding sites in sagittal sections of the rat brain. The abbreviations and the symbols used are: Cb, cerebellum; ChP, choroid plexus; CPu, caudate putamen; Cx, cortex; DG, dentate gyrus; GrC, granular layer of the cerebellum; HPC, hippocampus, pyramidal cell layer; MoC, molecular layer of the cerebellum; OB, olfactory bulb; Pn, pontine nuclei; SNC, substantia nigra, pars compacta; SNR, substantia nigra, pars reticulata; Th, thalamus; Tu, olfactory tubercle.

binding sites. In some areas like the substantia nigra, the pontine nuclei, the locus coeruleus, and the nucleus ruber, very low or even undetectable densities of (+)-[³H]PN200-110 binding sites are observed (Fig. 2; Cortés et al., 1984). These observations suggest that dopaminergic or noradrenergic neurons, at least in the areas of their cell bodies, are perhaps not the prime candidates for the investigation of a functional role of VDCC in brain.

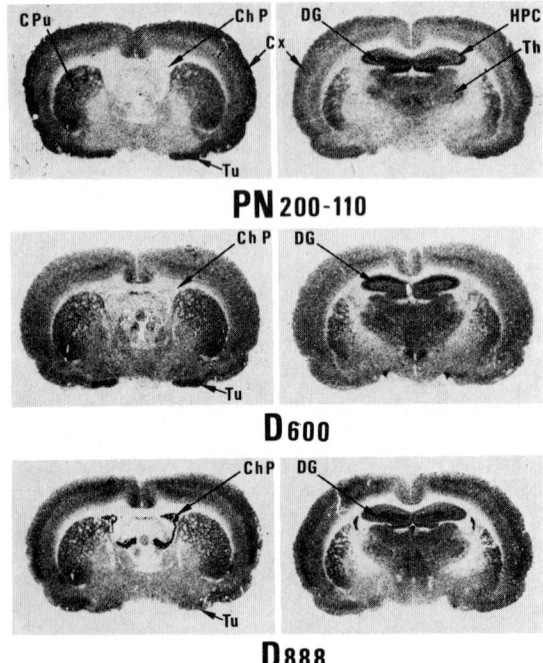

Fig. 3. Autoradiographic mapping of the distribution of (+)-[³H]PN200-110, (±)-[³H]D600 and (−)-[³H]D888 binding sites in coronal sections of the rat brain. The abbreviations and the symbols used are as described in legend to Fig. 2. On the left, autoradiograms derived from coronal sections at the level of the body of the caudate nucleus are shown. On the right the autoradiograms were obtained at the level of the thalamus.

(±)-[³H]D600 binding

(±)-[³H]D600 binding in all brain areas represents verapamil-sensitive sites as the binding can be completely blocked by coincubation with (±)-verapamil (10 μM) (not shown). The distribution of the specific (±)-[³H]D600 binding sites is very heterogenous in rat brain. High densities of (±)-[³H]D600 binding are found in hippocampus, olfactory bulb and in the substantia nigra (Figs. 2 and 3, Table 1). In the hippocampus, the highest density of (±)-[³H]D600 binding sites is observed mainly in the pyramidal cell layer, whereas the (+)-[³H]PN200-110 binding sites are most dense in the molecular layer of the dentate gyrus. Also the pontine nuclei and the inferior olive contain high levels of (±)-[³H]D600 binding whereas these brain areas only have a low density of (+)-[³H]PN200-110 binding sites (Table 1). These observations indicate that the pattern of distribution of the (±)-[³H]D600 binding sites differs from that of 1,4-dihydropyridine binding sites. Thus, (±)-[³H]D600 may label the phenylalkylamine drug receptor of VDCC and in addition other high affinity binding sites which perhaps are unrelated to VDCC. The latter sites appear to occur mainly in the midbrain, brainstem and medulla oblongata. However, it can-

TABLE 1

Microdensitometric determination of calcium antagonist binding sites in selected areas of the rat brain

Specific binding densities were measured by microdensitometry as described before (Cortés et al., 1983). Results are mean ± SEM of 2 (pontine nuclei) or of 3 animals (all other brain areas). Individual values were the mean value from 6 uni- or bilateral measurements

Tissue	Binding density in fmol/mg of protein (mean ± SEM)		
	(±)-[³H]D600	(+)-[³H]PN200-110	(−)-[³H]D888
Caudate putamen	93.7 ± 2.3	28.7 ± 4.4	91.9 ± 2.2
Dentate gyrus	80.0 ± 4.4	124.3 ± 2.0	148.1 ± 4.7
External plexiform layer of the olfactory bulb	90.7 ± 5.8	162.7 ± 10.0	169.6 ± 16.7
Choroid plexus	100.8 ± 12.5	21.3 ± 3.9	661.3 ± 42.1
Inferior olive	159.0 ± 3.5	28.7 ± 4.4	91.3 ± 6.7
Substantia nigra pars reticulata	82.0 ± 5.1	19.5 ± 6.6	122.7 ± 15.9
Inferior colliculus	92.0 ± 1.7	14.0 ± 4.9	126.0 ± 8.5
Pontine nuclei	87.5 ± 2.0	10.3 ± 0.9	84.0 ± 4.0

not be excluded that these sites may also occur in cerebral cortex where a better overlap in the distribution of ($\pm$)-[^{3}H]D600 binding and of (+)-[^{3}H]PN200-110 binding exists. This notion is supported by conventional binding studies in membrane fractions prepared from the cortex of rat brains. In these investigations we observed that the pharmacological properties of the ($\pm$)-[^{3}H]D600 binding sites to such membranes differ from those which are to be expected from the phenylalkylamine receptor of VDCC. For example ($\pm$)-[^{3}H]D600 binding is more sensitive to inhibition by (+)-verapamil and by (+)D600 than by (−)-verapamil of (−)D600 (Supavilai and Karobath, unpublished); this does not correlate with the calcium antagonistic properties of these drugs. Thus, the pharmacological properties as well as the pattern of the distribution of ($\pm$)-[^{3}H]D600 binding sites, as revealed by receptor autoradiography (Figs. 2 and 3, Table 1), are difficult to reconcile with the proposal (Reynolds et al., 1984) that ($\pm$)-[^{3}H]D600 can be used in all brain areas as a specific probe for the investigation of the phenylalkylamine drug receptors of VDCC.

(−)-[^{3}H]D888 binding

This ligand has recently been proposed by Ferry et al. (1984) as a label of the phenylalkylamine receptor of VDCC. Evidence for this was obtained by investigating the pharmacological properties of (−)-[^{3}H]D888 binding in guinea pig hippocampus homogenates which indicated the "right" stereospecific inhibition by the enantiomers of several phenylalkylamines. The potency series of phenylalkylamine calcium antagonists as inhibitors of (−)-[^{3}H]D888 binding correlated with the pharmacological actions of these drugs as calcium antagonists in peripheral tissue (Ferry et al., 1984). 1,4-Dihydropyridines regulate (−)-[^{3}H]D888 binding in a negative heterotropic allosteric manner. In addition, in microtome slices from guinea pig, the autoradiographic distribution of (−)-[^{3}H]D888 binding and of [^{3}H]nimodipine binding has been found to be very similar in the hippocampus, suggesting that in this species and this tissue (−)-[^{3}H]D888 labels the phenylalkylamine drug receptor of VDCC (Ferry et al., 1984).

Our results with membrane fractions from rat cerebral cortex support this concept (Supavilai and Karobath, unpublished). We therefore investigated the distribution of (−)-[^{3}H]D888 binding sites using receptor autoradiography. High densities of (−)-[^{3}H]D888 binding sites are found in all those brain areas such as the dentate gyrus of the hippocampus, the olfactory bulb, and the cerebral cortex, which contain also high densities of (+)-[^{3}H]PN200-110 binding sites (Figs. 2 and 3, Table 1). However, (−)-[^{3}H]D888 binding can also be found in high density in brain areas or tissues which contain low levels of (+)-[^{3}H]PN200-110 binding sites. These include the plexus choroideus, which has by far the highest density of (−)-[^{3}H]D888 binding sites, the substantia nigra, the pontine nuclei and the inferior colliculi (Fig. 2). The (−)-[^{3}H]D888 binding sites in all brain areas are sensitive to inhibition by coincubation with 10 μM ($\pm$)D600. A comparison of the distribution of (−)-[^{3}H]D888 binding and of ($\pm$)-[^{3}H]D600 binding reveals differences in their distribution which are most marked in the choroid plexus. Other brain nuclei which are localized in the midbrain, pons and medulla (Figs. 2 and 3, Table 1) exhibit a comparatively high density of (−)-[^{3}H]D888 binding and of ($\pm$)-[^{3}H]D600 binding, and a relatively low density of (+)-[^{3}H]PN200-110 binding (Figs. 2 and 3, Table 1) or of [^{3}H]PY108-068 binding (Cortés et al., 1984). These observations suggest that (−)-[^{3}H]D888 binding sites are found in those brain areas which contain 1,4-dihydropyridine binding sites and in addition in some other brain areas, where they are not apparently related to 1,4-dihydropyridine binding sites. Several possibilities need to be evaluated before these differences can be explained. For example, there is evidence that all three drug receptors of VDCC can be in high or in low affinity states (Glossmann et al., 1982). In our conditions for receptor autoradiography a low affinity state of a drug is most probably undetectable. Thus the observed differences in the distribution of (−)-[^{3}H]D888 binding and of (+)-[^{3}H]PN200-110 binding may be related to regional differences in the high affinity states of these binding sites. Alternatively, high affinity (−)-[³H]D888 binding sites may exist in some tissues and areas of the brain such as the choroid plexus or the mesencephalic nuclei, which are unrelated to the binding sites for 1,4-dihydropyridines and thus to conventional VDCC. A possible functional role of these (−)-[³H]D888 binding sites or of (±)-[³H]D600 binding in the mesencephalic nuclei is not known and the pharmacological properties of these binding sites are currently evaluated.

However, the observation that (−)-[³H]D888 binding sites can be detected in all those brain areas which contain high affinity binding sites for (+)-[³H]PN200-110 is in agreement with the concept, which has been derived mainly from binding studies with membrane fractions (Glossmann et al., 1982), that in the brain the supramolecular complex of VDCC exists which contains the three described drug receptors for 1,4-dihydropyridines, for phenylalkylamines and for diltiazem.

There appears to be no correlation in the distribution of the VDCC sites and that of published reports (Craigie, 1963) on the density of capillaries in different brain areas. This does not exclude that some VDCC-related drug receptors can occur also in the vascular system of the brain where they can mediate the cerebrovascular actions of organic calcium entry blockers (Kazda et al., 1982), although such actions have recently been questioned (Edvinsson et al., 1983). The anatomical distribution of VDCC-related drug receptors in rat brain suggests a rather heterogenous distribution in neurons with some areas which have been described as "receptor hot spots", containing high densities of these sites. A neuronal localization is also suggested from lesion experiments in the hippocampus. When the granule cells in this brain area are damaged by a local injection of colchicine, a depletion of the 1,4-dihydropyridine binding sites in the gyrus dentatus has been observed (Cortés et al., 1983) supporting the hypothesis that granule cells and their dendrites contain these sites.

References

Cortés, R., Supavilai, P., Karobath, M. and Palacios, J.M. (1983) The effects of lesions in the rat hippocampus suggest the association of calcium channel blocker binding sites with specific neuronal populations. *Neurosci. Lett.*, 42: 249–254.

Cortés, R., Supavilai, P., Karobath, M. and Palacios, J.M. (1984) Calcium antagonist binding sites in the rat brain: quantitative autoradiographic mapping using the 1,4-dihydropyridines [³H]PN200-110 and [³H]PY108-068. *J. Neural. Transm.*, 60: 169–197.

Craigie's Neuroanatomy of the rat (1963) *Academic Press*, New York.

Daniell, L.C., Barr, E.H. and Leslie, S.W. (1983) ⁴⁵Ca²⁺ uptake into rat whole brain synaptosomes unaltered by dihydropyridin calcium antagonists. *J. Neurochem.*, 41: 1455–1459.

Edvinsson, L., Johansson, B.B., Larsson, B., MacKenzie, E.T., Skärby, T. and Joung, A.R. (1983) Calcium antagonists: effects on cerebral blood flow and blood brain permeability in the rat. *Br. J. Pharmacol.*, 79: 141–148.

Ehlert, F.J., Roeske, W.L., Itoga, E. and Yamamura, H. (1982) The binding of ³H-nitrendipine to receptors for calcium channel antagonists in the heart, cerebral cortex, and ileum of rats. *Life Sci.*, 30: 2191–2202.

Ferry, D.R., Goll, A., Gadow, C. and Glossmann, H. (1984) (−)-³H-Desmethoxyverapamil labelling of Ca²⁺-antagonist drug receptor sites in brain. Autoradiographic distribution and allosteric coupling to 1,4-dihydropyridine and diltiazem sites. *Arch. Pharmac.*, 327: 183–187.

Freedman, S.B. and Miller, R.J. (1984) Calcium channel activation: a different type of drug action. *Proc. Natl. Acad. Sci. U.S.A.*, 81: 5580–5583.

Glossmann, H., Ferry, D.R., Lübbecke, F., Mewer, R. and Hofmann, T. (1982) Calcium channels. Direct identification with radioligand binding studies. *Trends Pharmacol. Sci.*, 3: 431–437.

Gould, R.J., Murphy, K.M.M. and Snyder, S.H. (1982) ³H-Nitrendipine labelled calcium channels discriminate inorganic calcium agonists and antagonists. *Proc. Natl. Acad. Sci. U.S.A.*, 79: 3657–3660.

Hoffmeister, F., Benz, V., Heise, A., Krause, H.P. and Neuser, V. (1982) Behavioural effects of nimodipine in animals. *Drug Res.*, 32: 347–360.

Janis, R.A. and Triggle, D.J. (1984) 1,4-Dihydropyridine Ca⁺⁺ channel antagonists and activations: a comparison of binding characteristics with pharmacology. *Drug Res.*, 4: 257–274.

Kazda, S., Gasthoff, B., Krause, H.P. and Schlossmann, K. (1982) Cerebrovascular effects of the calcium antagonist dihydropyridine derivative nimodipine in animal experiments. *Drug Res.*, 32: 331–338.

Miller, R.J. and Freedman, S.B. (1984) Are dihydropyridine binding sites voltage sensitive calcium channels? *Life Sci.*, 34: 1205–1221.

Murphy, K.M.M., Gould, R.J. and Snyder, S.H. (1982) Autoradiographic visualization of ^{3}H-nitrendipine binding sites in rat brain: localization to synaptic zones. *Eur. J. Pharmacol.*, 81: 517–519.

Murphy, K.M.M., Gould, R.J., Largent, B.L. and Snyder, S.H. (1983) A unitary mechanism of calcium antagonist drug action. *Proc. Natl. Acad. Sci. U.S.A.*, 80: 860–864.

Quirion, R. (1983) Autoradiographic localization of a calcium channel antagonist, ^{3}H-nitrendipine binding site in rat brain. *Neurosci. Lett.*, 36: 267–271.

Peroutka, S.J. and Allen, G.S. (1983) Calcium channel antagonist binding sites labeled by ^{3}H-nitrendipine in human brain. *J. Neurosurg.*, 59: 933–957.

Reynolds, I.J., De Souza, E., Gould, R.J. and Snyder, S.H. (1984) Visualization of ^{3}H-methoxyverapamil binding sites in rat brain. *Soc. Neurosci. Abstracts*, 10: p. 276.

Shoemaker, H., Lee, H., Roeske, W.R. and Yamamura, H. (1983) In vivo identification of calcium antagonist binding sites using ^{3}H-nitrendipine. *Eur. J. Pharmacol.*, 88: 275–276.

Supavilai, P. and Karobath, M. (1984) The interaction of ^{3}H-PY108-068 and of ^{3}H-PN200-110 with calcium channel binding sites in rat brain. *J. Neural. Transm.*, 60: 149–167.

A role for the mitochondrion in the protection of cells against calcium overload?

David G. Nicholls

Neurochemistry Laboratory, Department of Psychiatry, Ninewells Medical School, University of Dundee, Dundee DD1 9SY, Scotland, UK

Introduction

In addition to their ubiquitous role as the major synthesizers of ATP in aerobic cells (reviewed in Nicholls, 1982) mitochondria from virtually all sources possess a high capacity to transport Ca^{2+} across their inner membranes and to store it in their matrices (reviewed in Nicholls and Åkerman, 1982; Åkerman and Nicholls, 1983). Indeed, when presented with a free Ca^{2+} of 10 μM or more, isolated mitochondria will divert their entire respiratory capacity from ATP synthesis to the accumulation of the cation (reviewed in Nicholls and Åkerman, 1982). In this paper I shall describe the pathways which are responsible for mitochondrial calcium transport, discuss how these pathways act in concert to limit the extra-mitochondrial free Ca^{2+} concentration, $[Ca^{2+}]_e$, in in vitro models, and discuss the validity of the synaptosome as a model for studying the integration of mitochondrial and plasma membrane transport systems in the brain. Finally the extent to which these model systems provide an insight into the events during brain ischemia will be discussed.

Calcium transport pathways across the inner mitochondrial membrane

Mitochondrial Ca^{2+} transport must be considered within the context of the chemiosmotic theory (reviewed in Mitchell, 1976; Nicholls, 1982). Imbedded within the mitochondrial inner membrane is a protein complex termed the respiratory chain which functions as a linked series of three proton pumps. The respiratory chain conserves most of the energy made available from the transfer of electrons from respiratory substrates to oxygen by pumping protons out of the mitochondrial matrix. The expulsion of protons generates both an electrical gradient (membrane potential; $\Delta\psi_m$) and a proton concentration (ΔpH) gradient across the inner membrane which add together to give the total driving force for proton re-entry into the matrix, the proton electrochemical potential ($\Delta\mu_{H^+}$), by the relationship:

$$\Delta\mu_{H^+} = \Delta\psi_m - 60\Delta pH$$

The convention is that $\Delta\psi_m$ is positive when the matrix is negative with respect to the cytosol, and that ΔpH is positive when the matrix is acid with respect to the cytosol. The $\Delta\psi_m$ component of $\Delta\mu_{H^+}$ is nearly always dominant, and can account for 150–180 mV out of the total $\Delta\mu_{H^+}$ of 200–230 mV (Mitchell and Moyle, 1969; Nicholls, 1974; Rottenberg, 1975).

The proton electrochemical potential is utilized to drive an ATP-hydrolyzing proton pump in reverse. This pump, the proton-translocating ATPase or ATP synthase, would, in the absence of a $\Delta\mu_{H^+}$, simply hydrolyze mitochondrial ATP and pump protons out of the matrix. However, the existence of the large $\Delta\mu_{H^+}$ generated by the respiratory chain forces the ATP synthase to run in reverse, so that ATP is synthesized as protons force their way back into the matrix (Fig. 1a).

Ca^{2+} can be transported across the inner mito-

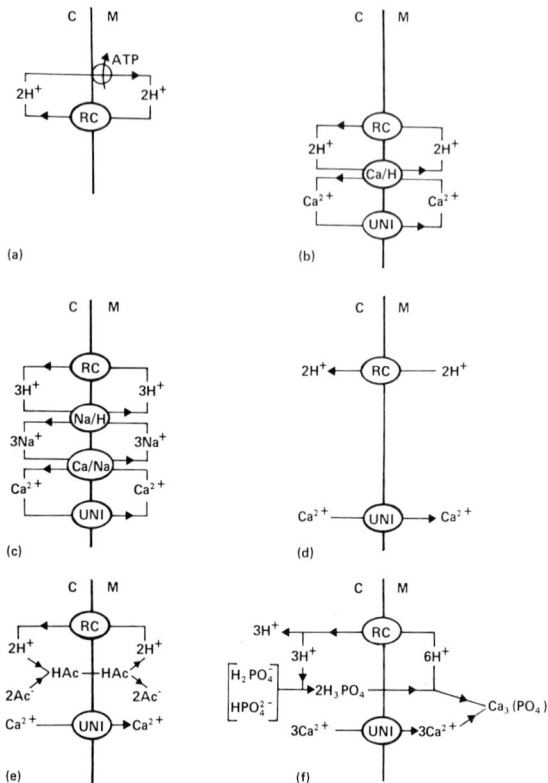

Fig. 1. Schematic representation of ion movements across the mitochondrial inner membrane. C, cytosol; M, matrix. (a) Proton circuit for the production of ATP, RC, respiratory chain; (b) cycling of Ca^{2+} between uniporter (UNI) and efflux pathway (Ca/H) in liver mitochondria; (c) cycling of Ca^{2+} between uniporter and Ca^{2+}/Na^+ exchanger in brain mitochondria, (Na/H) sodium/proton exchanger; (d) ion movements during the net uptake of Ca^{2+} in the absence of permeant anion; (e) ion movements during the net uptake of Ca^{2+} in the presence of acetate; (f) ion movements during the uptake of Ca^{2+} in the presence of phosphate — note the formation of a calcium phosphate complex in the matrix. (Adapted from Åkerman and Nicholls, 1983.)

potential. Since $\Delta\psi_m$ is in the range 150–180 mV, it follows that the gradient could attain a value of 100 000 to 1 000 000 if this pathway were the only means of transporting the cation across the inner membrane.

The electrical capacity of the mitochondrion is very small and the uptake of only about 1 nmol · min^{-1} · mg^{-1} protein of Ca^{2+} would be enough to discharge $\Delta\psi_m$ unless further proton extrusion by the respiratory chain occurred (Fig. 1d). However, since the pumping of protons out of the matrix to compensate for the charge of the accumulated Ca^{2+} would raise the pH of the matrix, there is a limit to the amount of Ca^{2+} which can be accumulated by mitochondria by simply pumping protons out through the respiratory chain. Thus the uptake of about 10 nmol · min^{-1} · mg^{-1} protein will increase the pH of the matrix by some 2 units (Mitchell and Moyle, 1969).

For more extensive Ca^{2+} accumulation to occur, there must be a parallel movement of a permeant anion into the matrix. Acetate is frequently used in experiments with isolated mitochondria (Fig. 1e), and its entry into the mitochondrion as the undissociated acetic acid allows it to carry in protons which exactly compensate for those pumped out by the respiratory chain. In the presence of acetate the capacity of mitochondria to accumulate Ca^{2+} is further increased by an order of magnitude to some 100 nmol · min^{-1} · mg^{-1} protein. With acetate as permeant anion, the matrix accumulates soluble calcium acetate which increases the internal osmolarity of the mitochondrion, leading to swelling, and this is the reason for the limitation in the accumulation capacity.

In the intact cell, the most likely anion to be accumulated with Ca^{2+} is phosphate. Calcium and phosphate do not remain osmotically active in the matrix, but form a complex (Fig. 1f). The chemical nature of this complex is not fully understood. It is not simply a precipitate, since this would be difficult to re-solubilize, whereas Ca^{2+} and phosphate can rapidly efflux in parallel but separately when the $\Delta\psi_m$ across the inner membrane is collapsed (Zoccarato and Nicholls, 1982). When precautions

chondrial membrane with two positive charges by a uniport mechanism, i.e. not involving co-transport or exchange of another ion (for review see Nicholls and Åkerman, 1982). It is the existence of the large $\Delta\psi_m$ across the inner membrane which provides the driving force for Ca^{2+} accumulation. If the uniport were allowed to accumulate Ca^{2+} until equilibrium were attained, the gradient of free Ca^{2+} concentration across the inner membrane would be ten-fold for every 30 mV of membrane are taken to incubate mitochondria in media approximating to the physiological cytosol in their Mg^{2+} and adenine nucleotide composition (Nicholls, D.G. and Scott, I.D., 1980), the capacity of mitochondria to accumulate Ca^{2+} from phosphate-containing media is almost unlimited, and can exceed 1000 nmol per mg (reviewed in Nicholls and Åkerman, 1982).

The kinetics of the uniporter are striking. The net rate of accumulation of Ca^{2+} increases as the cube of the extramitochondrial free Ca^{2+} and is only limited by the capacity of the respiratory chain to pump out protons to maintain $\Delta\psi_m$ (Zoccarato and Nicholls, 1982). With brain mitochondria the stage is soon reached where the entire capacity of the respiratory chain is diverted to the accumulation of Ca^{2+} (Nicholls, 1978) and it is this property of the Ca^{2+} uniporter which is the basis for the contention in this paper that one role of mitochondria in the intact cell is to limit the upper level which the free Ca^{2+} can attain in the cytosol.

First, however, there are two further aspects to be discussed, the mechanism by which Ca^{2+} gets out of the mitochondrial matrix, and whether Ca^{2+} transport by such an obviously aerobic organelle as the mitochondrion can have any relevance in the ischemic condition which is the subject of this volume.

Mitochondrial calcium cycling

The very potency of the Ca^{2+} uptake pathway of mitochondria was formerly used as an argument against the physiological significance of mitochondrial Ca^{2+} transport. Since the equilibrium gradient of Ca^{2+} across the inner membrane should approach 1 000 000 under respiring conditions, it was argued that the uniporter must be inactive in the cell, perhaps because of the low cytosolic Ca^{2+} concentrations, in order to prevent irreversible accumulation of all the cell's Ca^{2+} into the mitochondria. The discovery of an independent Ca^{2+}-efflux pathway in the mitochondrial inner membrane (Crompton et al., 1976) meant that these reservations had to be re-examined.

Heart (Crompton et al., 1976) and brain (Crompton et al., 1978; Nicholls, 1978) mitochondria possess, in addition to a Ca^{2+} uniporter, a pathway which exchanges Ca^{2+} for Na^+ (Fig. 1c). This pathway can most clearly be seen on adding ruthenium red, which is a specific inhibitor of the Ca^{2+} uniporter to mitochondria which have accumulated Ca^{2+}. A net efflux is seen, even though $\Delta\psi_m$ remains high (Nicholls, 1978). The activity of the efflux pathway is inversely related to the internal free phosphate concentration, and, in phosphate containing media, appears to be independent of the amount of Ca^{2+} accumulated in the matrix above about 20 $nmol \cdot min^{-1} \cdot mg^{-1}$ protein (Zoccarato and Nicholls, 1982).

This contrast between the kinetics of the uptake pathway, which is highly dependent on the cytosolic free Ca^{2+}, and the efflux pathway, which is essentially independent of the matrix Ca^{2+}, provides the basis for the steady-state regulation of the Ca^{2+} distribution across the membrane (reviewed in Nicholls and Åkerman, 1982). A steady state will be attained when uptake and efflux are equal and opposite (Fig. 2). With brain mitochondria in the presence of phosphate this balance is reached when the external Ca^{2+} is rather less than 1 μM (Nicholls and Scott, 1980). This is therefore a "set-point" to which the mitochondria will seek to restore $[Ca^{2+}]_e$ following a perturbation. Thus if $[Ca^{2+}]_e$ is raised — in an in vitro system by adding Ca^{2+} to the incubation, or in vivo perhaps by a Ca^{2+} influx across the plasma membrane, then the uniporter will respond by increasing its activity. There will be a net uptake of Ca^{2+} into the mitochondrion which will oppose the original change. Since the activity of the efflux pathway is independent of the total amount of Ca^{2+} accumulated in the matrix, the mitochondrion will accumulate Ca^{2+} until $[Ca^{2+}]_e$ falls to the initial set-point when uptake and efflux were in balance (Fig. 2). Conversely, when $[Ca^{2+}]_e$ falls the uniporter will be less active than the efflux pathway, and there will be a net efflux of Ca^{2+} from the matrix.

The level of the "set-point" depends on the kinetics of the two Ca^{2+}-transporting pathways —

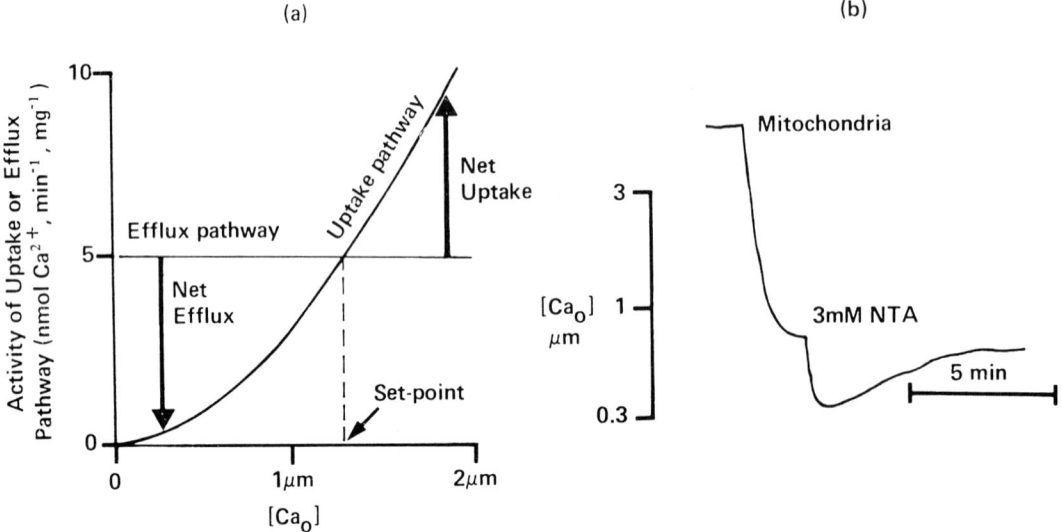

Fig. 2. Calcium cycling: the establishment of a set-point for $[Ca^{2+}]_e$. (a) Scheme for $[Ca^{2+}]_e$ regulation under conditions where the efflux pathway is constant. (b) The reversible maintenance of a set-point by liver mitochondria. $[Ca^{2+}]_e$ was monitored with a Ca^{2+}-selective electrode, while mitochondria were added to an incubation containing respiratory substrate and Ca^{2+}. Uptake of Ca^{2+} occurred until the $[Ca^{2+}]_e$ fell to 0.8 μM. Addition of the Ca^{2+}-chelator NTA caused an instantaneous decrease in the free Ca^{2+} concentration, and the mitochondria responded by a net efflux of Ca^{2+} to restore the initial set-point. (Adapted from Åkerman and Nicholls, 1983.)

an activation of the efflux pathway or an inhibition of the uniporter would both cause the set-point to be shifted towards a higher $[Ca^{2+}]_e$. This is shown in Fig. 3, where the addition of Na^+ to activate the efflux pathway of brain mitochondria leads to a stable redistribution of Ca^{2+} across the mitochondrial membrane to establish a new "set-point".

While isolated mitochondria are usually stable in

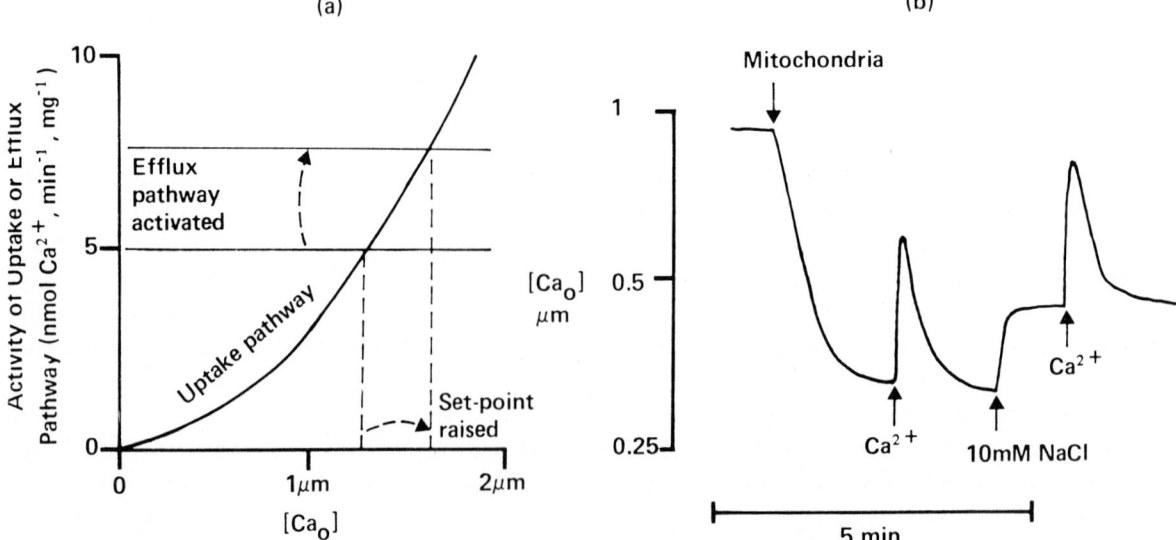

Fig. 3. Calcium cycling: the modulation of the set-point. (a) Scheme for raising the set-point by activating the efflux pathway. (b) Effect of activating the efflux pathway of brain mitochondria by raising $[Na^+]$. Mitochondria added to a Ca^{2+}-electrode chamber were given 25 nmol Ca^{2+} per mg protein at each addition. Note that addition of Na^+ causes a stable change in the set-point.

the presence of Ca^{2+} and phosphate as long as the incubation medium contains ATP (or ADP) and Mg^{2+}, there are conditions in vitro under which they can be induced to swell, collapse their membrane potential, release their Ca^{2+} and become irreversibly damaged. The mechanism of this Ca^{2+}-induced damage is far from understood. A number of apparently unrelated factors sensitize the mitochondria to this spontaneous discharge of the cation, which typically occurs 1–20 min after Ca^{2+} is added to the incubation. These factors include high Ca^{2+} itself, elevated phosphate, phosphoenolpyruvate, atractylate, palmitoyl CoA, diamide, decreased pH and unsaturated fatty acids (reviewed in Nicholls and Åkerman, 1982). It must, however, be emphasized that this uncontrolled and complete efflux of Ca^{2+} associated with collapse of the mitochondrial membrane potential is entirely distinct from the steady-state, Na^+-activated efflux pathway operative in the healthy mitochondrion.

This spontaneous discharge of Ca^{2+} is obviously not considered to be a normal physiological event, in view of the drastic effects on the mitochondrial integrity. It is, however, at first sight possible that what one is observing in vitro relates to cell death following ischemia, since a number of factors observed in vivo (increased Ca^{2+}, raised fatty acids, depleted cytosolic ADP and ATP, and lowered pH) would all conspire to induce these lethal changes in mitochondrial bioenergetic function. However, while mitochondria recovered from ischemic brain appear to have impaired rates of state-3 electron flow, consistent with exposure to low pH (Rehncrona et al., 1979; Hillered et al., 1984), their state-4 respiration is not elevated, indicating that the mitochondria in situ are able to avoid such irreversible damage for at least 30 min of ischemia.

Calcium transport by anaerobic mitochondria

It might be thought that Ca^{2+} transport by mitochondria could have no relevance to the anoxic condition, where the respiratory chain is unable to function. However, it must be recalled that the mitochondrion possesses two proton pumps, the second of which, the ATP-synthase, is reversible, so that it can hydrolyze ATP and pump protons out of the mitochondrion when not opposed by a high $\Delta\mu_{H^+}$ generated by the respiratory chain. The $\Delta\mu_{H^+}$ which can be generated by ATP hydrolysis in anaerobic mitochondria is the same as that produced by the respiratory chain under aerobic conditions (Nicholls, 1974). It has been long established that ATP can support mitochondrial Ca^{2+} transport under conditions where the respiratory chain is inhibited (for review see Nicholls and Åkerman, 1982). Thus if mitochondria are supplied with ATP in an anaerobic cell they will continue to perform their role as regulators of the upper limit of the $[Ca^{2+}]_e$.

There are conditions where the mitochondrion can utilize both its respiratory chain and ATP-synthase in parallel in order to deal with a massive influx of Ca^{2+} into the incubation. If mitochondria are exposed to a high $[Ca^{2+}]_e$, the influx of Ca^{2+} through the uniporter lowers $\Delta\psi_m$ to such an extent that the back pressure on the ATP-synthase is relieved, and the mitochondria will hydrolyze ATP, while still respiring in an attempt to restore the $\Delta\mu_{H^+}$ (reviewed in Nicholls and Åkerman, 1982). Thus, as first noted by Rossi and Lehninger (1964), under these conditions Ca^{2+} uptake by mitochondria can take precedence over ATP synthesis, and even utilize glycolytic ATP in the attempt to lower $[Ca^{2+}]_e$.

Because of this dual mechanism by which the mitochondrial membrane potential (and hence Ca^{2+} transport) is maintained, the inability of anaerobic glycolysis to maintain cytosolic ATP levels (rather than anoxia per se) will be the event which signals the inability of the mitochondria in situ to continue regulating the cytosolic free Ca^{2+}.

In vitro models for the mitochondrial response to cellular Ca^{2+} overload

In response to a continuous influx of Ca^{2+} into a mitochondrial incubation the $[Ca^{2+}]_e$ initially rises; this in turn allows the highly Ca^{2+}-dependent uniporter to operate more rapidly; a steady-state is soon attained where the net uptake of Ca^{2+} into the matrix exactly balances the influx of Ca^{2+} into the incubation (Zoccarato and Nicholls, 1982). $[Ca^{2+}]_e$ thus stabilizes for as long as the infusion continues, or until the very large capacity of the mitochondrion to sequester Ca^{2+} is exceeded. Because the activity of the uniporter increases as approximately the third power of the $[Ca^{2+}]_e$ (Nicholls and Zoccarato, 1982) even a rapid infusion of Ca^{2+} results in only a modest increase in $[Ca^{2+}]_e$. Thus, when liver mitochondria are infused with Ca^{2+} at a rate of 34 nmol $\cdot$ min^{-1} $\cdot$ mg^{-1} protein, $[Ca^{2+}]_e$ increases from the set-point of 1.6 μM to just 6 μM, at which level the mitochondria are able to sequester Ca^{2+} in their matrices as fast as it is supplied to the incubation (Zoccarato and Nicholls, 1982).

Fig. 3 also shows the response of isolated brain mitochondria to a series of pulsed additions of Ca^{2+} to the incubation (Nicholls and Scott, 1980). Each instantaneous rise in $[Ca^{2+}]_e$ is rapidly reversed as the mitochondria accumulate the cation.

The preceding sections thus show that the Ca^{2+} transport properties of isolated mitochondria are ideally suited to a role in limiting any increase in $[Ca^{2+}]_e$ which might otherwise damage the integrity of the cell, unless both oxidative phosphorylation and glycolysis are interrupted. The remainder of this paper will deal with the isolated nerve terminal as a model in which to study how the mitochondrial and plasma membrane transport properties are integrated in intact neuronal tissue.

Pathways for Ca^{2+} transport in the isolated nerve terminal

In neuronal tissue the plasma membrane, inner mitochondrial membrane and endoplasmic reticulum have each been implicated in the regulation of the cytosolic free Ca^{2+} concentration, $[Ca^{2+}]_c$ (reviewed in Nicholls and Åkerman, 1981; Åkerman and Nicholls, 1983). The complexity of possible Ca^{2+}-transport pathways which could in principle regulate $[Ca^{2+}]_c$ has been reviewed previously (Nicholls and Åkerman, 1981). In addition to the two mitochondrial pathways described above, Blaustein and colleagues (Blaustein et al., 1978) have emphasized the role of an ATP-dependent Ca^{2+}-sequestration mechanism in synaptosomal endoplasmic reticulum in the lowering of $[Ca^{2+}]_c$ following neurotransmission, although their preparation — from a hypotonic lysate of synaptosomes — has not been fully characterized to eliminate the possibility that the ATP-dependent Ca^{2+}-accumulating vesicles were in fact inverted plasma membrane vesicles. This possibility exists because other workers (e.g. Gill et al., 1981) have used a similar preparative procedure to purify plasma membrane vesicles containing both Ca^{2+}-transporting pathways and the $(Na^+ + K^+)$-dependent ATPase, a sure marker of plasma membranes.

At the plasma membrane of the synaptosome there may be up to four independent Ca^{2+}-transport mechanisms. Early studies with the intact synaptosome emphasized a role for Na^+/Ca^{2+} exchange in extruding Ca^{2+} from the cytosol (Swanson et al., 1974; Blaustein and Oborn, 1975; Blaustein and Ector, 1976). However, a Na^+-dependency for Ca^{2+} efflux could only be demonstrated in the non-physiological condition of external Ca^{2+}-depletion (Blaustein and Ector, 1976). Gill et al. (1981) have shown that isolated synaptosomal plasma membrane vesicles possess the exchange activity, and that it is localized in the same membrane population which has the $(Na^+ + K^+)$-dependent ATPase and a Ca^{2+}-ATPase activity. It is clear, however, that the synaptosome does not require the Na^+/Ca^{2+} exchanger in order to extrude Ca^{2+} across the plasma membrane, since when the Na^+ gradient across the plasma membrane is collapsed by the addition of ouabain to inhibit the $(Na^+ + K^+)$-dependent ATPase pump and veratridine to activate the voltage-dependent Na^+-channel the synaptosomes are still able to maintain a low $[Ca^{2+}]_c$, and to pump Ca^{2+} (Åkerman and Nicholls, 1981a; Snelling and Nicholls, 1985). It thus appears that the Ca^{2+}-ATPase is the most important mechanism for extruding Ca^{2+} from the isolated synaptosomes.

There are at least two pathways by which Ca^{2+}

enters the synaptosome, a basal leak, and a depolarization-activated pathway. Under steady-state conditions Ca^{2+} leaks into the synaptosomal cytosol (and is pumped out again) at a rate of about 0.4 nmol · min^{-1} · mg^{-1} protein (Snelling and Nicholls, 1985). Synaptosomes depolarized by ouabain plus veratridine can still achieve a steady-state Ca^{2+} distribution, in which case the influx and efflux are both elevated to about 0.9 nmol · min^{-1} · mg^{-1} protein. The elevated influx is due in part to the long-term activation of the voltage-dependent Ca^{2+} channel, since it can be blocked by the Ca^{2+}-channel inhibitor verapamil. The matching efflux of Ca^{2+} from the synaptosome is solely due to the Ca^{2+}-ATPase, since any Na^+/Ca^{2+} exchanger could not extrude Ca^{2+} when the Na^+ gradient is collapsed by ouabain plus veratridine.

The integration of mitochondrial and plasma membrane calcium transport pathways in the isolated nerve terminal

Under steady-state conditions, the mitochondria contain about half the total synaptosomal Ca^{2+} (Fig. 4). This can be determined by rapid fractionation of the synaptosomes (Åkerman and Nicholls, 1981b). If the hypothesis that the mitochondrion serves to sequester excess Ca^{2+} is true then it should be possible to observe an increased uptake of Ca^{2+} into the intra-synaptosomal mitochondria when plasma membrane Ca^{2+} influx is increased by depolarization-induced activation of the Ca^{2+} channel. This is shown in Fig. 4. Two modes of depolarization, by elevated potassium and by veratridine plus ouabain both cause a substantially increased total synaptosomal Ca^{2+} content (Åkerman and Nicholls, 1981b). In the case of potassium depolarization, the mitochondrial Ca^{2+} content increases by some 300%, accounting for virtually all the increase in transported Ca^{2+}. This therefore confirms that mitochondria in situ are capable of taking up the additional Ca^{2+} transported across the plasma membrane.

After depolarization by ouabain plus veratridine, the mitochondrial Ca^{2+} still increases, but the ex-

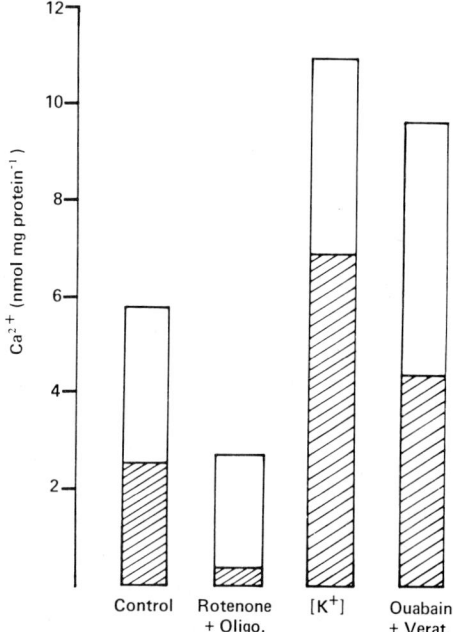

Fig. 4. Ca^{2+} content of synaptosomes and the extent of the mitochondrial pool. Synaptosomes were incubated in the presence of 1.3 mM Ca^{2+} under control conditions; in the presence of rotenone plus oligomycin to collapse the mitochondrial membrane potential, and hence abolish the capacity of the in-situ mitochondria to retain Ca^{2+}; in the presence of high potassium to depolarize the plasma membrane, and in the presence of veratridine plus ouabain to depolarize the plasma membrane and elevate the cytosolic free Na^+. The hatched part of the histogram represents the calcium recovered in the mitochondrial fraction after rapid synaptosomal fractionation. (Adapted from Scott et al., 1980, and Åkerman and Nicholls, 1981b.)

tent is less marked (Fig. 4). One reason for this might be the large Na^+ influx into the cytosol caused by veratridine. Since the Ca^{2+} efflux pathway at the mitochondrial inner membrane is activated by Na^+ (Fig. 3), the increased cytosolic Na^+, by activating the mitochondrial efflux pathway, would be predicted to shift the set-point at which the mitochondria maintain the cytosolic free Ca^{2+} to a higher value.

The bioenergetics of the anaerobic nerve terminal

The ability of mitochondria within nerve terminals to continue to regulate the upper limit of the cytosolic free Ca^{2+} in the ischemic state depends on their ability to maintain a high membrane potential. This in turn will be dependent on the ability of glycolysis to satisfy the ATP requirements of the synaptosome. We have examined the bioenergetics of the synaptosome under conditions where the anoxic state is mimicked by the addition of rotenone to inhibit electron flow through the respiratory chain (Scott and Nicholls, 1980). Under control conditions synaptosomes are able to maintain stable ATP and phosphocreatine levels. Simultaneous measurements of the plasma membrane potential ($\Delta\psi_p$) and in-situ mitochondrial membrane potential ($\Delta\psi_m$) give values of 60 mV for the former and 150 mV for the latter. Addition of rotenone to inhibit the respiratory chain results in a 40% decrease in ATP levels within 12 min, and a more extensive decrease in phosphocreatine. Under these conditions the total ATP demand of the synaptosome must now be born by glycolysis. There is only a slight drop in $\Delta\psi_m$, indicating that the ATP levels in anoxia are adequate to maintain a large measure of the mitochondrial potential. As a control, the addition of oligomycin (to inhibit the mitochondrial ATP synthase) in addition to rotenone now causes a complete collapse of $\Delta\psi_m$ since both mitochondrial proton pumps are now inhibited. Under conditions of low energy demand, anaerobic glycolysis thus appears adequate to maintain the ATP demands of the synaptosome, including the polarization of the mitochondrial membrane which is a prerequisite for its ability to accumulate and regulate Ca^{2+} in the cytosol.

A more stringent test is to examine the competency of anaerobic glycolysis to maintain synaptosomal energy levels under conditions of elevated energy demand. This may most readily be accomplished by inducing a dissipative Na^+ cycle at the plasma membrane by the addition of veratridine to activate the Na^+ channel, resulting in Na^+ cycling rapidly across the plasma membrane between the ($Na^+ + K^+$)-dependent ATPase and the Na^+ channel. Under these conditions the fall in ATP induced by rotenone is more extensive, and a complete depletion of phosphocreatine rapidly occurs (Scott and Nicholls, 1980). The mitochondrial membrane potential collapses to an unmeasurably low level, indicating that insufficient ATP is present for the normal functioning of the ATP synthase.

Thus the anoxic nerve terminal, while apparently being able to survive as long as glucose continues to be available, and as no elevated ATP demands are made on it, experiences problems when the ATP demand is elevated by ion movements at the plasma membrane such as might be expected to occur during neuronal activity. However, in vivo, the catastrophic drop in ATP within 5 min of ischemia (Lowry et al., 1964; Yoshida et al., 1984) indicates that any ability of the mitochondria to continue to regulate cytosolic Ca^{2+} is very short term.

Conclusions

Mitochondria are equipped with Ca^{2+} transport pathways which make it very likely that, when faced with an elevation in cytosolic Ca^{2+}, the organelles divert some or all their respiratory capacity to the uptake of that Ca^{2+} and to restoring a low $[Ca^{2+}]_c$. In their matrices they are able to complex the accumulated Ca^{2+} with phosphate in such a way that the normal functioning of the mitochondrion is not affected. The Ca^{2+} is not irreversibly sequestered within the matrix, since lowering of the $[Ca^{2+}]_e$ below the "set-point" at which uptake and efflux balance leads to a net loss of Ca^{2+} from the matrix. Thus the plasma membrane Ca^{2+}-ATPase, by lowering $[Ca^{2+}]_c$ below the set-point could ultimately deplete the mitochondrion of its Ca^{2+} and pump it out across the plasma membrane.

In the intact nerve terminal the mitochondria and the plasma membrane Ca^{2+}-ATPase are the main means by which Ca^{2+} can be removed from the cytosol. The mitochondrion has a high rate of Ca^{2+} accumulation. Indeed since it can divert all its energy production to Ca^{2+} uptake, it follows that no other ATP-dependent Ca^{2+}-transport process could be appreciably faster. However the plasma membrane Ca^{2+}-ATPase of the synaptosome appears to be able ultimately to lower $[Ca^{2+}]_c$ to substantially below the approximately micromolar "set-point" for the mitochondria. Thus, judged by the fluorescence of the cytosolic Ca^{2+}-indicator quin-2 (Ashley et al., 1984) or the absorbance of arsenazo III (Åkerman and Heinonen, 1983) the resting $[Ca^{2+}]_c$ is about 0.2 μM.

In the anoxic synaptosome glycolytic ATP is still adequate to maintain the mitochondrial membrane potential (and hence the ability of the mitochondrion to protect against Ca^{2+}-overload) under conditions of low energy demand. However, when the energy demand of the anoxic terminal is increased, for example by rapid ion transport at the plasma membrane, the inadequacy of glycolytic ATP becomes apparent, the mitochondrial membrane potential collapses and the ability of the mitochondrion to retain Ca^{2+} will be lost.

The in vivo situation differs from that with the isolated synaptosome in two respects. Firstly ischemia interrupts the supply of glucose to the cell, and this may be a factor potentiating the catastrophic drop in ATP within 5 min of ischemia (Lowry et al., 1964; Yoshida et al., 1984). Secondly the build up of lactic acid and free fatty acids is likely to be much more pronounced in vivo than in the much more dilute system of the isolated synaptosome.

The physiological significance of mitochondrial Ca^{2+} transport has frequently been questioned. However, even if the sole role of the process were the protection of the cell against damage due to Ca^{2+} overload, this would place it on a par with other protective mechanisms such as the immune system and the blood clotting cascade in ensuring the survival of the organism in response to pathological disturbances.

Acknowledgment

Work from our laboratory has been supported by the Medical Research Council.

References

Åkerman, K.E.O. and Nicholls, D.G. (1981a) Calcium transport by intact synaptosomes: the voltage-dependent Ca^{2+} channel and a re-evaluation of the role of Ca^{2+}/Na^+ exchange. Eur. J. Biochem., 117: 491–497.

Åkerman, K.E.O. and Nicholls, D.G. (1981b) Intra-synaptosomal compartmentation of calcium during depolarization: induced calcium uptake across the plasma membrane. Biochim. Biophys. Acta, 645: 41–48.

Åkerman, K.E.O. and Nicholls, D.G. (1983) Physiological and bioenergetic aspects of mitochondrial calcium transport. Rev. Physiol. Biochem. Pharmacol., 95: 149–201.

Åkerman, K.E.O. and Heinonen, E. (1983) Qualitative measurements of cytosolic calcium ion concentration within isolated guinea-pig nerve endings using entrapped arsenazo III. Biochim. Biophys. Acta, 732: 117–121.

Ashley, R.H., Brammer, M.J. and Marchbanks, R. (1984) Measurement of intra-synaptosomal free calcium by using the fluorescent indicator quin-2. Biochem. J., 219: 149–158.

Blaustein, M.P. and Oborn, C.J. (1975) The influence of Na^+ on Ca^{2+} fluxes in pinched-off nerve terminals in vitro. J. Physiol. (London), 247: 657–686.

Blaustein, M.P. and Ector, A.C. (1976) Carrier-mediated Na^+-dependent and Ca^{2+}-dependent Ca^{2+} efflux from pinched-off presynaptic nerve terminals (synaptosomes) in vitro. Biochim. Biophys. Acta, 419: 295–308.

Blaustein, M.P., Ratzlaff, R.W. and Schweitzer, E.S. (1978) Calcium buffering in presynaptic nerve terminals: kinetic properties of the non-mitochondrial calcium sequestration mechanism. J. Gen. Physiol., 72: 43–64.

Crompton, M., Capano, M. and Carafoli, E. (1976) The Na^+-induced efflux of Ca^{2+} from heart mitochondria. Eur. J. Biochem., 69: 453–462.

Gill, D.L., Grollman, E.F. and Kohn, L.D. (1981) Calcium transport mechanisms in membrane vesicles from guinea-pig brain synaptosomes. J. Biol. Chem., 256: 184–192.

Hillered, L., Ernster, L. and Siesjö, B.K. (1984) Influence of in vitro lactic acidosis and hypercapnia on respiratory activity of isolated rat brain mitochondria. J. Cereb. Blood Flow Metabol., 4: 430–437.

Lowry, O.H., Passonneau, J.V., Hasselberger, F.X. and Schulz, D.W. (1964) Effect of ischaemia on known substrates and cofactors of the glycolytic pathway in brain. J. Biol. Chem., 239: 18–30.

Mitchell, P. (1976) Vectorial chemistry and the molecular mechanism of chemiosmotic coupling. Biochem. Soc. Trans., 4: 399–430.

Mitchell, P. and Moyle, J. (1969) Estimation of membrane potential and pH difference across the cristae membrane of rat liver mitochondria. Eur. J. Biochem., 7: 430–471.

Nicholls, D.G. (1974) The influence of respiration and ATP hydrolysis on the proton electrochemical gradient across the inner membrane of liver mitochondria as determined by ion distribution. Eur. J. Biochem., 50: 305–315.

Nicholls, D.G. (1978) Calcium transport and proton electrochemical potential in mitochondria from cerebral cortex and heart. *Biochem. J.,* 170: 511–522.

Nicholls, D.G. (1982) *Bioenergetics, an Introduction to the Chemiosmotic Theory,* Academic Press, London.

Nicholls, D.G. and Scott, I.D. (1980) The regulation of brain mitochondrial calcium transport: the role of ATP in the discrimination between kinetic and membrane potential dependent calcium efflux mechanisms. *Biochem. J.,* 186: 833–839.

Nicholls, D.G. and Åkerman, K.E.O. (1981) Biochemical approaches to the study of cytosolic calcium regulation in nerve endings. *Phil. Trans. Soc. Lond. B.,* 296: 115–122.

Nicholls, D.G. and Åkerman, K.E.O. (1982) Mitochondrial calcium transport. *Biochim. Biophys. Acta,* 683: 57–88.

Rehncrona, S., Mela, L. and Siesjö, B.K. (1979) Recovery of brain mitochondrial function in the rat complete and incomplete cerebral ischaemia. *Stroke,* 10: 437–446.

Rossi, C.S. and Lehninger, A.L. (1964) Stoichiometry of respiratory stimulation, accumulation of calcium and phosphate and oxidative phosphorylation in rat liver mitochondria. *J. Biol. Chem.,* 239: 3971–3980.

Rottenberg, H. (1975) The measurement of transmembrane electrochemical proton gradients. *Bioenergetics,* 7: 61–74.

Scott, I.D. and Nicholls, D.G. (1980) Energy transduction in intact synaptosomes: influence of plasma membrane depolarization on the respiration and membrane potential of internal mitochondria determined in situ. *Biochem. J.,* 186: 21–33.

Scott, I.D., Åkerman, K.E.O. and Nicholls, D.G. (1980) Calcium ion transport by intact synaptosomes: intrasynaptosomal compartmentation and the role of the mitochondrial membrane potential. *Biochem. J.,* 192: 873–880.

Snelling, R. and Nicholls, D.G. (1985) Calcium efflux and cycling across the synaptosomal plasma membrane. *Biochem. J.,* 226: 225–231.

Swanson, P.D., Anderson, L. and Stahl, W.L. (1974) Uptake of calcium ions by synaptosomes from rat brain. *Biochim. Biophys. Acta,* 356: 174–183.

Yoshida, S., Harik, S.I., Busto, R., Santiso, M., Martinez, E. and Ginsberg, M. (1984) Free fatty acids and energy metabolites in ischaemic cerebral cortex with noradrenaline depletion. *J. Neurochem.,* 42: 711–717.

Zoccarato, F. and Nicholls, D.G. (1982) The role of phosphate in the regulation of the calcium efflux pathway of liver mitochondria. *Eur. J. Biochem.,* 127: 333–338.

Regulation of calcium transport in rat hippocampal mitochondria during development and following denervation

Michel Baudry and Gary Lynch

Center for the Neurobiology of Learning and Memory, U. C., Irvine, CA 92717, USA

Introduction

The role of calcium in cell death is now well documented for a variety of conditions and tissues (Schanne et al., 1979; Farber, 1981), although the precise mechanism underlying the toxic effect of this cation is not yet understood. The recent identification in a variety of cells of calcium-dependent proteases which are activated by micromolar concentrations of calcium and which preferentially degrade protein required for the integrity of the cell cytoskeleton (e.g. microtubules and neurofilament) (De Martino, 1981; Murachi et al., 1981; Zimmerman and Schlaepfer, 1982; Siman et al., 1983), suggests a mechanism through which prolonged increases in intracellular calcium concentration result in atrophy, degeneration, and ultimately lead to cell death. In fact, such a mechanism has been proposed to underly muscle atrophy and peripheral neuron degeneration (Libby and Goldberg, 1978; Schlaepfer and Hasler, 1979; Salpeter et al., 1982). Accordingly, it is of obvious importance to obtain a better appreciation of the regulation of intracellular concentration of calcium and of its changes under different experimental conditions. While calcium concentrations in extracellular fluids are in the millimolar range, intracellular concentrations are generally estimated to be between 10^{-7} and 10^{-6} M. Various intracellular organelles or systems are used by the cells to maintain this low concentration, among which are the mitochondria, the endoplasmic reticulum and various energy-driven pumps (Erulkar and Fine, 1979). Although the question of the relative contribution of these different systems is still a matter of debate (Somlyo, 1984), it is very likely that disturbances in the regulation of any of them will have profound consequences for the functioning of cells. Although mitochondria were for a long time thought to have a transport system for calcium with an affinity too low to be of functional significance, several observations indicate that mitochondria play a major role in the buffering of calcium concentration. For instance, Rose and Lowenstein (1975) showed that the diffusion of calcium injected into the cytosol of the salivary gland cells is normally quite restricted but becomes extensive following treatment with cyanide, a mitochondrial poison. Similarly, the inhibition of mitochondrial electron transport or oxidative phosphorylation is accompanied by an increase in neurotransmitter release at the neuromuscular junction and by the depolymerization of microtubules (which is known to be linked to free intracellular calcium concentrations) (Rahamimoff et al., 1978; Maro and Bornens, 1982). Moreover, recent biochemical experiments provide evidence that mitochondria have a much greater affinity for calcium than previously suspected (Browning et al., 1981a). Mitochondria also have a tremendous storage capacity for calcium, something which is probably not true for the other buffering devices found in brain cells (Blaustein et al., 1978). This, coupled with their high affinity, raises the possibility that mitochondria are critically important for calcium regulation especially during periods in which unusually high concentrations are experienced by the cell, as for example is thought to occur during repetitive synaptic activation (Morris et al., 1983) or ischemia and hypoxia (Siesjö, 1981).

In fact, it has been suggested that mitochondria provide a unique mechanism for the protection of cells against calcium overload (Nicholls, 1985). Unfortunately, the mechanism by which mitochondrial calcium transport is accomplished is far from being totally understood. There is general agreement that the driving force consists of a proton electrochemical gradient generated across the inner mitochondrial membrane by the electron transport system and oxidative phosphorylation (Bygrave, 1977; Saris and Åkerman, 1980). Since the central nervous system is critically dependent on glucose and the glycolytic pathway as an energy source (McIlwain and Bachelard, 1971), we previously advanced the hypothesis that disturbances at the level of the rate-limiting enzyme of mitochondrial metabolism, pyruvate dehydrogenase (PDH), trigger degenerative processes by disturbing mitochondrial contributions to calcium regulation (Baudry et al., 1982a; Lynch and Baudry, 1983). The present chapter will review this hypothesis. We will first summarize experimental data indicating that calcium transport in mitochondria is tightly linked to PDH activity and then describe the effects of certain types of denervation (which cause dendritic atrophy) on this enzyme and mitochondrial calcium transport. We will also present data indicating that the regulation of mitochondrial calcium transport changes dramatically during development and suggests that mitochondria in immature brain possess biochemical mechanisms to provide energy sources to fuel calcium transport that are absent in the adult. The possibility that these might be involved in the different responses of brain to injury or other insults found at different ages will be discussed.

Pyruvate dehydrogenase activity and mitochondrial calcium transport

Pyruvate dehydrogenase (PDH) is a key step in mitochondrial metabolism; by converting pyruvate and coenzyme A into acetyl CoA this complex enzyme, located in the inner mitochondrial matrix, fuels the Krebs cycle and the oxidative phosphorylation machinery of the cell (Lehninger, 1975). This enzyme is regulated by a variety of allosteric factors as well as by the phosphorylation-dephosphorylation of its α-subunit, the enzyme being inactive when the α-subunit is phosphorylated (Linn et al., 1969). The kinase and phosphatase responsible for this phosphorylation-dephosphorylation reaction are also associated with the multi-enzyme complex, thus allowing rapid changes in the state of phosphorylation of the α-subunit and therefore in PDH activity. The link between PDH activity and mitochondrial calcium transport was studied by using two different techniques to evaluate calcium transport. First we determined the rate and amount of ^{45}Ca taken up by crude mitochondrial fractions from rat brain. By using Ca-EGTA buffers and pyruvate, succinate, or ATP as an energy source, it was possible to identify the existence in rat brain mitochondria of a high-affinity transport system with an apparent affinity for calcium of about 1.5 μM (Browning et al., 1981a). Calcium sequestration was completely inhibited by mitochondrial poisons or calcium ionophores. As expected, pyruvate-supported calcium transport was found to be tightly coupled to PDH activity; thus the apparent affinity for pyruvate of the calcium transport was found to be about 35 μM while the apparent K_m of pyruvate for PDH was found to be about 30 μM. More importantly, modifying the state of phosphorylation of α-PDH by inhibiting PDH kinase with the inhibitor dichloracetate (DCA) (Whitehouse et al., 1974) resulted in parallel changes in PDH activity and pyruvate-supported calcium transport. Moreover, the concentration of DCA giving half-maximal stimulation of calcium transport (0.4 mM) was close to those at which it stimulated PDH activity (0.3 mM) and inhibited the phosphorylation of α-PDH (0.2 mM). Under these conditions, inhibiting α-PDH phosphorylation induced an increase in the maximal calcium accumulation, without changes in the apparent affinity for calcium of the calcium transport (Fig. 1), suggesting that the extent of calcium transport in brain mitochondria is partly regulated by the state of phosphorylation of α-PDH. In addition, these effects of DCA were specific since succinate- and ATP-supported calcium transport were not modified by this compound.

The second approach consisted in following the changes in free calcium by the use of a calcium-sensitive electrode when mitochondria were incubated in the presence of calcium and various mitochondrial substrates (Baudry et al., 1983). Under these conditions, mitochondria sequester calcium until its free concentration reaches very low values (about 0.5 μM), defined as a set-point. At this concentration, it is assumed that release of calcium is equilibrated with uptake. Presumably, ATP synthesis then takes place as long as calcium levels remain at this low level. Under normal conditions, the mitochondria will again very rapidly accumulate any excess of free calcium as demonstrated by applying successive pulses of calcium. Increasing PDH activity by decreasing the phosphorylation state of α-PDH with DCA, not only increased the rate at which calcium is transported but also decreased the value of the set-point (Fig. 2). Conversely, increasing PDH phosphorylation by blocking PDH phosphatase with potassium fluoride had the opposite effects. In addition, potassium fluoride induced a marked increase in the rate of inactivation of the pyruvate-supported transport following successive additions of calcium.

Thus both techniques provided clear evidence that changing the state of phosphorylation of α-PDH results in the predicted changes in pyruvate-supported calcium transport in mitochondria. Inhibiting PDH kinase induces a decrease in α-PDH phosphorylation, a stimulation of PDH activity and an increase in the rate and extent of pyruva-

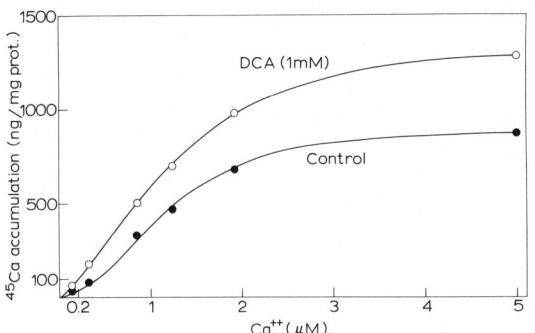

Fig. 1. Effect of dichloroacetate (DCA) on high-affinity calcium transport in purified mitochondria from rat brain. Brain mitochondria were purified according to the procedure of Clark and Nicklas (1970) and ^{45}Ca accumulation supported by 0.1 mM pyruvate and 1 mM ADP was measured in the absence or presence of 1 mM DCA as described by Browning et al. (1981a). Values are the means of 3-4 experiments (Browning et al., 1981a).

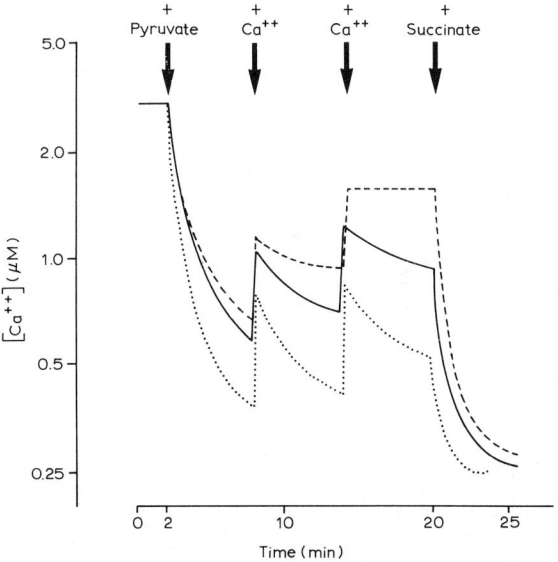

Fig. 2. Effect of dichloroacetate and potassium fluoride on calcium transport by rat brain mitochondria. Forebrain mitochondria were purified according to Clark and Nicklas (1970) and were incubated at room temperature under control conditions (———) or in the presence of 5 mM DCA (·······) or 10 mM potassium fluoride (– – –). Concentration of free calcium was evaluated with a calcium-sensitive electrode calibrated with Ca-EGTA buffers. After a 2 min preincubation, 0.5 mM pyruvate was added in the presence of 1 mM ADP. At the time indicated by arrow, calcium chloride (25 nmol/mg protein) was added. Succinate (5 mM) was added after 20 min of incubation. Data are from a typical experiment which was replicated with similar results 3 times (Baudry et al., 1983).

te-supported calcium accumulation. Conversely, inhibiting PDH phosphatase induces an increase in PDH phosphorylation, a decrease in PDH activity and a decrease in the rate and extent of pyruvate-supported calcium accumulation. This suggests that physiologically-induced changes in PDH phosphorylation can modulate the ability of mitochondria to regulate intracellular free calcium concentration.

To obtain some information concerning the rate of turnover of the phosphate group carried by the α-subunit of PDH we performed a number of manipulations using the hippocampal slice preparation which offers the advantage of exhibiting most of the physiological properties of the intact animal as well as a rapid way of changing the composition of the extracellular fluids (Lynch and Schubert, 1980). A series of observations have indicated that brief trains of high frequency electrical stimulation of the Schaffer-commissural pathways modified the state of phosphorylation of a protein with a M_r of 40 000 daltons (Browning et al., 1979). The change in phosphorylation was detected with a back-titration assay and indicated that the endogenous state of phosphorylation of this protein was rapidly but reversibly increased. Subsequent experiments revealed that this protein was the α-subunit of PDH (Morgan and Routtenberg, 1980; Browning et al., 1981b), and these experiments were therefore the first to suggest that the state of α-PDH phosphorylation could be rapidly altered by physiological stimulation. We next determined the effect of DCA on α-PDH phosphorylation and PDH activity in hippocampal slices (Blaudry et al., 1982b). As previously found with mitochondrial fractions, incubating hippocampal slices with DCA resulted in a rapid increase in ^{32}P-incorporation in α-PDH when performing a back-titration assay as well as in an increase in PDH activity (Fig. 3). The increase represented almost a total activation of PDH and occurred in about 5 minutes. This suggested that DCA in the slices effectively inhibited PDH kinase activity reducing its state of phosphorylation in situ thus allowing more labelled phosphate groups to be incorporated in the back-titration assay. This also indicated that the turnover of the phosphate group carried by the α-subunit in situ is very rapid under

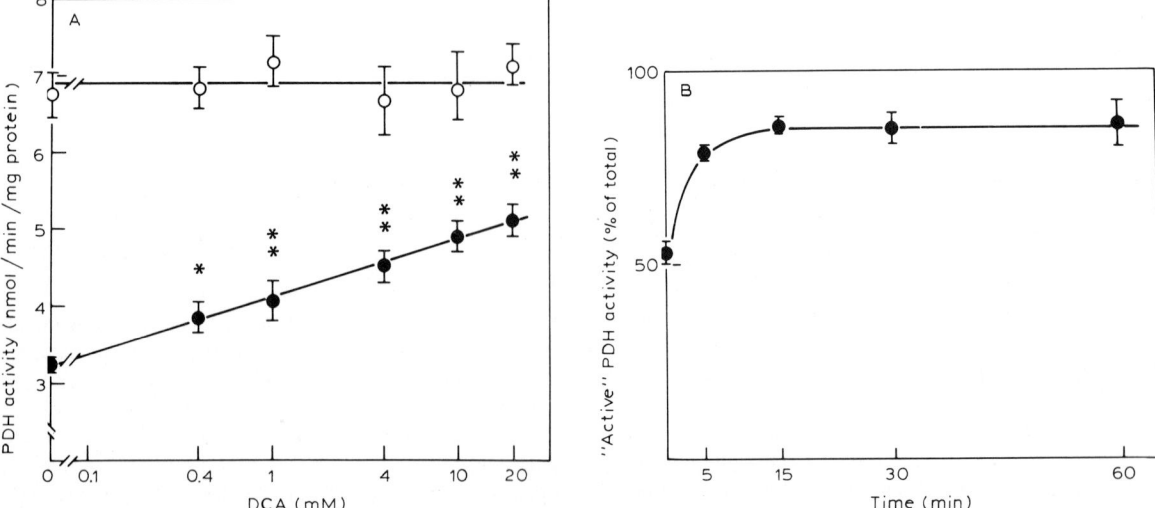

Fig. 3. Effect of dichloroacetate (DCA) on pyruvate dehydrogenase activity in hippocampal slices. Transverse hippocampal slices (0.4 mm thick) were preincubated for 30 min at 35°C in Krebs-Ringer bicarbonate under a constant stream of $O_2:CO_2$ (95:5). Various concentrations of DCA were then added and the incubation continued for 30 min (A). In another set of experiments 5 mM DCA was added and the incubation continued for various periods of time (B). Slices were then homogenized and active and total PDH activity was determined. Data are the means ±SEM of 4–5 experiments. * $p < 0.01$. ** $p < 0.001$ (Student's t test) (Baudry et al., 1982b).

normal conditions and suggested therefore that alterations in PDH kinase or phosphatase activity are likely to rapidly modify PDH phosphorylation and activity.

Effect of denervation on mitochondrial calcium transport in hippocampus

Because the morphologic changes which follow destruction of the primary afferents to the hippocampus are well described, the effects on mitochondrial calcium transport of hippocampal deafferentation were investigated.

Unilateral lesions of the major input to the hippocampus, the entorhinal cortex, initiate the following sequence of events in denervated dendrites: (1) a disruption of the cytoskeleton, (2) a loss of spines and synapses and (3) a severe retraction of the dendritic tree (Parnavelas et al., 1974; Matthews et al., 1976; Lee et al., 1977). These effects are complete by 5 days post lesion and are accompanied by hypertrophy of the astroglial cells (Rose et al., 1976), and a proliferation of the microglial cells (Gall et al., 1978). Beyond 5 days post lesion, the remaining inputs to the deafferented neurons begin emitting new branches (sprouting) and these partially reinnervate the dendritic zones which have lost contacts (Lynch et al., 1975, 1976; Lee et al., 1977); despite this, the dendritic tree remains severely atrophic for months after the lesion (Lynch and Gall, 1982). This well-described set of events provided a suitable model with which to study the involvement of changes in calcium regulation in various aspects of cell growth and degeneration.

We found that entorhinal cortex lesions caused a rapid and severe decrease in pyruvate-supported calcium transport by mitochondria in the hippocampus ipsilateral to the lesion as compared to the hippocampus contralateral to the lesion (it is important to note that no difference was found in calcium transport in the hippocampus contralateral to the lesion as compared to control rats) (Baudry et al., 1982a). This effect was present as soon as 24 hours after the lesions, reached its maximum by 5 days post lesion and was still present up to 6 months later (Fig. 4). Thus the decrease in calcium transport by hippocampal mitochondria precedes any light or electron-microscopic evidence of pre- or post-synaptic degeneration. These results also suggest that some irreversible modification in the regulatory processes governing calcium transport is produced by denervation. The activity and in vitro phosphorylation of PDH were also significantly reduced following lesions of the entorhinal cortex, indicating that denervation altered the endogenous state of phosphorylation of α-PDH, possibly by decreasing PDH phosphatase activity, therefore resulting in higher levels of phosphorylation of the enzyme in situ. Furthermore, the decrease in PDH activity across animals correlated remarkably well with the decrease in pyruvate-supported calcium uptake. These effects are probably not due to a generalized impairment of mitochondrial functions, since ATP-supported calcium uptake was only marginally affected by the lesion and cytochrome oxidase activity was not modified. Succinate dehydrogenase activity and succinate-supported calcium uptake were also reduced by the lesions but not to

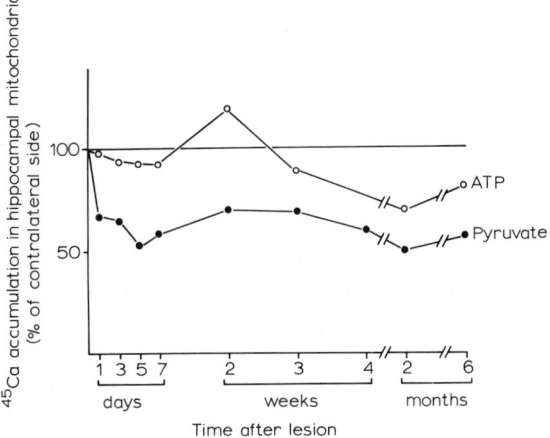

Fig. 4. Effects of unilateral entorhinal cortex lesions on hippocampal mitochondrial calcium transport. At various times following unilateral entorhinal cortex lesions, ^{45}Ca accumulation supported by pyruvate or by ATP was measured in hippocampal crude mitochondrial fractions. Results are means of 3–6 experiments and are expressed as percent of ^{45}Ca accumulation found in the contralateral hippocampus (Baudry et al., 1983).

the same extent that was observed for PDH and pyruvate-supported uptake. The decrease in calcium transport was present in both synaptic and non-synaptic mitochondria, indicating that the effects of the lesions were not restricted to a specific population of mitochondria and in particular were not due to the elimination of a significant portion of nerve terminals. Lesions of the commissural pathway also resulted in a decrease in pyruvate-supported calcium transport whereas lesions of the septo-hippocampal pathway were without effect (Baudry et al., 1983). This suggested that the effect requires the loss of a significant number of afferent projections since the septal inputs provide only a minor portion of terminals in the hippocampus. In addition, since both the perforant pathway and the commissural pathway are excitatory and are likely to use an excitatory amino acid as a transmitter (presumably L-glutamate) (Storm-Mathisen, 1977) these results suggest that the loss of an excitatory transmitter is responsible for the denervation-induced decrease in PDH activity and calcium transport. In this regard it is interesting to note that incubation of slices with L-glutamate results in an increase in PDH activity (Baudry and Lynch, unpublished data), possibly indicating that the release of glutamate by presynaptic elements maintains PDH in a high state of activity.

The denervation-induced changes in pyruvate-supported calcium transport were not as marked in the period from 5 days to 3 weeks after the lesions. This coincides with the period of axonal sprouting in the mature hippocampus (McWilliams and Lynch, 1979), suggesting that sprouting might be accompanied by either an increase in the amount of mitochondria or an increased functional activity of existing mitochondria.

Using the calcium-sensitive electrode to study the kinetics of calcium transport in hippocampal mitochondria allowed us to better define the alteration in calcium transport and to evaluate potential consequences of the denervation in the target dendrites (Baudry et al., 1983). As previously described, mitochondria from denervated hippocampi were incubated with calcium and various substrates and the concentration of free calcium was followed with the calcium-sensitive electrode. Lesions of the entorhinal cortex resulted not only in a decreased rate of calcium accumulation, but also in an increase in the value of the set point to which mitochondria buffer free calcium and, more importantly, in a marked increase in the rate of inactivation of the pyruvate-supported calcium transport following successive pulses of calcium. This latter effect resulted in a considerable amplification of the differences between mitochondria prepared from control and lesioned sides (Fig. 5). Since this effect was very similar to that seen when control mitochondria were incubated in the presence of a phosphatase inhibitor, these results are consistent with the idea that denervation results in a decrease in PDH phosphatase activity and therefore in an increase in the state of phosphorylation of α-PDH in situ corresponding to a lower PDH activity and pyruvate-supported calcium transport. This also suggests that intracellular calcium levels could increase markedly in the dendrites and cell bodies of the denervated neurons as a result of successive influxes

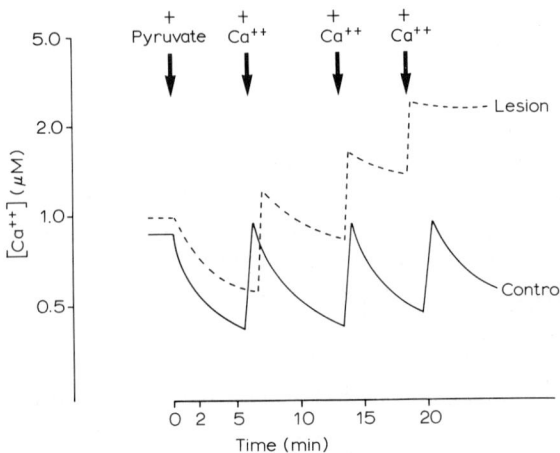

Fig. 5. Effects of unilateral entorhinal cortex lesions on hippocampal mitochondrial calcium transport. One week after unilateral lesion of the entorhinal cortex pyruvate-supported calcium transport was measured in purified mitochondrial fractions from the contralateral (control) and ipsilateral (lesion) hippocampi, using a calcium-sensitive electrode. Pyruvate (0.5 mM) and calcium chloride (25 nmol/ng protein) were added at the times indicated by arrows (Baudry et al., 1983).

of calcium resulting from the synaptic activity in the remaining terminals.

Elevations of intracellular calcium concentrations would then activate a host of calcium-dependent processes normally quiescent in the denervated dendrites, and in particular of calcium-dependent proteases acting on several proteins constituting the cytoskeleton. This mechanism could be responsible for the initial atrophy, loss of spines and dendritic shrinkage which follows denervation in the initial stage. It is worth noting that several degenerative diseases in the CNS are accompanied by decreases in PDH activity (Blass and Gibson, 1978; Blass, 1979). In particular, different groups have reported decreases in PDH activity in post-mortem brain of Alzheimer's patients (Perry et al., 1980; Sorbi et al., 1983). In addition there was a good correlation between the severity of the disease and the decrease in PDH activity.

Taken together these data provide experimental support for the idea that disturbances at the level of PDH lead to alterations in regulation of intracellular calcium levels which can initiate a series of biochemical events ultimately resulting in activation of calcium-dependent processes and in degenerative processes.

Changes in regulation of calcium transport during development

While it was already known that two forms of sprouting are present during the postnatal period, one of these disappearing after the second postnatal week, McWilliams and Lynch (1983) discovered that the rate of synaptic replacement following lesions exhibits a dramatic change between the juvenile and young adult period. Whereas young adult rats (about 90 days old) require over 2 months to replace synapses lost as a result of a lesion, juvenile rats (30 days old) need less than 1 week to reach such a stage. In both cases, the sprouting of intact afferents responsible for synaptic replacement is initiated only after a delay of 5 days following the lesions, indicating that juvenile rats have a tremendous capacity to form new synaptic connections.

Possibly related to this, preliminary experiments indicate that entorhinal cortex lesions in juvenile rats produce only a transient reduction in mitochondrial calcium transport, a result that stands in marked contrast to the lasting change found after similar lesions in older animals. This result suggested that some aspects of the link between denervation and mitochondrial calcium transport were clearly different between juvenile and young adult rats. Since the regulation of brain metabolism exhibits dramatic changes during the developmental period, it was of interest to determine if changes in the link between PDH and mitochondrial calcium transport alo occurred during this period.

Pyruvate-supported calcium transport was very high in the first 10 postnatal days, increased slightly between postnatal days 8 and 16, but dramatically decreased between postnatal days 16 and 24, without further changes up to the adult period (Fig. 6). In contrast the succinate- and ATP-supported calcium transport remained relatively constant during the whole developmental period. Expressed as a ratio of pyruvate over succinate or pyruvate over ATP-supported calcium transport, the data indicate a very sharp decrease occurring between postnatal days 16 and 22 (Fig. 7). This result was somewhat surprising since PDH activity increases progressively during the developmental period and reaches its adult values only after a month (Land et al., 1977).

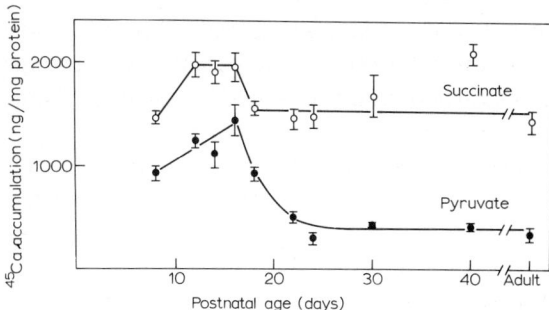

Fig. 6. Changes in pyruvate- and succinate-supported ^{45}Ca accumulation at various postnatal times in rat hippocampus. ^{45}Ca accumulation supported by pyruvate (0.1 mM) or succinate (5 mM) was determined in crude mitochondrial fractions from hippocampus of rats of different postnatal ages. Results are means ± SEM of 4–6 experiments.

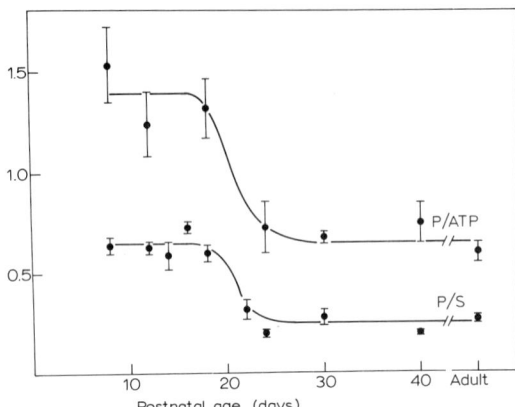

Fig. 7. Changes in mitochondrial calcium transport at various postnatal times in rat hippocampus. ^{45}Ca accumulation supported by pyruvate (0.1 mM), succinate (5 mM) or ATP (1 mM) was determined in crude mitochondrial fractions from hippocampus of rats of different postnatal ages. Results are expressed as the ratios of pyruvate over succinate (P/S) or pyruvate over ATP (P/ATP) ^{45}Ca accumulation and are means ± SEM of 4–6 experiments.

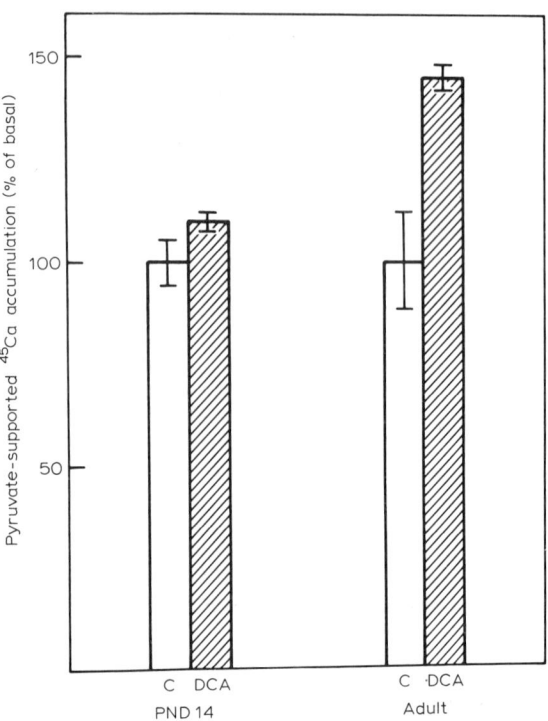

Fig. 8. Effect of dichloroacetate (DCA) on pyruvate-supported ^{45}Ca accumulation in forebrain mitochondria in neonatal and adult rat. Purified mitochondrial fractions were prepared from the forebrain of neonatal rats (14 days) and adult rats, and ^{45}Ca accumulation was measured in the presence of pyruvate (0.1 mM) and ADP (1 mM) with and without 1 mM DCA. Results are expressed as percentages of values measured in the absence of DCA and are means ± SEM of 4 experiments.

In addition, PDH has been reported to be fully activated up to postnatal day 20 and only thereafter to become partially inactive, possibly due to the progressive phosphorylation of the α-subunit (Land et al., 1977). In agreement with this, we found that DCA, while stimulating PDH activity and pyruvate-supported calcium transport in adult hippocampal mitochondria, was ineffective in mitochondria from young animals (Fig. 8). However, considering the size of the differences in PDH activity between young and adult animals, this result cannot by itself explain the difference in pyruvate-supported calcium transport found between mitochondria from young and adult rats.

These results indicate that some fundamental changes in the regulation of mitochondrial calcium transport occur during the developmental period. Interestingly, the time-course of the changes in pyruvate-supported calcium transport corresponds quite well with changes in pyruvate metabolism during brain development. In the developing rat brain, the main utilization of pyruvate is through the formation of oxaloacetate via the enzyme pyruvate carboxylase, which is activated by the high levels of acetyl CoA generated from the ketone bodies provided by the high fat content of dietary milk (Henning, 1981). In turn, oxaloacetate is converted to citrate and is used mainly for the synthesis of fatty acids. Pyruvate carboxylase, a key enzyme in this sequence, exhibits a maximum activity at 20 days postnatal in the rat brain, and declines rather abruptly to about 50% of this value (Land and Clark, 1975). It is interesting that postnatal day 20 represents not only the peak of pyruvate carboxylase activity but also the time at which rats are generally weaned and shift from a high fat to a low fat diet; in fact our results on the changes in pyruvate over succinate-supported calcium transport parallel very closely those reported by Page et al. (1971) for the level of ketone bodies in blood plasma. Together these developmental events redirect the utilization of pyruvate through acetyl CoA and the Krebs cycle via PDH. However, the potential for utilization of ketone bodies remains present even though the concentration of ketone bodies in blood plasma appears to increase only in case of glucose deprivation.

Although major changes in mitochondrial metabolism occur between postnatal days 18 and 22, it is likely that further modifications continue to be made during the transition between the juvenile and young adult period. For instance, acetyl CoA is formed in the mitochondria both by the PDH system and by the enzyme aceto-acetyl CoA thiolase. While PDH activity increases 6-fold between postnatal day 5 and adulthood, the activity of the thiolase is maximal by postnatal day 20, remains constant between days 20 and 30 and decreases in the adult. Thus the ratio of the activities of aceto-acetyl CoA thiolase and PDH remains relatively constant between postnatal days 10 and 30 and decreases 3-fold thereafter (Cremer et al., 1975). These results raise the possibility that the high levels of pyruvate-supported calcium transport found until postnatal day 18 in the hippocampus, reflect a higher contribution of pyruvate carboxylase in providing carbon atoms to the Krebs cycle. Thereafter, as the diet shifts to a low fat content and the levels of ketone bodies decrease, resulting in a decrease in the levels of acetyl CoA, the concomitant decrease in the levels of pyruvate carboxylase and the increase in PDH activity might contribute to the tight coupling of pyruvate-supported calcium transport with PDH activity (Fig. 9). It is also possible to speculate that this shift in regulation of calcium transport permits a more rapid, calcium-dependent regulation of calcium transport since calcium has been shown to activate PDH phosphatase activity (Denton et al., 1972). This could occur at a time when most synapses become functional (at least in the hippocampus) and might therefore explain the differential effect of lesions performed at different ages.

Because regulation of energy metabolism has

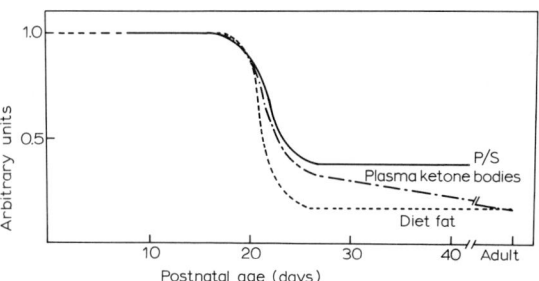

Fig. 9. Changes in diet fat, plasma ketone bodies and hippocampal mitochondrial calcium transport during postnatal development in rat. The ratios of pyruvate-over-succinate-supported ^{45}Ca accumulation in hippocampal mitochondrial fractions (P/S) are from Fig. 7; the data for diet fat are from Dymsza et al. (1964) and for plasma ketone bodies from Page et al. (1971).

been shown to differ between different brain structures, it was of interest to study mitochondrial calcium transport in the presence of various substrates in different regions of the rat brain. Although the absolute values for pyruvate-, succinate- and ATP-supported calcium accumulation varied among different brain subdivisions, a clear distinction between telencephalic and non-telencephalic structures emerged on the basis of the ratios pyruvate- over succinate-supported calcium transport (Table 1). These values were about 3-fold lower in

TABLE 1

Pyruvate- and succinate-supported ^{45}Ca accumulation in mitochondria prepared from different regions of the rat brain

Regions	Pyruvate	Succinate	Pyruvate/succinate
Cerebellum	1728 ± 213	3066 ± 304	0.56 ± 0.05
Pons-medulla	788 ± 180	1684 ± 355	0.49 ± 0.01
Mesencephalon	1089 ± 227	2267 ± 239	0.47 ± 0.04
Hippocampus	470 ± 89	2597 ± 350	0.18 ± 0.02
Striatum	447 ± 80	1674 ± 242	0.26 ± 0.02
Cortex	890 ± 182	2877 ± 386	0.31 ± 0.04

^{45}Ca accumulation was measured in crude mitochondrial fractions prepared from different regions of the rat brain. Mitochondria were fueled with 0.1 mM pyruvate or 5 mM succinate (in the presence of 1 mM ADP and 0.1 mM CoA). Results are expressed in ng ^{45}Ca accumulated/mg protein and are mean ± SEM of 3 experiments.

telencephalic structures than in non-telencephalic ones. This agrees will with a recent report showing that PDH kinase activity is higher in telencephalic structures than in non-telencephalic ones, suggesting that PDH might be more phosphorylated and therefore less active in the former than in the latter regions (Sheu et al., 1984). Alternatively, it is possible that non-telencephalic structures maintain, even in the adult, some capacity to use the same mechanism for calcium transport as that employed in the neonatal brain, a point that merits testing.

Conclusion

The regulation of intracellular calcium concentration is clearly the resultant of multiple regulatory processes and we have focused our studies only on the mitochondrial calcium transport on the assumption that this organelle is the only one which has a very large capacity for calcium and therefore that disturbance of this system is likely to have profound consequences for the normal functioning of cells in general and neurons in particular. This assumption is reinforced by the fact that the levels of PDH activity in the brain have been reported to be only minimally sufficient to maintain a normal flux of pyruvate through the oxidative pathway (Cremer and Teal, 1974; Blass and Gibson, 1978), and that brain energy metabolism is almost totally dependent on glucose. In addition pyruvate dehydrogenase activity is regulated by a multiplicity of factors, including a phosphorylation-dephosphorylation reaction which itself is dependent on calcium concentration (Cate and Roche, 1978). Under resting conditions, when calcium concentrations are low, the enzyme exists under two configurations, i.e. phosphorylated and non-phosphorylated corresponding to inactive and active states, and the conversion of pyruvate into acetyl CoA leads to the generation of ATP. When calcium levels rise the enzyme is activated by dephosphorylation and the conversion of pyruvate leads to the transport of calcium into the mitochondria. Our studies clearly showed that the rate and extent of calcium transport are critically dependent on the state of phosphorylation of PDH. However, following denervation some aspect of the regulation of PDH phosphorylation becomes irreversibly modified such that the enzyme remains more phosphorylated and therefore less active. The exact site of this modified regulation is not clear at the moment. One possibility could be a decrease in PDH phosphatase activity which could be the consequence of the removal of a factor normally provided by the presynaptic afferents. The factor could be an excitatory transmitter or a modulatory peptide. There is evidence that the interaction of insulin with its plasma membrane receptor induces the release of a peptide which stimulates PDH activity by activating PDH phosphatase (Seals and Jarret, 1980; Seals and Czech, 1980). In addition, since the fibers of the perforant path have been shown to contain a variety of neuropeptides (Gall et al., 1981), it is tempting to speculate that some of these participate indirectly in the regulation of calcium levels in the target dendrites by a similar mechanism. Another candidate which could play a role in the regulation of PDH activity consists in a polybasic factor, since it has recently been shown that polyamines such as spermine, spermidine and putrescine stimulate PDH phosphatase activity (Damuni et al., 1984).

Whatever the mechanism, denervation appears to decrease the ability of mitochondria to buffer calcium levels in target dendrites and cell bodies and thus may allow calcium levels to remain elevated for extended periods of time, and thereby to activate various calcium-dependent processes. Among these processes are those resulting in the dissolution of microtubules and microfilaments, events that might well be responsible for the morphological alterations seen after partial denervation and in various degenerative conditions. Current studies are directed at testing some of these ideas by determining the effect of PDH manipulation on the morphological and biochemical consequences of partial denervation. The idea that PDH alteration following partial denervation is involved in the resulting morphological alteration receives further support from the observations that denervation during the developmental period results in a totally different pattern of morphological alterations and that during this period mitochondrial calcium transport appears to be regulated by mechanisms distinctly different from those found in the adult. It seems very likely that during the developmental period mitochondrial metabolism does not depend on PDH activity but rather on pyruvate carboxylase. Since this enzyme is regulated mainly by acetyl CoA it should be less susceptible to transient alteration in calcium concentrations and should not respond in the same way as PDH to denervation. This might also explain why young animals are much less sensitive to ischemia than adult animals. The progressive increase in PDH activity and decrease in pyruvate carboxylase and acetyl CoA levels might then allow a more precise regulation of mitochondrial metabolism by increasing the number of factors regulating pyruvate metabolism. In addition there is the possibility that the capacity for pyruvate metabolism via pyruvate carboxylase remains present and differentially distributed in the adult rat brain and that under certain conditions mitochondria can shift back to a more immature mode of functioning. This might also contribute to the differential sensitivity of specific regions of brain to hypoxia and hypoglycemia.

Acknowledgements

This study was supported by Grant NS-18 427, to Michel Baudry.

The authors wish to thank Denise Arst for her skillful technical assistance and Jackie Porter for the preparation of the manuscript.

References

Baudry, M., Fuchs, J., Kessler, M., Arst, D. and Lynch, G. (1982a) Entorhinal cortex lesions induce a decrease in calcium transport in hippocampal mitochondria. *Science*, 216: 411–413.

Baudy, M., Kessler, J., Smith, E.K. and Lynch, G. (1982b) The regulation of pyruvate dehydrogenase activity in rat hippocampal slices: effect of dichloroacetate. *Neurosci. Lett.*, 31: 41–46.

Baudry, M., Gall, C., Kessler, M., Alapour, H. and Lynch, G. (1983) Denervation-induced decrease in mitochondrial calcium transport in rat hippocampus. *J. Neurosci.*, 3: 252–259.

Blass, J.P. (1979) Disorders of pyruvate metabolism. *Neurology*, 29: 280–286.

Blass, J. and Gibson, G. (1978) Studies of the pathophysiology of pyruvate dehydrogenase deficiency. *Adv. Neurol.*, 21: 181–194.

Blaustein, M.P., Ratzlaff, R.W., Kendrick, N.C. and Schwertzer, E.S. (1978) Calcium buffering in presynaptic terminals. I. Evidence for involvement of a non-motochondrial ATP-dependent sequestration mechanism. *J. Gen. Phys.*, 72: 15–41.

Browning, M., Dunwiddie, T., Bennett, W., Gispen, W. and Lynch, G. (1979) Synaptic phosphoproteins: specific changes after repetitive stimulation of the hippocampal slice. *Science*, 203: 60–62.

Browning, M., Baudry, M., Bennett, W. and Lynch, G. (1981a) Phosphorylation-mediated changes in pyruvate dehydrogenase activity influence pyruvate-supported calcium accumulation by brain mitochondria. *J. Neurochem.*, 36: 1932–1940.

Browning, M., Bennett, W., Kelly, P. and Lynch, G. (1981b) The 40 000 M_r brain phosphoprotein influenced by high frequency synaptic stimulation is the alpha subunit of pyruvate dehydrogenase. *Brain Res.*, 218: 255–266.

Bygrave, F. (1977) Mitochondrial calcium transport. *Curr. Top. Bioenerg.*, 6: 259–318.

Cate, R. and Roche, T. (1978) A unifying mechanism for stimulation of mammalian pyruvate dehydrogenase (a) kinase by reduced nicotinamide adenine dinucleotide, dihydrolipoamide, acetyl coenzyme A, or pyruvate. *J. Biol. Chem.*, 253: 496–503.

Clark, J. and Nicklas W. (1970) The metabolism of rat brain mitochondria. *J. Biol. Chem.*, 245: 4724–4731.

Cremer, J. and Teal, H. (1974) The activity of pyruvate dehydrogenase in rat brain during postnatal development. *FEBS Lett.*, 39: 17–20.

Cremer, J.E., Teal, H.M. and Heath, D.F. (1975) Regulatory factors in glucose and ketone body utilization by the developing brain. In: F. A. Hommes and C. J. van den Berg (Eds.), *Normal and Pathological Development of Energy Metabolism*. Academic Press, New York.

Damuni, Z., Humphreys, J.S. and Reed, L.J. (1984) Stimulation of pyruvate dehydrogenase activity by polyamines. *Biochem. Biophys. Res. Comm.*, 124: 95–99.

De Martino, G.N. (1981) Calcium-dependent proteolytic activity in rat liver: identification of two proteases with different calcium requirements. *Arch. Biochem. Biophys.*, 211: 253–257.

Denton, R., Randle, P. and Martin B. (1972) Stimulation by calcium ions of pyruvate dehydrogenase phosphate phosphatase. *Biochem. J.*, 123: 161–163.

Dymsza, H.A., Czajka, D.M. and Miller S.A. (1964) Influence of artificial diet on weight gain and body composition of the neonatal rat. *J. Nutrit.*, 84: 100–106.

Erulkar, S.D. and Fine, A. (1979) Calcium in the nervous system. *Rev. Neurosci., Vol. 4.* New York, Raven Press, pp. 197–232.

Farber, J.L. (1981) The role of calcium in cell death. *Life Sci.*, 29: 1289–1295.

Gall, C., Rose, G. and Lynch, G. (1978) Proliferative and migratory activity of glial cells in the deafferented hippocampus. *J. Comp. Neurol.*, 183: 539–550.

Gall, C., Brecha, N., Chang, T. and Karten, H. (1981) Localization of enkephalines in rat hippocampus. *J. Comp. Neurol.*, 198: 335–350.

Gall, C., Ivy, G. and Lynch, G. (1985) Neuroanatomical plasticity: its role in the organization and reorganization of the central nervous system. In: J.M. Tanner and F. Falkner (Eds.), *Human Growth, a Comprehensive Treatise*, 2nd Edn. Plenum Press, New York, in press.

Henning, S.J. (1981) Postnatal development: coordination of feeding, digestion, and metabolism. *Am. J. Physiol.*, 241: G199–214.

Land, J.M. and Clark, J.B. (1975) The changing pattern of brain mitochondrial substrate utilization during development. In: F.A. Hommes and C.J. van den Berg (Eds.), *Normal and Pathological Development of Energy Metabolism*. Academic Press, New York, pp. 155–165.

Land J.M., Booth, R.F.G., Berger, R. and Clark, J.B. (1977) Development of mitochondrial energy metabolism in rat brain. *Biochem. J.*, 164: 339–348.

Lee, K., Stanford, E., Cotman, C.W. and Lynch, G.S. (1977) Ultrastructural evidence for bouton sprouting in the adult mammalian brain. *Exp. Brain Res.*, 29: 475–485.

Lehninger, A.L. (1975) *Biochemistry*, 2nd Edn. Worth, Publ. Inc., New York.

Libby, P. and Goldberg, A.L. (1978) Leupeptin, a protease inhibitor, decreases protein degradation in normal and diseased muscles. *Science*, 199: 534–536.

Linn, T., Pettit, F. and Reed, L. (1969) Alpha-beta and dehydrogenase complexes. X. Regulation of the activity of the pyruvate dehydrogenase complex from beef kidney mitochondria by phosphorylation and dephosphorylation. *Proc. Natl. Acad. Sci. USA*, 62: 234–241.

Lynch, G. and Schubert, P. (1980) The use of in vitro brain slices for multidisciplinary studies of synaptic function. *Ann. Rev. Neurosci.*, 3, 1–22.

Lynch, G. and Baudry, M. (1983) Origins and manifestations of neuronal plasticity in the hippocampus. In: W. Willis (Ed.), *Clinical Neurosciences, Vol. 5.* Churchill-Livingston, Publ., Edinburgh, pp. 171–202.

Lynch, G., Rose, G., Gall, C. and Cotman, C.W. (1975) The response of the dentate gyrus to partial deafferentation. In: M. Santini (Ed.), *Golgi Centennial Symposium Proceedings.* Raven Press, New York, pp. 305–317.

Lynch, G., Gall, C., Rose, G. and Cotman, C.W. (1976) Changes in the distribution of the dentate gyrus associational system following unilateral or bilateral entorhinal lesion in the adult rat. *Brain Res.*, 110: 57–71.

Maro, B. and Bornens, M. (1982) Reorganization of Hela cell cytoskeleton induced by an uncoupler of oxidative phosphorylation. *Nature*, 295: 334–336.

Matthews, D.A., Cotman, C. and Lynch, G. (1976) An electron microscopic study of lesion-induced synaptogenesis in the dentate gyrus of the adult rat. I. Magnitude and time course of degeneration. *Brain Res.*, 115: 1–21.

McIllwain, H. and Bachelard, H. (1971) *Biochemistry and the Nervous System*, 4th Edn. Churchill-Livingston, Edinburgh.

McWilliams, J.R. and Lynch, G.S. (1979) Terminal proliferation in the partially deafferented dentate gyrus. Time courses for the appearance and removal of degeneration and the replacement of lost terminals. *J. Comp. Neurol.*, 187: 191–198.

McWilliams, J.R. and Lynch, G. (1983) Rate of synaptic replacement in denervated rat hippocampus declines precipitously from the juvenile period to adulthood. *Science*, 221: 574–575.

Morgan, D.G. and Routtenberg, A. (1980) Evidence that a 41 000 dalton brain phosphoprotein is pyruvate dehydrogenase. *Biochem. Biophys. Res. Comm.*, 95: 569–576.

Morris, M.E., Krnjevic, K. and Ropert, N. (1983) Changes in free Ca recorded inside hippocampal pyramidal neurons in response to fimbrial stimulation. *Neurosci. Abstr.* 9: 395.

Murachi, T., Hatanaka, M., Yasumoto, Y., Nakayama, N. and Tanaka, K. (1981) A quantitative distribution study on calpain and calpastatin in rat tissues and cells. *Biochem. Int.*, 2: 651–656.

Nicholls, D.G. (1985) A role for the mitochondrion in the protection of cells against calcium overload? *This volume*, pp. 97–106.

Page, M.A., Krebs, H.A. and Williamson, D.H. (1971) Activities of enzymes of ketone-body utilization in brain and other tissues of suckling rats. *Biochem. J.*, 121: 49–53.

Parnavelas, J.G., Lynch, G., Brecha, W., Cotman, C.W. and Globus, A. (1974) Spine loss and regrowth in hippocampus following deafferentation. *Nature*, 248: 71–73.

Perry, E.K., Perry, R.H., Tomlinson, B.E., Blessed, G. and Gibson, P.H. (1980) Coenzyme A acetylating enzymes in Alzheimer's disease: possible cholinergic compartment of pyruvate dehydrogenase. *Neurosci. Lett.*, 18: 205–110.

Rahamimoff, R., Erulkar, S.D., Lev-Tov A. and Meiri, H. (1978) Intracellular and extracellular calcium ions in transmitter release at the neuromuscular synapse. *Ann. NY Acad. Sci.*, 307: 583–597.

Rose, B. and Loewenstein, W.R. (1975) Calcium ion distribution in cytoplasm visualized by aequorin: diffusion in cytosol restricted by energized sequestering. *Science*, 190: 1204–1206.

Rose, G., Cotman, C.W. and Lynch, G.S. (1976) Hypertrophy and redistribution of astrocytes in the deafferented hippocampus. *Brain Res. Bull.*, 1: 87–92.

Salpeter, M., Leonard, J.P. and Kasprzak, H. (1982) Agonist-induced postsynaptic myopathy. *Neurosci. Comment.*, 1: 73–83.

Saris, N.E. and Åkerman, K.E.O. (1980) Uptake and release of bivalent cations in mitochondria. *Curr. Top. Bioenerg.,* 10: 103–179.

Schanne, F.A.X., Kane, A.B., Young, E.E. and Farber, J.L. (1979) Calcium dependence of toxic cell death: a final common pathway. *Science,* 206: 700–702.

Schlaepfer, W.W. and Hasler, M.B. (1979) Characterization of the calcium-induced disruption of neurofilaments in rat peripheral nerve. *Brain Res.,* 168: 299–309.

Seals, J.R. and Czech, M.P. (1980) Evidence that insulin activates an intrinsic plasma membrane protease in generating a secondary chemical mediator. *J. Biol. Chem.,* 255: 6529–6531.

Seals, J.R. and Jarret, L. (1980) Activation of pyruvate dehydrogenase by direct addition of insulin to an isolated plasma membrane/mitochondrial mixture: evidence for generation of insulin's second messenger in a subcellular system. *Proc. Natl. Acad. Sci. USA,* 77: 77–81.

Sheu, K.F.R., Lai, J.C.K. and Blass, J.P. (1984) Properties and regional distribution of pyruvate dehydrogenase kinase in rat brain. *J. Neurochem.,* 42: 230–236.

Siesjö, B.K. (1981) Cell damage in the brain: a speculative synthesis. *J. Cereb. Blood Flow Metabol.,* 1: 155–185.

Siman, R., Baudry, M. and Lynch, G. (1983) Purification from synaptosomal plasma membranes of calpain I, a thiol-protease activated by micromolar calcium concentration. *J. Neurochem.,* 41: 950–956.

Somlyo, A.P. (1984) Cellular site of calcium regulation. *Nature,* 309: 560–561.

Sorbi, S., Bird, E.D. and Blass, J.P. (1983) Decreased pyruvate dehydrogenase complex activity in Huntington and Alzheimer brain. *Ann. Neurol.,* 13: 72–78.

Storm-Mathisen, Jr. (1977) Localization of transmitter candidates in the brain: the hippocampal formation as a model. *Prog. Neurobiol.,* 8: 119–181.

Whitehouse, S., Cooper, R. and Randle, P. (1974) Mechanism of activation of pyruvate dehydrogenase by dichloroacetate and other halogenated carboxylic acids. *Biochem. J.,* 141: 761–774.

Zimmerman, U.J.P. and Schlaepfer, W.W. (1982) Characterization of a brain calcium-activated protease that degrades neurofilament proteins. *Biochemistry,* 21: 3977–3983.

Acid-base homeostasis in the brain: physiology, chemistry, and neurochemical pathology

Bo K. Siesjö

Laboratory for Experimental Brain Research, University of Lund, Lund, Sweden

Introduction

Although changes in extracellular pH (pH_e) of brain tissues have attracted the attention of research workers from several different fields, mainly those studying central regulation of pulmonary ventilation and of cerebral blood flow (CBF), the literature on intracellular pH (pH_i) is less extensive. In fact, it is not until recently that the subject has come into the focus of more general interest. There are many reasons for this slow development, and for the current surge of interest. First, the subject of tissue acid-base metabolism has been burdened with conceptual controversies and complexities which may have discouraged many potential students. Second, development of suitable methodologies has been slow, and changes in pH_i during pathological states have remained largely elusive. Third, it was only recently that results emerged suggesting a role for changes in pH_i in the development of irreversible brain damage, notably in ischemia and hypoxia, thus forcing a larger group of research workers to approach the subject.

During the last decade, a wealth of information has amassed on the regulation of pH_i, particularly in isolated cells. This information has been discussed in a comprehensive and authorative review article (Roos and Boron, 1981), and new information is constantly being added (e.g. Moody, 1981; Rink et al., 1982; Boron and Boulpaep, 1983; Grinstein et al., 1984). To a large extent, this development has been made possible by the advent of new methodologies, e.g. the construction of micro pH electrodes sufficiently small to allow measurement inside invertebrate and vertebrate cells (Thomas 1974; Amman et al., 1981). It is also of importance that some experimental methods have been successfully adopted for use in patients (Syrota et al., 1983; Buxton et al., 1984; Brooks et al., 1984), and that the non-invasive ^{31}P-NMR (nuclear magnetic resonance) technique yields information on pH_i (Thulborn et al., 1982; Prichard et al., 1983; Hilberman et al., 1984). Another important advent is the definition of membrane ion exchangers which achieve translocation of H^+ from intra- to extracellular fluids, probably constituting the molecular devices for pH_i regulation (see Roos and Boron, 1981; Vigne et al., 1982; Grinstein et al., 1984). Although the cellular heterogeneity of the brain, and the fragility of its neuronal elements to electrode impalement, still hamper elucidation of changes in pH_i, the methodological and conceptual advents open up new ways of approaching the basic problems.

The present article attempts to summarize current information on brain acid-base metabolism in health and disease. It consists of four main sections. In the first, I will try to clarify some of the conceptual difficulties of applying acid-base theory to systems having the composition of extra- and intracellular fluids. The following section will be devoted to features of cellular acid-base regulation in extracerebral tissues, and to current information on the corresponding regulation of extra- and intracellular pH in the brain. In the third section data will be briefly discussed which bear on changes in brain pH_e and pH_i in disease. In the last one, finally, I will consider possible molecular mechanisms whereby acidosis could cause or aggravate cell injury.

Acid-base metabolism: theory and concepts

A simple acid-base model

The essential features of acid-base regulation in an isolated system which can exchange gases with the environment were clearly described by Siggaard-Andersen (1966). As Fig. 1 shows, the system has two independent and one dependent variable. One of the independent variables is P_{CO_2}, i.e. the partial pressure of CO_2, and the other is the excess of non-volatile acid or base added. The dependent variable is pH. Some of the terms require definition and clarification.

In an open system in diffusion equilibrium with a gas phase the P_{CO_2} of the system, be it a fluid or a solid tissue, is by definition that of the gas phase. Addition of acid or base can be viewed as changes in buffer base (BB) concentration, or as causing a Base Deficit/Base Excess. To take an example, if strong acid is added to a final concentration of 5 $mmol \cdot l^{-1}$, the BB concentration has decreased by 5 $mmol \cdot l^{-1}$, or there is now a Base Deficit of 5 $mmol \cdot l^{-1}$ (this is to say that Base Excess is -5

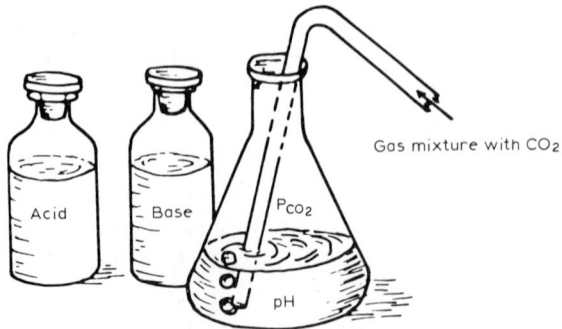

Fig. 1. This simple analogy illustrates the fact that pH (a dependent variable) varies with P_{CO_2} and buffer base concentration (two independent variables). (Reproduced with permission from Siggaard-Andersen, 1966.)

$mmol \cdot l^{-1}$). We note that in this open system a change in P_{CO_2} will not alter [BB], or vice versa. Thus, P_{CO_2} and BB are not only independent variables in the sense that they are changes imposed on the system from the outside, but also independent of each other unless the system is subject to "regulation" (see below).

An acid can be conveniently defined as a substance which, when added to a system at constant P_{CO_2}, lowers the pH of the system (see Nahas, 1966; Stewart, 1981). The term strong acid stands for acids that ionize completely (or almost completely) into H^+ ions and the corresponding anion (e.g. hydrochloric, sulfuric, or lactic acid). A base is defined in a corresponding manner. Some bases ionize into a cation and OH^- (e.g. NaOH). However, others increase pH by removing H^+ according to the reaction $[NH_3^+] + [H^+] \rightleftharpoons [NH_4^+]$. Such compounds are usually called "add-on bases" (e.g. Stewart, 1981).

Controversy has long revolved around the term pH, defined as $pH = -\log[H^+]$, where $[H^+]$ is the hydrogen ion concentration (more accurately: the hydrogen ion activity). Little advantage is gained by abandoning the pH term. Besides, as emphasized by some authorities, many biological processes in which H^+ is involved are proportional, not to H^+ concentration, but to its logarithm (Van Slyke, 1922; Davis, 1967). It should be emphasized that neither pH nor $[H^+]$ can be precisely defined, and that the operational definition of pH rests on the measurement of differences in electrochemical potential between an unknown solution and that of certain standard solutions (Roos and Boron, 1981).

In summary, the resultant of any acid-base perturbation in a closed system in equilibrium with a gas phase is pH (or the H^+ concentration). Changes in this dependent variable are brought about by alterations in P_{CO_2} or BB concentration, the two independent variables.

An extended acid-base model

Clearly, cells are open systems which can exchange, not only CO_2, but also H^+ (and HCO_3^-) with the

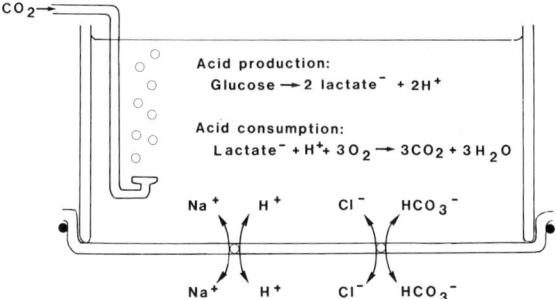

Fig. 2. An extended acid-base model which illustrates that changes in buffer base concentration in intracellular fluids are caused either by production/consumption of metabolic acids or transmembrane ion fluxes via electroneutral cation and anion exchangers.

surroundings. The complexities introduced by this fact can be covered by an extended model, which has two additional features (Fig. 2). First, it is endowed with a membrane which allows fluxes of either H^+ or HCO_3^- between the system and its surroundings. We will later return to the membrane devices allowing such fluxes and provisionally state that outflux of H^+ is synonymous with influx of HCO_3^-, and vice versa. Furthermore, for reasons given below we will assume that transmembrane fluxes of H^+ and HCO_3^- occur as Na^+/H^+ and Cl^-/HCO_3^- exchanges. The molecular devices facilitating such exchanges ("antiport" systems) are assumed to be electroneutral, and to catalyze exchange in any direction, dependent on the chemical gradient of the coupled exchange. The second feature of our model system is that it is capable of forming metabolic acids, as exemplified by production of lactic acid and its ionization into H^+ and lactate anions (la^-). Obviously, since lactic acid is a relatively strong acid (pK' about 3.9) such production will lead to a stoichiometrical decrease in buffer base concentration. We also note that if lactate anions should be metabolized to CO_2 and H_2O, a corresponding amount of H^+ will be removed (increase in BB concentration). It is clear, therefore, that changes in [BB] can be induced by two means: production/consumption of acids and transmembrane fluxes of H^+ or HCO_3^-. However, the basic principles are the same: the two independent variables (P_{CO_2} and BB concentration) determine the dependent one (pH).

The quantitative approach

A simulated extracellular fluid

A better understanding of acid-base changes in biological systems requires a quantitative approach, as realized decades ago (e.g. Van Slyke, 1922; Edsall and Wyman, 1958). It seems profitable to begin by considering a simple Na^+, Cl^-, HCO_3^- system with an ionic strength of 0.16 mol·l^{-1}, equilibrated with CO_2 at a temperature of 38°C. For such a system, in itself a good approximation of extracellular fluid (and CSF), the acid-base relations are described by four equations:

$$[H^+] \cdot [OH^-] = K'_w \quad (1)$$

$$[H_2CO_3] \cdot K^* = P_{CO_2} \cdot S \cdot K'_1 = [H^+] \cdot [HCO_3^-] \quad (2)$$

$$[HCO_3^-] \cdot K'_2 = [H^+] \cdot [CO_3^{2-}] \quad (3)$$

$$[Na^+] + [H^+] = [Cl^-] + [OH^-] + [HCO_3^-] + 2[CO_3^{2-}] \quad (4)$$

The first of these equations describes the ionization of water, the second and third the ionization of H_2CO_3 and HCO_3^-, respectively, and the fourth the requirement for electrical neutrality. K'_w, K'_1 and K'_2 are ionization constants. For the system under study they have the following values (with the dimensions omitted): $K'_w = 10^{-13.6}$, $K'_1 = 10^{-6.1}$, $K'_2 = 10^{-9.8}$. We note that since H_2CO_3 is proportional to the amount of CO_2 dissolved ($[CO_2]$), and the latter to P_{CO_2}, it is permissable to express the H_2CO_3 concentration as $P_{CO_2} \cdot S$ where S is a solubility coefficient, having a value of $3.1 \cdot 10^{-5}$ mol·l^{-1}·mmHg^{-1}. When this is done, a K'_1 value of $10^{-6.1}$ should be used (K^* is larger). In equation (4) the molar concentration of CO_3^{2-}, a divalent ion, has been multiplied by two to give the charge contribution.

Equation (4) can be expanded to include also other strong cations than Na^+ (e.g. K^+, Ca^{2+}) and other strong anions than Cl^- (e.g. SO_4^{2-}, $lactate^-$). The term "strong" then simply means that these ions remain uncombined, i.e. they do not participate in acid-base events by combining with H^+, OH^-, HCO_3^-, or CO_3^{2-}. Following substitution of terms the equation can then be written as

$$[Cat^+] - [An^-] = \frac{K_w}{[H^+]} - [H^+] + \frac{P_{CO_2} \cdot S \cdot K_1'}{[H^+]} \left(1 + \frac{2 \cdot K_2'}{[H^+]}\right) \quad (5)$$

At pH values between 6 and 8 the term $K_w/[H^+] - [H^+]$, which expresses the difference $[OH^-] - [H^+]$, can be neglected without significant loss of accuracy. Since the term $[Cat^+] - [An^-]$ is equal to the buffer base concentration the equation simplifies into

$$[BB] = \frac{P_{CO_2} \cdot S_1 \cdot K_1'}{[H^+]} \left(1 + \frac{2 \cdot K_2'}{[H^+]}\right) \quad (6)$$

This was the equation given in one previous publication (Siesjö, 1972). The equation describes the influence of the two independent variables (P_{CO_2} and BB) on the dependent one (H^+, or pH). We note that the right hand term is equal to $[HCO_3^-]$ plus $[CO_3^{2-}]$ and that at pH < 7.8, the latter is less than 2% of $[HCO_3^-]$. As a fair approximation, therefore, one can neglect the CO_3^{2-} concentration at pH values below 8. Equation (6) then simplifies into

$$[BB] = [HCO_3^-] = \frac{P_{CO_2} \cdot S \cdot K_1'}{[H^+]} \quad (7)$$

In other words, addition of strong acid will cause a mole to mole decrease in HCO_3^- concentration or, stated differently, the deviation of $[HCO_3^-]$ from normal adequately describes the number of moles of acid or base added.

A simulated intracellular fluid

For such a fluid, equations (1)–(3) are still valid, and we must be able to write an equation expressing the requirement for electrical neutrality (4). However, intracellular fluids (and blood) differ from extracellular fluids (ECF) by containing other buffers than the H_2CO_3/HCO_3^- system. Such buffers, which usually are weak acids, comprise free or bound phosphate, and protein groups which ionize at physiological pH values (e.g. imidazole groups). We neither know the exact concentrations nor the pK_{Ha} values of these acids. However, it seems reasonable to conclude that the pK values cover a relatively large range of pH values around 7.0.

In order to describe the acid-base behavior of our simulated intracellular fluid, we need two additional equations, describing the ionization of a weak acid (Ha), and the conservation of mass, i.e. the constancy of total buffer concentration (C). We then get

$$[Ha] \cdot K_{Ha}' = [H^+] \cdot [a^-] \quad (8)$$

$$C = [Ha] + [a^-] \quad (9)$$

By substitution of terms we can now expand equation (6) to give the following equation

$$[BB] = \frac{P_{CO_2} \cdot S \cdot K_1'}{[H^+]} \left(1 + \frac{2K_2'}{[H^+]}\right) + \frac{C \cdot K_{Ha}}{[H^+] + K_{Ha}} \quad (10)$$

As described previously (Siesjö and Messeter, 1971; Siesjö, 1973), the equation can be properly expanded to include several buffer systems (C_1, C_2, C_3 etc.), with their appropriate K_{Ha} values. As a puristic approach, it can also be expanded to include the terms for H^+ and OH^- as in equation (5). If we neglect these, and the CO_3^{2-} concentration, we can write

$$[BB] = [HCO_3^-] + [a^-]_1 + \ldots\ldots [a^-]_n \quad (11)$$

Thus, the BB concentration is now equal to the sum of the concentrations of HCO_3^- and all anions of buffer acids. What is, then, a buffer acid and how does it differ from a strong acid? A buffer acid, and its anion, participate in acid-base reactions, releasing or combining with H$^+$ ions. Its participation in such reactions depends on the K_{Ha} value. At pH values <8 an acid with a K_{Ha} value of 10^{-10} will be more than 99% undissociated, and remain so, and at pH values >6 an acid with $K_{Ha} = 10^{-4}$ will be more than 99% dissociated. Thus, the terms strong and weak are relative. However, for all practical purposes buffer acids can be defined as those having K_{Ha} values in the range 10^{-5} to 10^{-9} and, as will be described below, only those having K_{Ha} values in the range 10^{-6} to 10^{-8} function efficiently as buffers at normal pH$_i$ values, the efficacy of any given buffer being maximal when pK_{Ha} = pH.

To exemplify the acid-base behavior of extra- and intracellular fluids we will now consider changes in pH and [HCO$_3^-$] induced by alterations in buffer base concentration and in P$_{CO_2}$. For both fluids we assume a starting P$_{CO_2}$ of 45 mmHg. The extracellular fluid (ECF) has a starting pH of 7.3 and, therefore, a [HCO$_3^-$] of 22 mmol · l^{-1}. The intracellular fluid (ICF) is assumed to have a pH of 7.0. At a P$_{CO_2}$ of 45 mmHg this gives [HCO$_3^-$] = 11 mmol · l^{-1}. Previous results suggest that the cellular buffer capacity can be reproduced if the system is endowed with a total buffer concentration (C) of 0.050 mol · l^{-1} (Siesjö and Messeter, 1971). In some examples given below I have used five K_{Ha} values ($10^{-6.4}$, $10^{-6.7}$, $10^{-7.0}$, $10^{-7.3}$, $10^{-7.6}$), each buffer having a concentration of 0.010 mol · l^{-1} but, in others, the pK of a single acid has been set equal to the starting pH. In all instances, I calculated H$^+$ and HCO$_3^-$ for different values of P$_{CO_2}$ and [BB], using an iterative procedure with a program adopted for a Basic desk computer with a 28K memory. In these calculations, all relevant equations were included, and the terms [OH$^-$], [H$^+$] and [CO$_3^{2-}$] were retained in the equations for electrical neutrality.

Fig. 3 shows how pH and [HCO$_3^-$] vary with the buffer base concentration (left panels) and with P$_{CO_2}$ (right panels). Some changes observed are those expected. For example, decreases or increases in P$_{CO_2}$ give larger pH changes in ECF than in ICF, i.e. the latter is better "buffered". Intuitively, we

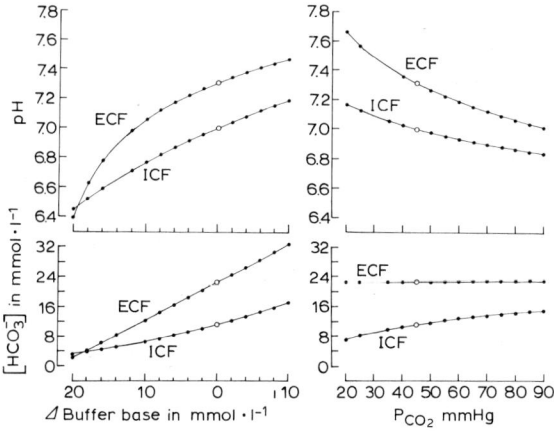

Fig. 3. Changes in pH and HCO$_3^-$ concentration of simulated extracellular fluid (ECF) and intracellular fluid (ICF) with changes in buffer base concentration (left panels) or in P$_{CO_2}$ (right panels). Initial conditions were: P$_{CO_2}$ = 45 mmHg, pH$_e$ = 7.3, pH$_i$ = 7.0. ICF was assumed to contain non-bicarbonate buffers in a concentration of 0.050 mol · l^{-1} (five acids, pK_{Ha} 6.4–7.6).

ascribe this to the presence of non-bicarbonate buffer systems. As a corollary, the HCO$_3^-$ concentration of ECF remains essentially unchanged while that of ICF varies with P$_{CO_2}$.

In the left panel we observe that, as expected, Δ [BB] = Δ [HCO$_3^-$] for ECF, while Δ [BB] > Δ [HCO$_3^-$] for ICF. Unexpectedly, in the [BB] range ± 10 mmol · l^{-1}, the pH changes are very similar in ECF and ICF, demonstrating similar buffer capacities to addition of strong acid or base, and it is first when more than 20 mmol · l^{-1} of acid is added that ECF pH falls precipitously. We note that at Δ [BB] = -19 mmol · l^{-1}, pH$_{ECF}$ = pH$_{ICF}$.

The Stewart approach

Stewart (1981) has recently given a detailed account of acid-base equilibria in fluids mimicking those of biological origin. In his penetrating treatise, Stewart distinguishes between several independent and dependent variables. As independent variables he lists P$_{CO_2}$, the Strong Ion Difference (SID), and A_{Tot}, and as dependent variables pH (or [H$^+$]), [HCO$_3^-$] and [CO$_3^{2-}$], as well as [a$^-$] and [Ha], i.e. the anions and acids of buffer systems. He arrives at equations identical to equations (5) and (10) above, the terms for [H$^+$] and [OH$^-$] being included. The only difference is, therefore, that Stewart prefers the term SID instead of BB (or Base Excess/Base Deficit), and that he emphasizes the independent nature of A_{Tot} ($= C$ in the equations given above).

Stewart's terminology has been adopted by workers discussing extra- and intracellular acid-base events (e.g. Kraig et al., 1983, 1985; Fencl, 1985). Although I find his approach useful in its rigorous adherence to basic principles, two of the main postulates are potentially misleading. First, since SID is one of two independent variables (A_{Tot} or C is usually constant in the systems under study) Stewart emphasizes that changes in pH (or $[H^+]$) at constant P_{CO_2} are due to accumulation or loss of strong cations or anions, and not of H^+ (or HCO_3^-). This has led to confusing statements, e.g. that pH changes are due to fluxes of lactate anions. Second, when setting the initial conditions for a given acid-base system Stewart (1981) gives it a value for SID, as calculated from the equation [SID] = $[Cat^+]$ − $[An^-]$. For example, he derives [SID] for an intracellular fluid by considering only K^+, Na^+, and Cl^- concentrations, neglecting the presence of cationic and anionic charges on amino acids or other macromolecules. This is one reason why he arrives at such biologically dubious statements that the presence of buffers in a solution can *decrease* its ability to resist changes in pH. I will attempt clarifying these issues by discussing in turn sources or sinks for H^+ at constant P_{CO_2}, and buffering. In the latter section, it will be emphasized that one commonly used buffer term is conceptually misleading, or indeed erroneous.

Changes in buffer base — sources and sinks for H^+

Inspection of Fig. 2 (see above) reveals that a decrease in [BB] (or [SID]) can be due to two events. First, if we let the system represent an intracellular fluid, it may be caused by the production of a certain amount of strong acid, e.g. lactic acid. Since the acid is strong it ionizes "completely" according to the equation Hla → H^+ + la^-. It is of course correct to state that Δ [BB] = Δ [SID] = Δ [la^-]. However, it is equally correct to conclude that the amount of H^+ added is the same, i.e. the molar amount of H^+ added corresponds to the alteration of [BB] or [SID].

The other cause of a pH change is the efflux/influx of a certain amount of H^+ ions or the influx/efflux of an equal amount of HCO_3^- ions. Stewart is correct in stating that such fluxes *per se* would not change [SID], which is defined as $[Cat^+]$ − $[An^-]$. However, H^+ and HCO_3^- can only be translocated across the membrane together with a counterion, or in exchange for it, to maintain electrical neutrality. For example, the influx of H^+ must occur with an anion (e.g. Cl^-), or there must be counter-transport of another cation (e.g. Na^+). As Fig. 2 indicates, major transmembrane fluxes of H^+ and HCO_3^- seem to occur by antiport ion transport which allow coupled Na^+/H^+ and Cl^-/HCO_3^- exchange. Acidification of any of the two compartments by the Na^+/H^+ or the Cl^-/HCO_3^- antiporter involves loss of strong cation or gain of strong anion, and the amounts of Na^+ or Cl^- translocated quantitatively determine Δ [SID] or Δ [BB]. However, equal amounts of H^+ or HCO_3^- have traversed the membrane. Thus, it is equally correct to state that when [SID] or [BB] have changed by a given amount, the same amount of H^+ has been added, or removed. Clearly, if Na^+ leaves in exchange for K^+ (or Ca^{2+}), or if Cl^- enters in exchange for e.g. $lactate^-$, [SID] or [BB] do not change. Thus, fluxes of strong ions lead to changes in pH only if the counterions are H^+ or HCO_3^-.

One special mode of acidifying ECF is that due to acid production in the ICF. Suppose that la^- left ICF and ended up in the ECF. This could only occur if la^- passed the membrane with a cation, or in exchange for an anion. If the cation were K^+ or Na^+, or the anion Cl^-, [BB] or [SID] would not change, nor would pH. Clearly, acidification of ECF can only occur if la^- enters ECF together with H^+, i.e. as lactic acid. This seems to occur by "nonionic diffusion" (see Roos and Boron, 1981). Thus, although we regard lactic acid as a strong acid it exists to a very small extent as unionized acid and since this is much more permeable than the anion, it leaks out, acidifying the ECF. In other words, it is lactic acid and not lactate which reduces the pH of both ICF and ECF.

Stewart's emphasis on strong ion changes as determinants of pH has led to the dubious statement that H^+ and HCO_3^- concentrations in one compartment cannot *per se* influence the corresponding concentrations of another compartment. This statement is wrong, since H^+ and HCO_3^- concentrations enter as thermodynamic determinants of ionic flux, catalyzed by the Na^+/H^+ and Cl^-/HCO_3^- exchanges (see below).

In summary, although [BB] (or [SID]) is the dependent variable altering pH at constant P_{CO_2}, a change in [BB] (or [SID]) implies that a corresponding amount of H^+ has been added or removed. We also note that transmembrane loss or gain of H^+ is synonymous with a corresponding gain or loss of HCO_3^-, and that such fluxes cause pH to change in opposite direction in the two fluids separated by the membrane.

Buffers and buffering

The buffer capacity of a solution to addition of strong acid or base is unequivocal. In 1922, Van Slyke discussed the buffer value (β), defined as

$$\beta = \frac{\Delta B}{\Delta pH} \quad (12)$$

in which β is the amount of strong base (plus sign) or strong acid (minus sign) added. β is thus the amount of acid or base required to cause a unit change in pH. As pointed out by Roos and Boron (1981), it is inappropriate to give β in units of "Slykes" since expression (12) was defined before Van Slyke (1922) by Koppel and Spiro (1919).

These early publications clearly demonstrate that β for a solution containing a buffer acid and its anion depends on C (the total buffer concentration), K_{Ha}, and pH. Thus, at any given pH, β varies linearly with C. Furthermore, at any given C, β is maximal when pH = pK_{Ha}. When pK_{Ha} deviates from pH by 1 unit, β is reduced to 33% of the maximal value, and when it deviates by 2 units, β is only 4% of the maximal value. Thus, buffer acids with pK_{Ha} values lower than 5 or values higher than 9 should play a very little role in buffering tissue fluids with pH values in the range 6.5–7.5.

In order to illustrate buffering against changes in [BB], we consider two solutions, each having a P_{CO_2} of 45 mmHg. One of them has a starting pH of 7.3 (equal to that of ECF) and the other a pH of 7.0 (equal to that of ICF). If we add to each of them a non-bicarbonate buffer at concentrations of 0.0125, 0.025, and 0.050 M, respectively, and let pK_{Ha} = pH (maximal buffer capacity), we obtain the curves of Fig. 4. Two results emerge. First, the buffer capacities of the solutions are proportional to C, the concentration of the non-bicarbonate buffer. Second, at a starting pH of 7.3, the influence of such buffers is indeed moderate but, at pH 7.0, it is pronounced.

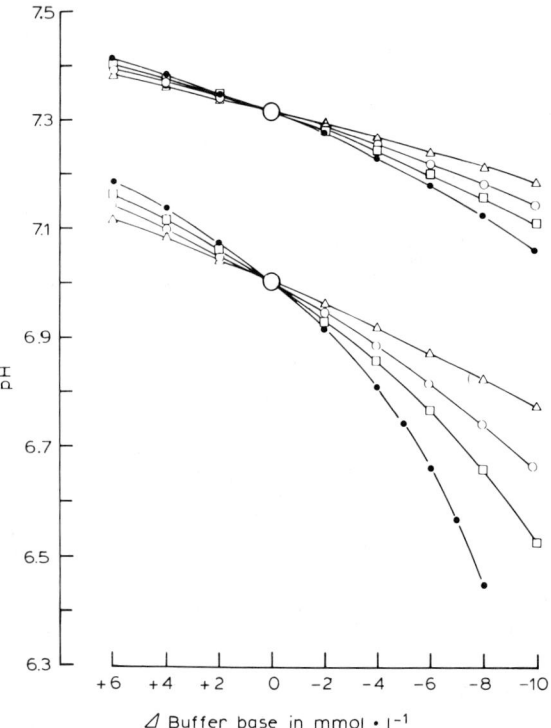

Fig. 4. Influence of non-bicarbonate buffers on buffer capacity ($\Delta B/\Delta$ pH) of a system with P_{CO_2} of 45 mmHg and a starting pH of either 7.3 or 7.0. The concentrations of non-bicarbonate buffers (one buffer acid, pK_{Ha} = pH) were the following: 0 (●—●), 0.0125 mol · l^{-1} (□—□), 0.025 mol · l^{-1} (○—○), and 0.050 mol · l^{-1} (△—△).

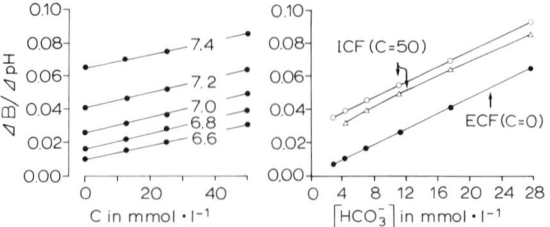

Fig. 5. Dependence of the buffer capacity ($\Delta B/\Delta$ pH) on total buffer concentration (C), and on HCO_3^- concentration. The P_{CO_2} was held at 45 mmHg throughout. The left panel shows that, at each initial pH studied, $\Delta B/\Delta$ pH is linearly related to C (one buffer acid, pK_{Ha} = pH), and that at each C value studied, $\Delta B/\Delta$ pH increases with pH. The reason for this is given in the right panel which shows that $\Delta B/\Delta$ pH varies linearly with $[HCO_3^-]$. In ECF, $\Delta B/\Delta$ pH decreases towards zero with $[HCO_3^-]$. In ICF, the presence of non-bicarbonate buffers gives the system a buffer capacity, proportional to $[C]$, even at $[HCO_3^-] = 0$. If C is maintained at 0.050 mol·l^{-1}, but distributed over five buffer systems (each with $C = 0.010$ mol·l^{-1}, pK_{Ha} = 6.4–7.6), $\Delta B/\Delta$ pH is reduced (triangles).

The behavior of the two solutions is explained by the data of Fig. 5. We observe from the left panel that at any given pH, β is linearly dependent on C. Furthermore, although β varies with pH, the dependence is not linear. The right hand panel shows, though, that at any given C value β is linearly dependent on the HCO_3^- concentration. In an unbuffered solution, i.e. when $C = 0$, β becomes infinitesimally small when $[HCO_3^-]$ is reduced to zero. At a total buffer concentration of 0.050 mol·l^{-1}, one observes the same, linear dependence of β upon $[HCO_3^-]$. However, when the latter is reduced to zero, β is 0.029 mol·l^{-1}. If the total buffer concentration is the same but the buffers are composed of five acids with different K_{Ha} values ($10^{-6.4}$, $10^{-6.7}$, $10^{-7.0}$, $10^{-7.3}$, and $10^{-7.7}$) β is somewhat lower, and its dependence on $[HCO_3^-]$ deviates somewhat from linearity.

For equal concentrations of $[HCO_3^-]$ and C the former has a much larger influence on β. In fact, if the P_{CO_2} is held constant, HCO_3^- has 2.3 times the buffer value of non-volatile, non-bicarbonate buffers (Woodbury, 1965; see also Roos and Boron, 1981). This is why normal ECF ($C = 0$, $[HCO_3^-] = 0.023$ mol·l^{-1}) has a larger buffer capacity than ICF ($C = 0.050$ mol·l^{-1}, $[HCO_3^-] = 0.011$ mol·l^{-1}). It is now also apparent why the buffer capacity of ECF becomes very low when $[HCO_3^-]$ approaches zero, and why ICF retains a significant buffer capacity at very low pH values.

The conclusions drawn from Figs. 4 and 5 are obviously at variance with those of Stewart (1981) who states that addition of a weak acid to a Na^+, Cl^- or a Na^+, Cl^-, HCO_3^- solution *decreases* the buffer capacity. The discrepancy arises because Stewart makes the comparisons at widely different pH values and HCO_3^- concentrations, defining instead a starting [SID] value. In discussing the biological advantage of buffers it seems to be more reasonable to make the comparison at the existing pH and $[HCO_3^-]$ values. When this is done it becomes obvious that the presence of buffers does indeed decrease the pH change for a given addition of acid or base. However, we recognize that the advantage gained is larger at the pH of intracellular fluids (pH $\approx$ 7.0) than at that of extracellular fluids (pH $\approx$ 7.3).

The conceptual meaning of β is clear: it gives the change in the dependent variable (Δ pH) for a defined alteration in one of the independent ones (Δ BB). Controversy revolves around corresponding expressions for Δ pH as a function of the other independent variable, i.e. P_{CO_2}. Some authors have exploited the fact that the relationship between log P_{CO_2} and pH is close to linear, expressing CO_2 as

$$\beta_{CO_2} = \frac{\Delta \log P_{CO_2}}{\Delta \text{ pH}} \qquad (13)$$

(e.g. Siggaard-Andersen, 1966; Siesjö and Messeter, 1971). Since the expression is not ideal a more unambiguous one was suggested, the "percent pH regulation" (Siesjö, 1971). The designation of the Δ log P_{CO_2}/Δ pH ratio as a buffer "capacity" has been criticized (Karman and Held, 1972). However, this is a semantic problem, not a conceptual one. A more important controversy revolves around the use of the ratio $\Delta [HCO_3^-]/\Delta$ pH to express buffering against CO_2. The expression was suggested by Woodbury (1965) who based it on Van Slyke's discussion of buffering in CO_2-containing media (Van Slyke, 1922). This misinterpretation has unfortunately been perpetuated in subsequent publications and caused considerable confusion (e.g. Karman and Held, 1972; Thomas, 1976; see also Roos and Boron, 1981). It seems necessary, therefore, to discuss in some more detail buffering against changes in P_{CO_2}.

In his article from 1922, Van Slyke attempted to calculate the buffer value ($\Delta B/\Delta$ pH) for normal blood, having access to data on pH and $[HCO_3^-]$ at varying P_{CO_2} values. He reasoned that, in considering titration of buffers other than the HCO_3^-/H_2CO_3 system, $\Delta B = \Delta [HCO_3^-]$. This follows from equation (11) above. In other words, since [BB] was not altered $\Delta [HCO_3^-]$ must be numerically equal to $\Delta [a^-]$. Therefore, Van Slyke could calculate β *for the non-bicarbonate buffers* by assuming that $\Delta [HCO_3^-]$ was equivalent to the amount of strong acid or base which had to be added to give the observed change in $\Delta [a^-]$. In this way, he arrived at a value of for the non-bicarbonate buffers of 0.021 mol · l^{-1}. Inspection of Fig. 5 (see above) shows that this value is reasonable for a non-bicarbonate buffer system with $C = 0.04$ mol · l^{-1}. However, Van Slyke did not suggest that the $\Delta [HCO_3^-]/\Delta$ pH ratio could be used to express buffering against changes in P_{CO_2}.

This is where the error arose. In addition, Woodbury (1965; see also Karman and Held, 1972) reasoned that when P_{CO_2} is increased the amount of H$^+$ "added" stems from H_2CO_3 whose ionization gives rise to equal amounts of H$^+$ and HCO_3^-. Accordingly, $\Delta [HCO_3^-]$ was assumed to express the amount of H$^+$ "titrating" the solution. There are several awkward implications of this assumption. *First*, the expression $\Delta [HCO_3^-]/\Delta$ pH gives the change in one dependent variable (pH) as a function of another dependent one, i.e. $[HCO_3^-]$. *Second*, the expression leads to dubious conclusions with respect to the amount of acid added. Suppose that P_{CO_2} is increased by 10 mmHg in our model ECF and ICF solutions. In the former, $[HCO_3^-]$ is not measurably altered but pH falls by 0.087 units. In the latter, $[HCO_3^-]$ increases by 1.1 mmol · l^{-1}, and pH falls by 0.050 units. Using the concept of $\Delta [HCO_3^-]/\Delta$ pH, we thus arrive at the conclusion that addition of an infinitesimally small amount of acid gives a larger change in pH than addition of a larger amount of acid does. *Third*, if the expressions $\Delta B/\Delta$ pH and $\Delta [HCO_3^-]/\Delta$ pH were really comparable it would be possible to increase the P_{CO_2}, calculate the amount of acid added as $\Delta [HCO_3^-]$, and bring pH back to normal by adding a stoichiometrical amount of strong base. This is of course not possible, as any calculation shows.

Stewart's (1981) strict adherence to basic chemical principles made him emphasize that the only satisfactory way of expressing buffering against CO_2 is by using the expression $\Delta P_{CO_2}/\Delta$ pH, i.e. the change in the dependent variable pH as a function of the independent variable P_{CO_2} (cf. $\Delta \log P_{CO_2}/\Delta$ pH). I agree with him that this is the most sensible approach. In Fig. 6, pH has been given as a function of P_{CO_2} in solutions with starting pH values of 7.4, 7.0, and 6.6, each being either unbuffered ($C = 0$) or endowed with a single buffer with concentrations of 0.0125, 0.025, and 0.050 mol · l^{-1}, and with pK_{Ha} set equal to pH (maximal buffering). The following results emerge. First, in unbuffered solutions ($C = 0$), the curves are identical at different pH values, i.e. buffering is independent of pH. We note, though, that at each starting pH, the buffering capacity decreases at low and increases at high CO_2 tensions. Second, addition of a non-bicarbonate buffer increases the buffer capacity. However, the effect is most pronounced at low pH values (and BB concentrations). Third, at low pH values and high buffer capacity the relationship between P_{CO_2} and pH is not far from being linear, at least in the P_{CO_2} range 45–75 mmHg.

Fig. 7 (left panel) gives β_{CO_2} as a function of C at different initial pH values. We note that at these pH values β_{CO_2} of unbuffered solutions is 100, i.e. the solutions have a finite buffer capacity. However, this decreases if P_{CO_2} is lowered (see Fig. 6 above). Fig. 7 also shows that at any initial pH value, β_{CO_2} is linearily related to C. Finally, at any given C value, β_{CO_2} increases with decreasing pH. For comparison, Fig. 7 (right panel) gives

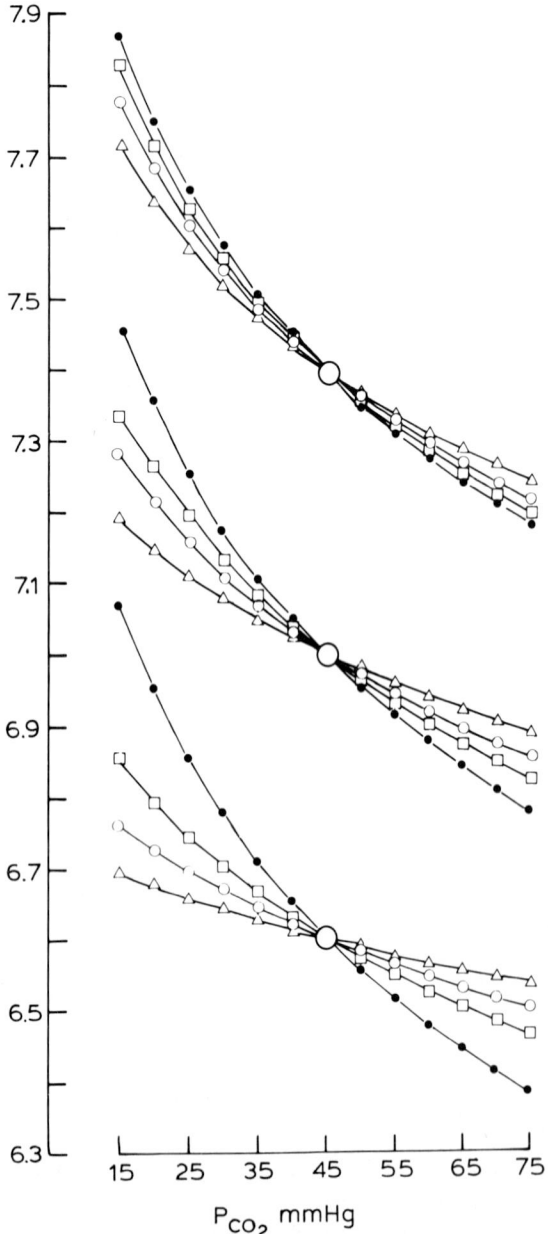

Fig. 6. Influence of non-bicarbonate buffers on buffer capacity of a system towards changes in $P_{CO_2}(\Delta P_{CO_2}/\Delta\,pH)$. Starting pH was 7.4, 7.0, or 6.6. The concentrations of non-bicarbonate buffers were the following: 0 (●—●), 0.0125 mol · l^{-1} (□—□), 0.025 mol · l^{-1} (○—○), and 0.050 mol · l^{-1} (△—△).

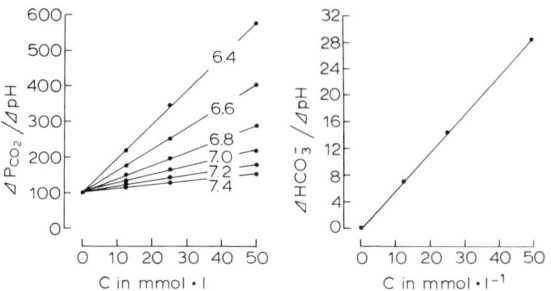

Fig. 7. Dependence of the buffer capacity towards changes in $P_{CO_2}(\Delta P_{CO_2}/\Delta\,pH)$ on the concentration of non-bicarbonate buffers (C). The left panel shows that at any given initial pH, $\Delta P_{CO_2}/\Delta\,pH$ is linearly dependent on C. The expression $\Delta\,[HCO_3^-]/\Delta\,pH$, which has erroneously been used to express buffering towards CO_2, is also linearly dependent on C; however, it does not vary with pH (right panel).

$\Delta\,[HCO_3^-]/\Delta\,pH$ as a function of C. A comparison between this curve, and one given previously (see Fig. 5 above), shows that the values for $\Delta\,[HCO_3^-]/\Delta\,pH$ are identical to the $\Delta B/\Delta\,pH$ values for solutions with $[HCO_3^-] = 0$. In other words, the data support Van Slyke's (1922) suggestion that derived values for $\Delta\,[HCO_3^-]/\Delta\,pH$ reflect the buffer capacity ($\Delta B/\Delta\,pH$) of non-bicarbonate buffers. If this expression were used to quantitate buffering against CO_2, though, two erroneous conclusions would arise. First, one would have to conclude that β_{CO_2} is zero at P_{CO_2} 45 mmHg in solutions lacking non-bicarbonate buffers. Second, we would have to conclude that β_{CO_2} does not vary with pH at constant C. Clearly, the expression $\Delta\,[HCO_3^-]/\Delta\,pH$ is untenable.

As emphasized by Stewart (1981) the buffer capacities against changes in [BB] and P_{CO_2} are incomparable since the dimensions are dissimilar. This author has suggested that a comparison can be made by calculating equal percentage changes in [SID] and P_{CO_2}, i.e. % ΔSID versus % ΔP_{CO_2}, the change in pH then being compared. There is an obstacle, though, since the comparison requires that [SID] is known. For intracellular fluid, this is not the case. Stewart (1981) derives [SID] from the concentrations of major intracellular cations and anions, and arrives at a value of 0.13 mol · l^{-1}. This is clearly an erroneous figure since the author ignores the cationic and anionic charges on macromolecules, and the fact that the latter predominate. If equation (11) is solved for $P_{CO_2} = 45$ mmHg, pH

= 7.0, and $C = 0.050$ mol $\cdot$ l^{-1} (five acids, pK_{Ha} 6.4–7.6), [SID] becomes 0.036 mol $\cdot$ l^{-1}, i.e. less than one third of Stewart's value. Clearly, the value 0.036 mol $\cdot$ l^{-1} is an approximation, serving the purpose of a fictitious value useful for derivation of acid-base events resulting from a *change* in [BB]. In view of the uncertainty with respect to the absolute value it seems adventurous to calculate % ΔBB.

Acid-base regulation

Transmembrane distribution of H^+ and HCO_3^-

Before we discuss regulation of pH in extracerebral and cerebral tissues, it seems justified to recall current information on absolute pH values, and on the non-equilibrium distribution of H^+ and HCO_3^-.

Ever since Fenn and Maurer (1936) and Wallace and Hastings (1942) calculated pH$_i$ in skeletal muscle from the HCO_3^- distribution, it has been clear that pH$_i$ of most cells in the body is close to 7.0. Thus, although Conway and Fearon (1944) questioned the validity of the CO$_2$ method, and Carter et al. (1967) obtained pH$_i$ values of close to 6 in skeletal muscle, it now seems established that these values were erroneous (see Roos and Boron, 1981). In the brain, similar values for pH$_i$ (about 7.0) have been obtained with the DMO and the CO$_2$ methods (Roos, 1965, 1971; Messeter and Siesjö, 1971b; Siesjö et al., 1972; Arieff et al., 1976; Pellegrino et al., 1981a). Values for pH$_i$ of around 7.0 have also been obtained by direct electrode measurements in invertebrate neurons (see below). We may use the data of Fig. 8, therefore, to illustrate H^+ and HCO_3^- distribution across nerve cell membranes. The value for the membrane potential (-60 mV) was chosen to facilitate calculations. The true values may vary between -60 and -90 mV. Some of the other variables require comment.

At an arterial P_{CO_2} of about 40 mmHg, the mean tissue CO$_2$ tension is considered to be around 45 mmHg. More precisely, tissue P_{CO_2} should be 0.5–1 mmHg higher than the arithmetic mean of the arterial and the cerebrovenous CO$_2$ tensions (Pontén and Siesjö, 1966; Siesjö, 1972). This is the

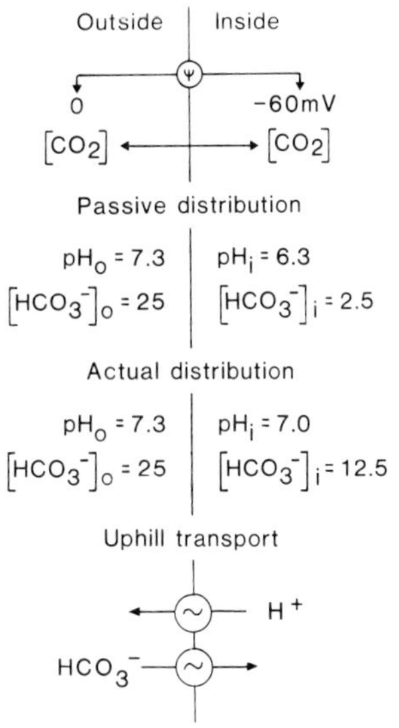

Fig. 8. Non-equilibrium distribution of H^+ and HCO_3^- between extra- and intracellular fluids. At a membrane potential of -60 mV passive distribution of H^+ and HCO_3^-, as calculated from the Nernst equation, gives much lower values for $[HCO_3^-]_i$ and pH$_i$ than those measured. Accordingly, one must postulate the existance of molecular devices which translocate H^+ out, or HCO_3^- in, at the expense of energy ($\sim$).

P_{CO_2} which can be calculated from diffusion theory, and which also can be measured with a surface tissue CO$_2$ electrode, or by using cisternal CSF as a "tonometer". Claims have been made that tissue P_{CO_2} is higher (Davies et al., 1973). However, these claims have not been substantiated. We conclude, therefore, that the tissue CO$_2$ tension is only slightly higher than the arithmetric mean of the arterial and cerebrovenous P_{CO_2} values. It follows from this that two major factors determine tissue P_{CO_2}: the arterial P_{CO_2}, and the CBF, changes in metabolic rate having but small effects (see Pontén and Siesjö, 1966). For all practical purposes, the extra- and intracellular P_{CO_2} values are identical.

The values for pH$_e$ and $[HCO_3^-]_e$ are lower than those measured in cisternal CSF (for data in rats, see Messeter and Siesjö, 1971a; Siesjö et al., 1972; MacMillan and Siesjö, 1973). Results reported in goats suggest that $[HCO_3^-]_{CSF}$ and $[HCO_3^-]_e$ are identical (Fencl et al., 1966; Fencl, 1985). However, since microelectrode pH$_e$ measurements have consistently given values around 7.3 (Kraig et al., 1983; Mutch and Hansen, 1984; Siesjö et al., 1985a), we will assume that these are correct. Accordingly, calculated $[HCO_3^-]_e$ is around 22 mmol · l^{-1}.

The numbers of Fig. 8 demonstrate that H^+ and HCO_3^- are not passively distributed in the electrical field across the membrane. If this were the case, and if the membrane potential (ψ) is 60 mV (inside being negative) the Nernst equation predicts a pH_i of 6.3, and a $[HCO_3^-]_i$ of 2 mmol · l^{-1}. The actual distribution is generally thought to reflect active transport of H^+ (out) or HCO_3^- (in), the forces favoring influx of H^+ or outflux of HCO_3^- being given by the equations

$$\Delta\mu H^+ = \frac{RT}{F} \ln \frac{[H^+]_i}{[H^+]_e} + \psi \qquad (14)$$

$$\Delta\mu HCO_3^- = \frac{RT}{F} \ln \frac{[HCO_3^-]_e}{[HCO_3^-]_i} - \psi \qquad (15)$$

However, these equations are valid only if H^+ and HCO_3^- would move across the membrane carrying a charge (conductive flux). If the major part of these fluxes occurs as electrosilent Na^+/H^+ and Cl^-/HCO_3^- exchanges, the driving forces are given by the equations (see Cala, 1983)

$$\Delta\mu_{Na^+ - H^+} = RT \ln \frac{[Na^+]_i}{[Na^+]_o}$$

$$- RT \ln \frac{[H^+]_i}{[H^+]_o} \qquad (16)$$

$$\Delta\mu_{Cl^- - HCO_3^-} = RT \ln \frac{[Cl^-]_i}{[Cl^-]_o}$$

$$- RT \ln \frac{[HCO_3^-]_i}{[HCO_3^-]_o} \qquad (17)$$

If these are the mechanisms the membrane potential plays little role for the net translocation of H^+ or HCO_3^- across the membrane. Furthermore, one cannot make predictions about the direction of H^+ or HCO_3^- flux unless the Na^+ and Cl^- gradients are known. Clearly, membranes must contain pores which allow some conductive flux of H^+ along the electrochemical gradient of that ion. However, such flux may be small, especially since the chemical gradients are miniscule. Suppose that H^+ flux almost exclusively occurs via a Na^+/H^+ antiporter. Since the normal gradient for Na^+ is about 10:1 (extra- to intracellular fluid) one must then conclude that the normal Na^+/H^+ gradient favors *outflux* of H^+. In fact, this may well constitute the major mechanism for H^+ extrusion (Fig. 9). Thus, we can envisage that Na^+ extrusion via an ATP-driven Na^+/K^+ exchange creates the force (the Na^+ gradient) which expels H^+ in exchange

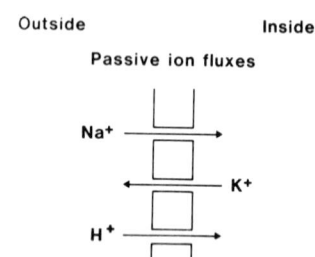

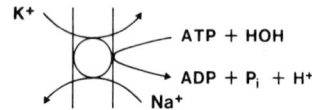

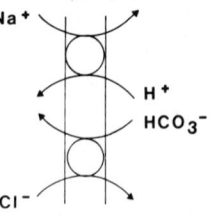

Fig. 9. Proposed mechanisms of acid extrusion from cells, and for back leakage of H^+ into the cells. The dissipative ("passive") fluxes of K^+ and Na^+ activate the Na^+-K^+-dependent ATPase, which maintains the ionic gradients at the expense of ATP energy. The Na^+ gradient, so created, allows Na^+ to enter by another dissipative pathway, one which is electroneutral and allow a 1:1 exchange between Na^+ and H^+. Back leakage of H^+ into the cell is assumed to occur by HCO_3^- efflux via a Cl^-/HCO_3^- ion exchanger.

for Na^+ when the latter leaks back into the cell. How is the H^+ gradient then dissipated? As will be discussed below, one possibility is that influx of H^+ occurs as HCO_3^- loss via a Cl^-/HCO_3^- antiporter. We recognize that this exchange is favored by the normal extra- to intracellular Cl^- gradient (10:1). Although such coupled exchanges seem likely, the issue is complicated by claims that *influx* of HCO_3^- occurs during pH regulation and that it may, at least under some circumstances, be driven by metabolic energy (see below).

Regulation of pH_i

Brain tissues

The mere fact that H^+ and HCO_3^- are not passively distributed across cell membranes suggests that pH_i should be subject to regulation. However, conclusive evidence was not obtained until 1971, when it was shown that hypercapnia initially leads to a clear decrease in pH_i which is then gradually altered towards normal values (Messeter and Siesjö, 1971b; Siesjö and Messeter, 1971). On the basis of the results obtained it was postulated that three mechanisms contribute to this regulation (Siesjö and Messeter, 1971; Siesjö, 1971, 1973):
(a) physicochemical buffering;
(b) consumption of metabolic acids; and
(c) transmembrane transport of H^+/HCO_3^-.

The importance of physicochemical buffering is obvious. Consider a system with a P_{CO_2} of 45 mmHg and a pH of close to 7.0. If P_{CO_2} is raised by 40 mmHg, and the system contains no non-bicarbonate buffers, pH should decrease by 0.28 units, but if it contains non-bicarbonate buffers at a concentration of $0.05\ mol \cdot l^{-1}$, Δ pH is limited to about 0.15 units. In the experiments quoted (see Messeter and Siesjö, 1971b) the Δ pH was 0.13, 0.09, and 0.03 after 15, 45, and 180 min, respectively. It seemed likely that already after 15 min, some mechanism other than physicochemical buffering had limited the fall in pH, a mechanism which achieved consumption of H^+ ions, or their translocation from intra- to extracellular fluids. Subsequent results reinforced the need to invoke such mechanisms. Thus, Ahmad and Loeschcke (1982) reported that in the first minutes of hypercapnia, $ECF[HCO_3^-]$ rose with a corresponding fall in $[Cl^-]$, suggesting that HCO_3^- was lost from parenchymal (glial?) cells in exchange for Cl^- (observe that this should lead to a *reduction* in intracellular BB concentration). Our results defined an acid consumption of sufficient magnitude to account for a large part of the pH_i regulation during the first 45 min of hypercapnia. As Fig. 10 shows, this entails reduction of the tissue concentrations of metabolites distal to the phosphofructokinase step, including glycolytic metabolites, citric acid cycle intermediates, and associated amino acids. Since most of these carbohydrate metabolites exist as anions of metabolic acids, their oxidation should lead to a stoichiometrical removal of H^+, and a similar effect should result from the oxidation of diprotic amino acids (glutamate and aspartate).

The mechanism proposed is perhaps more easy to grasp if we consider changes occurring during hypocapnia. It had been known for some time that a reduction in tissue CO_2 tension triggers increased production of lactic acid (e.g. Weyne et al., 1968; Kjällqvist et al., 1969), and it soon became clear that tissue concentrations of other acids also increased (MacMillan and Siesjö, 1973). Essentially, therefore, hypocapnia represents the opposite situation to hypercapnia. Evidence accumulated that such acid production limited the rise in pH_i and that, at very low CO_2 tensions, pH_i returned to normal, or subnormal values (Fig. 11). One could envisage, therefore, that the cell responds to hypercapnia with consumption of metabolic acids, and to hypocapnia with production of such acids, and that the effects are elicited by modulation of the rate of delivery of carbon skeletons from glucose (or glycogen). Presumably, the signal is a change in pH, exerting its main effect at the phosphofructokinase step (see Folbergrová et al., 1975; Miller et al., 1975; Norberg, 1976). One must then assume, though, that an *acid* shift of pH in extreme hypocapnia occurs by an additional modulation of phosphofructokinase activity by impending tissue hypoxia, caused by the reduced CBF (MacMillan and

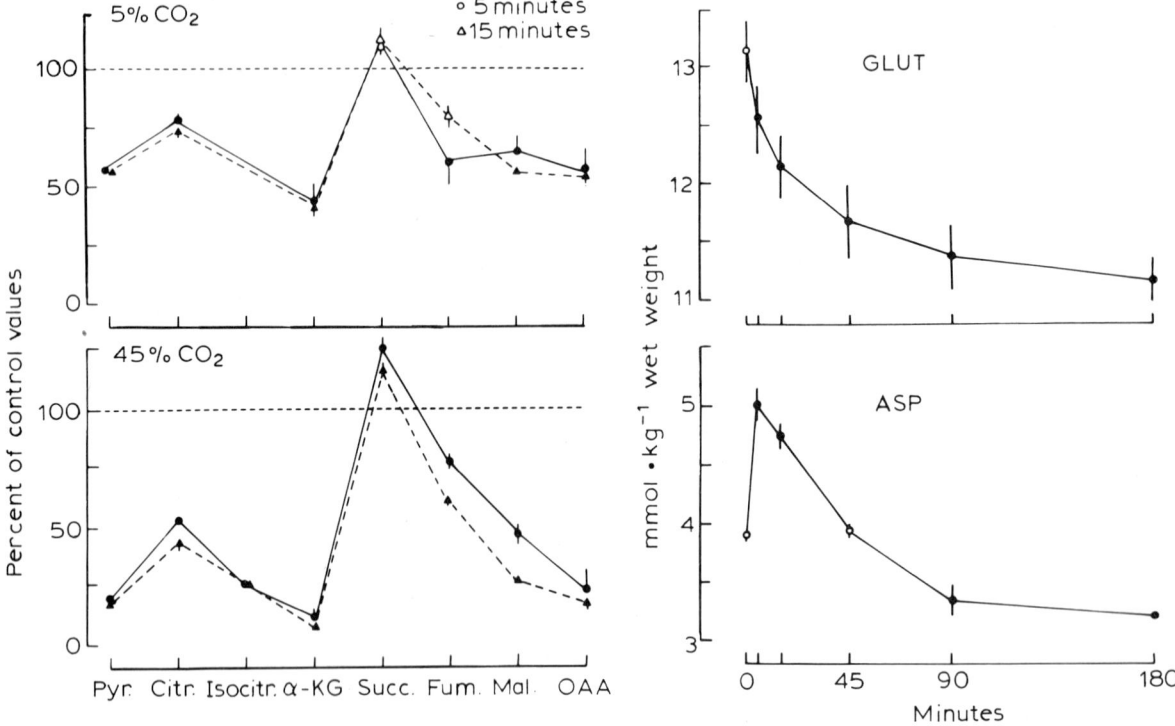

Fig. 10. Consumption of metabolic acids during hypercapnia. The panels to the left (A) demonstrate reductions in tissue concentrations of pyruvate and of all citric acid cycle intermediates except succinate. The "acid consumption", which is proportional to the degree of hypercapnia, is maximal within the first 5–15 min. The panels to the right (B) demonstrate a slower reduction in the tissue concentrations of diprotic amino acids. (Slightly modified after Folbergrová et al., 1972, 1975.)

Siesjö, 1973; however, see also Arieff et al., 1976; Pelligrino et al., 1981a).

Our results led us to conclude that some of the regulation at 45 min of hypercapnia, and most of it occurring thereafter, was due to acid extrusion from cells. However, the evidence for regulation of pH_i by transmembrane fluxes of H^+ or HCO_3^- came later, and had to await the development of new methods.

Isolated cells

With the advent of microelectrode techniques it became feasible to measure intracellular pH of isolated nerve and muscle cells, and to ionophoretically inject acids and bases. Most of this literature has been reviewed by Roos and Boron (1981). In the following, I will discuss selected data obtained on isolated neurons, treating in turn pH changes caused by CO_2 exposure and those caused by addition of strong acid or base. When justified, results obtained on non-neuronal tissues will be recalled for comparison.

It is obvious that direct intracellular pH measurements offer a number of advantages in the pursuit of mechanisms of regulation, especially since they can often be combined with measurements of membrane potential, of intracellular Na^+ and Cl^- activities, and with insertion of electrodes for injection of acid or base. However, it must be kept in mind that the procedures have certain drawbacks. One such drawback is that measurements of intracellular metabolites become difficult (indeed, such measurements have not been performed). As a consequence, it has not been possible to separate events ascribed to buffering or transmembrane fluxes of H^+/HCO_3^- from those involving consumption

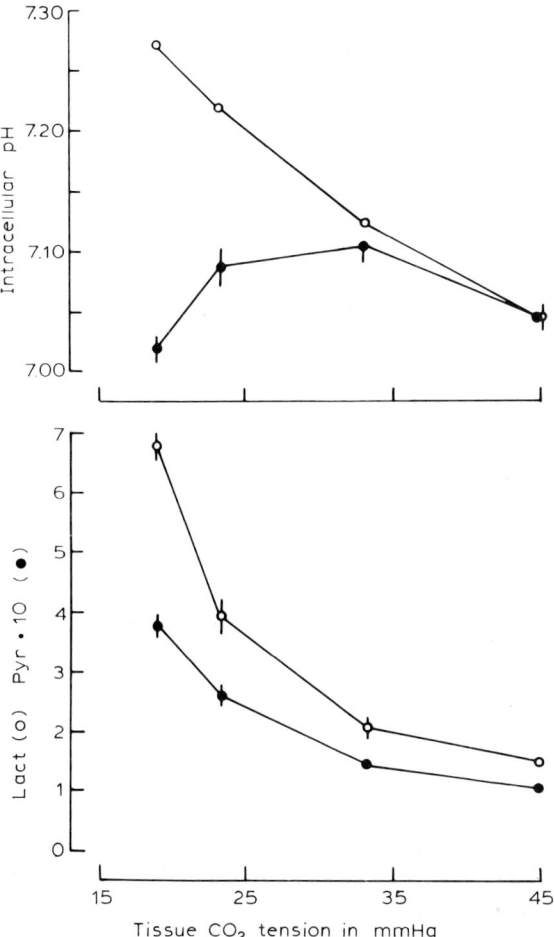

Fig. 11. Regulation of pH$_i$ during hypocapnia by acid production. The upper panel compares actual pH$_i$ values, derived for an ECF volume of 15% (●—●), and those calculated on the assumption that physicochemical buffering alone would regulate pH$_i$ (○—○). The difference between the two curves reflects a decrease in [BB]. The lower panel demonstrates that one likely mechanism is production of metabolic acids. The intracellular lactate and pyruvate concentrations were calculated from the tissue, CSF, and blood contents. (Data from MacMillan and Siesjö, 1973.)

or production of acids. Unfortunately, many experiments have also been conducted under unphysiological conditions, e.g. in the absence of CO_2/HCO_3^-, at reduced temperatures, or at pH$_e$ values of 7.5–8.0. Finally, difficulties of interpretation arise because changes in P_{CO_2} have been induced at constant pH$_e$, i.e. with corresponding al-

terations in $[HCO_3^-]_e$. For all those reasons, one should view the experiments conducted as manipulations aimed at unravelling mechanisms of regulation rather than as examples of physiological regulation.

Regulation of pH$_i$ in response to *changes in* P_{CO_2} has been studied in snail and crayfish neurons (Thomas, 1974, 1976, 1977; Moody, 1981). Fig. 12 (upper panel) shows that although CO_2 exposure leads to an initial acidification, pH$_i$ is quickly regulated towards control values, with a posthypercapnic overshoot in the alkaline direction (Thomas, 1976). The middle panel hints the mechanisms involved (Thomas, 1977). Regulation was virtually completely blocked when intracellular Cl$^-$ was depleted by soaking the cell in Cl$^-$-poor fluids (left) and when extracellular Na$^+$ was replaced by bis(2-hydroxyethyl) dimethylammonium chloride

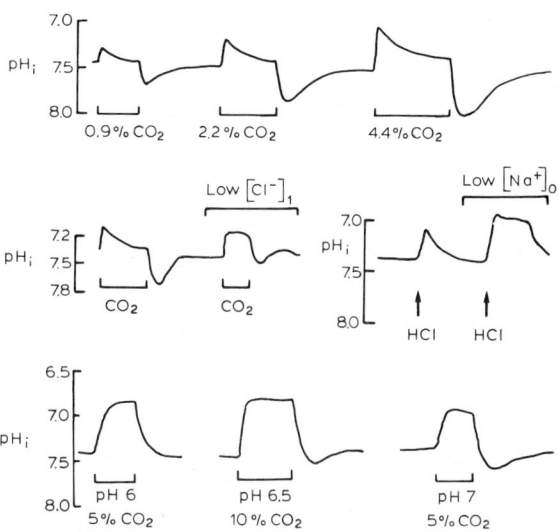

Fig. 12. Regulatory changes in pH$_i$ of *Aplysia* neurons following CO_2 exposure or HCl injection. The upper panel shows that exposure to CO_2 is followed by initial acidification, rapid regulation, and post-exposure alkalosis. The graphs of the middle panel hint at the mechanisms involved. Thus, since regulation during CO_2 exposure was markedly decreased by prior reduction of [Cl$^-$]$_i$, and regulation following HCl injection by depletion of [Na$^+$]$_o$, the results suggest that Cl$^-$/HCO$_3^-$ and Na$^+$/H$^+$ exchanges were involved. The lowermost panel shows that regulation is absent at pH$_o$ = 6.0 and 6.5, and sluggish at pH$_o$ = 7.0. Figures constructed from data reported by Thomas (1974, 1976, 1977).

(right). Since the results also showed that regulation was accompanied by a decreased intracellular chloride concentration and, at least during regulation following intracellular HCl injection, by raised $[Na^+]_i$, it seemed likely that pH_i regulation involved Na^+/H^+ and Cl^-/HCO_3^- exchange, with both H^+ and HCO_3^- moving against their own electrochemical gradients (Thomas, 1977).

These results should be interpreted with some caution, though. For example, as Fig. 12 (lower panel) shows little regulation occurs if the CO_2 transient is instituted at a pH_o of 6.5, rather than 7.5 and, at pH_o values of close to 7.0 it is sluggish (Thomas, 1974). We recall that, in the brain, P_{CO_2} is close to 45 mmHg and pH_o is around 7.3. If P_{CO_2} is increased to 80 mmHg, pH_o will fall below 7.1, at constant $[HCO_3^-]_o$. Clearly, this situation is different from that usually employed *in vitro*. The results reported by Thomas (1974, 1976, 1977) and Moody (1981, his Fig. 7) do not, therefore, unequivocally demonstrate that fast and extensive regulation of pH_i would occur under physiological conditions. Furthermore, the results obtained *in vitro* suggest that at a pH_o of 7.5 hypercapnia may cause net *alkalosis* once the acid transient has subsided (Thomas, 1976). Probably, such effects arose because, at the induction of hypercapnia, $[HCO_3^-]_o$ was increased from nominally zero to values giving a pH_o of 7.5 at the CO_2 concentration employed (at 4.4% CO_2, $[HCO_3^-]_o$ was raised to 40 mM). The question arises, therefore, if HCO_3^-/Cl^- exchange would achieve inward translocation of HCO_3^- under physiological conditions (see below).

Since P_{CO_2} was altered and pH_i measured in these experiments it should be possible to derive β_{CO_2}. Unfortunately, data obtained in such experiments have been expressed as $\Delta[HCO_3^-]/\Delta pH$ ratios. This has led to misunderstandings. Sufficient data are not at hand to allow recalculation, and those existing have resulted from the procedure of raising P_{CO_2}, not from the normal value of the species studied, but from a control value of nominally zero. For these reasons, intracellular buffer capacities should be judged from experiments in which intracellular buffer base concentrations were altered by ionophoretic injections.

Two main procedures have been used to induce *intracellular buffer base changes:* intracellular injection of H^+/HCO_3^-, or extracellular application of ammonium salts. The first of these appears unambiguous. Thus, injection of HCl will decrease [BB] in proportion to the Cl^- delivered, and injection of $NaHCO_3$ or $KHCO_3$ will increase [BB] in proportion to the increase in the cation concentration. However, some problems arise. Thus, apart from the fact that quantification of acid or base released from the current delivered requires knowledge of the transport number (see Thomas, 1976), the rate of diffusion and the final distribution of the injected species within the cell are poorly known; hence regulation by transmembrane transport becomes correspondingly difficult to assess.

The second procedure (Boron and de Weer, 1976a; see also Roos and Boron, 1981) is an elegant way of repeatedly inducing initial alkalosis (NH_3 entry), plateau phase acidification (presumed to be due to NH_4^+ entry), and post-exposure acidosis, the latter allowing studies of mechanisms of acid extrusion. There are problems of quantifying the acid-base transients, though. For example, it becomes difficult to describe the behavior of the NH_3 and NH_4^+ species in terms of the independent and dependent variables discussed above, especially since P_{NH_3} cannot be measured as P_{CO_2} can, and since the counterion for NH_4^+ entry has not been defined. Furthermore, any increase in pH_i should elicit fast and extensive acid production. In the brain, increases in tissue ammonia concentrations (NH_3 plus NH_4^+) to only 2–3 $\mu mol \cdot g^{-1}$ cause the lactate concentration to rise to values of 8–10 $\mu mol \cdot g^{-1}$, effectively preventing pH_i from increasing (Hindfeldt and Siesjö, 1971). For these reasons, I will regard transient exposure of cells to ammonium salts as a qualitative means of inducing low pH_i, useful for unravelling mechanisms of regulation.

Before discussing evidence bearing on membrane translocation of HCO_3^- during pH_i regulation in response to an acid load, it seems justified to consider the regulatory event involving Na^+/H^+ exchange.

Work on CO_2 exposure, ammonia loading, and HCl injection showed that pH_i regulation was strongly inhibited by removal of extracellular Na^+, and that such regulation was accompanied by increased intracellular Na^+ concentration (Thomas, 1976; Moody, 1981). Obviously, these results suggest that pH_i regulation in response to an acid load involves extrusion of H^+ in exchange for Na^+. This may well constitute a general mechanism for pH_i regulation, as results obtained in many different tissues demonstrate. It may serve our purpose to take an example from a non-neural tissue. Recently, Grinstein et al. (1984) studied acid extrusion in isolated thymocytes suspended in HCO_3^--free media so as to avoid any contribution from Cl^-/HCO_3^- exchange. They acid-loaded the cells by exposing them to the ionophore nigericin, and measured pH_i by the carboxylated fluorescein derivative DCF (Rink et al., 1982). Several interesting results were reported. First, normal pH_i was close to 7.0, and the intracellular buffer capacity ($\Delta B/\Delta pH$) was 0.025 $mol \cdot l^{-1} \cdot pH^{-1}$. Second, acid extrusion (maximal values about 10 $mmol \cdot l^{-1} \cdot min^{-1}$) was indirectly related to pH_i and directly related to pH_o (Fig. 13). Third, its mediation via Na^+/H^+ exchange was obvious. Thus, pH_i regulation was accompanied by intracellular accumulation of Na^+ and by acidification of the external medium, and it was inhibited by amiloride, a known inhibitor of Na^+/K^+ exchange (Benos, 1982). Interestingly, in this preparation H^+ extrusion ceased at pH_i values of 6.9.

In summary, results from both neuronal and non-neuronal cells demonstrate that intracellular acidification results in activation of an electrosilent Na^+/H^+ exchange wich causes H^+ extrusion by Na^+ influx. The energy source of this extrusion is the Na^+ gradient created by the Na^+, K^+-dependent ATPase (cf. Fig. 9 above). It follows from this that regulation should cease when the sum of the electrochemical gradients for Na^+ and H^+ approaches zero (for a numerical example, see

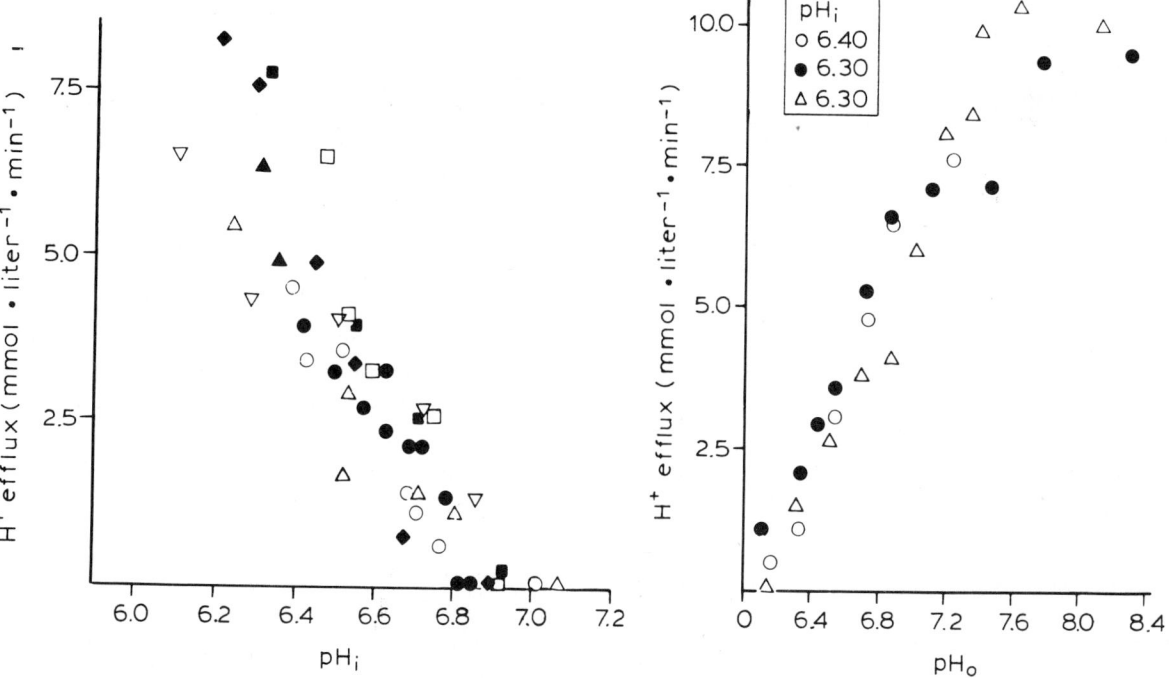

Fig. 13. Effect of pH_i and pH_o on Na^+-induced H^+ efflux from thymocytes. H^+ extrusion rates were calculated from ΔpH_i changes on the assumption that $\Delta B/\Delta pH_i$ is 0.025 $mol \cdot l^{-1}$. The experiments were carried out in the absence of added CO_2 and HCO_3^-. (Reproduced with permission from Grinstein et al., 1984.)

Moody, 1981). For a given Na^+ gradient, the rate of H^+ extrusion should be proportional to the H^+ gradient. Thus, all other things being equal, the rate of flux should increase with decreasing pH_i. Furthermore, at any given pH_i H^+ extrusion should increase with pH_o. It must be recalled, though, that the rate of Na^+/H^+ exchange is probably not a simple function of the electrochemical gradients for Na^+ and H^+ since the antiporter must be subject to regulation by hormonal and other influences, which probably modulate the affinity of the external and internal sites for Na^+ and H^+, respectively. To take one example, Na^+/H^+ exchange in muscle tissue has been proposed to be enhanced by insulin (Moore, 1983). Furthermore, I wish to recall the evidence suggesting that agonist-receptor interactions which in some cells activate phospholipase C and, via the formation of diacylglycerides, the C-kinase system, can increase the activity of the Na^+/H^+ exchanger with a resultant increase in pH_i (Berridge, 1984). As Fig. 14 shows, the results of an increased Na^+/H^+ exchange may serve as signals to cell proliferation. Thus, we can envisage situations in which changes in Na^+/H^+ exchange are brought about, or at least modulated by, factors which enhance (or inhibit) the activity of the antiporter even though the Na^+-H^+ gradient does not change.

Thomas' (1976) results on HCl-injected snail neurons provided important information on the roles played by the HCO_3^-/H_2CO_3 buffer system. First, the data showed that this system increases the buffer capacity of the cell. In the absence of HCO_3^-/H_2CO_3, the author could calculate a $\Delta B/\Delta pH$ value of 0.011 mol $\cdot$ l^{-1} $\cdot$ pH^{-1} but, at a CO_2 concentration of 2.2% and $[HCO_3^-]_o = 20$ mmol $\cdot$ l^{-1}, the value increased to 0.032 mol $\cdot$ l^{-1} $\cdot$ pH^{-1}. The first value was similar to that obtained following $NaHCO_3$ ionophoresis. The increase in the buffer value by CO_2 exposure reflects, as has been discussed above, the contribution by intracellular HCO_3^-.

The results reported by Thomas (1976, 1977) and by Boron and de Weer (1976b) established that the rate of pH_i regulation following intracellular acidification is increased when P_{CO_2} is increased, and HCO_3^- is added to ECF. Similar results were obtained by Moody (1981). In calculating the rate of H^+ extrusion the authors assumed an intrinsic buffer value ($\Delta B/\Delta pH$) of 0.021 mol $\cdot$ l^{-1} $\cdot$ pH^{-1}, adding that due to HCO_3^- as 2.3 $[HCO_3^-]_i$. As the results of Fig. 15 show, the rate of extrusion of H^+ was proportional to the deviation of pH_i from the normal. Interestingly, at a given ΔpH_i, and at constant pH_o, extrusion rate was directly proportional to $[HCO_3^-]_o$. Results demonstrating that both pH_o and $[HCO_3^-]_o$ influence the rate of acid extrusion have also been obtained in barnacle muscle (Boron et al., 1979).

These results suggest that regulation of pH_i involves HCO_3^-/Cl^- exchange, with HCO_3^- entering the cell against its own electrochemical gradient, and Cl^- leaving. Three further results support this notion. First, the intracellular Cl^- concentration

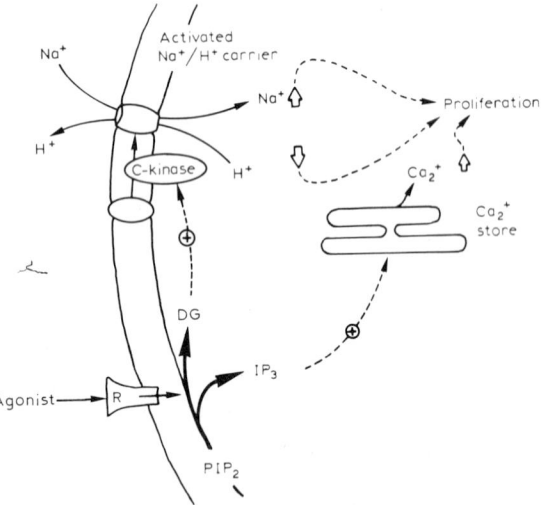

Fig. 14. Model to illustrate the proposed coupling between agonist-receptor interaction, activation of phospholipase C, activation of C-kinase, and activation of Na^+/H^+ exchange. The model, proposed by Berridge (1984), demonstrates that enzymatic cleavage of phosphatidylinositol 4,5-bisphosphate (PIP_2) to diacylglycerol (DG) and inositol 1,4,5-triphosphate (IP_3) activates two parallel messenger systems, one of which (the C-kinase system) may enhance Na^+/H^+ exchange. Berridge (1984) further proposes that increased Na^+ and Ca^{2+} concentrations, and decreased $[H^+]_i$, act to stimulate proliferative processes (cf. activation of C-kinase by phorbol esters). (Slightly modified after Berridge, 1984.)

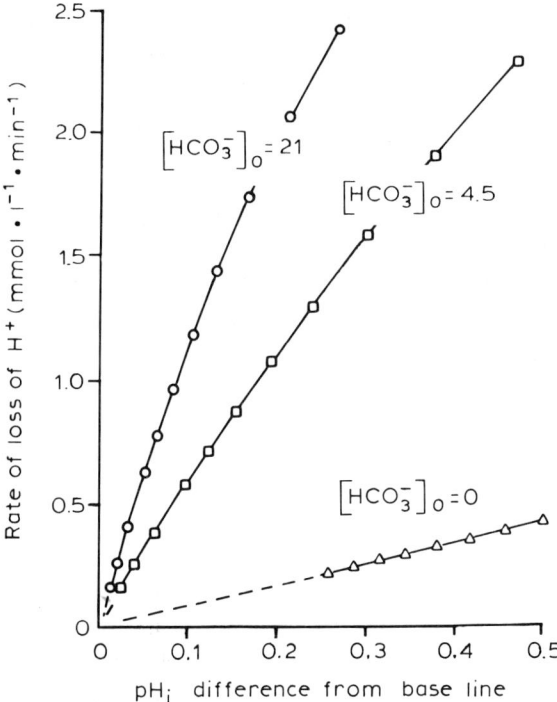

Fig. 15. Dependence of acid extrusion on $[HCO_3^-]_o$ in *Aplysia* neurons. The cells were ionophoretically injected with HCl, and acid extrusion calculated from the rate of change of pH_i at three different $[HCO_3^-]_o$ values. Note that since pH_o was held constant (at 7.5) both P_{CO_2} and $[HCO_3^-]_o$ were altered. (Redrawn from a Figure published by Thomas, 1976.)

was found to decrease during pH_i regulation following acid loading (Thomas, 1977; Moody, 1981). Second, as was the case during CO_2 exposure, depletion of intracellular $[Cl^-]$ markedly retarded pH_i regulation (Thomas, 1977). Third, application of SITS, a disulfonic stilbene derivative which retards anion exchange, was found to block (Thomas, 1977) or markedly slow down (Moody, 1981) pH_i regulation following HCl injection. It was also shown that SITS blocked that part of H^+ extrusion which was induced by HCO_3^- (Moody, 1981). As a final point, I wish to recall that, in squid axons, regulatory uptake of HCO_3^- via a Cl^-/HCO_3^- antiporter is driven by ATP energy (Boron and de Weer, 1976b). No such evidence has been obtained for other tissues, and Thomas (1977) suggested that Cl^-/HCO_3^- exchange is energetically coupled to Na^+ influx.

The question arises, though, whether the anion exchanger normally functions to transport HCO_3^- inwards, i.e. against the electrochemical gradient of this ion. In a previous part of this article, I have assumed that the opposite is true, i.e. that HCO_3^- leaks out from the cell in exchange for Cl^-. Let us examine the thermodynamic forces involved. A dissipative, conductive flux of HCO_3^-, i.e. one in which HCO_3^- diffuses in the direction of its own electrochemical gradient, would normally be from intra- to extracellular fluids. The same would be true for electroneutral HCO_3^- flux via a Cl^-/HCO_3^- antiporter. Thus, with a $[Cl^-]_o/[Cl^-]_i$ ratio of 10 and a $[HCO_3^-]_o/[HCO_3^-]_i$ ratio of 2, the thermodynamic gradient predicts that spontaneous Cl^- influx will drive HCO_3^- efflux. In some cells, Cl^- is distributed at equilibrium which, at a membrane potential of -60 mV, gives a 10:1 ratio. An electroneutral antiporter which exchanges Cl^- for HCO_3^- has the peculiar characteristics that, although it does not require ATP, it displaces the "leading" ion (i.e. Cl^-) away from equilibrium. This behavior is consistent with results obtained in e.g. sheep-heart Purkinje fibres, which demonstrate that Cl^- is "actively" accumulated in the cell by an electroneutral Cl^-/HCO_3^- exchanger which is reversible in the sense that it catalyzes flux in either direction, depending on the Cl^- and HCO_3^- gradients (Vaughan-Jones, 1979).

In view of these considerations I tentatively conclude that the normal operation of the antiporter involves efflux of HCO_3^-, i.e. that it serves as a H^+ leak. Obviously, this interpretation is not supported by the results obtained in snail and crayfish neurons since these show that $[Cl^-]_i$ *decreases* during pH_i regulation in response to an acid load (Thomas, 1977; Moody, 1981). However, since the CO_2 exposures in these experiments involved a sudden increase in $[HCO_3^-]_o$ from nominally zero to 21 or 50 mmol·l^{-1} it is possible that flux via the anion exchanger was reversed. It is also possible that the role of the exchanger differs between tissues (and between cells in the brain), the variability being dictated by the requirements for control of intracellular Cl^- concentration (see Vaughan-Jones, 1979;

Moody, 1981). For example, at some synapses inhibition is mediated by conductive influx of Cl^-, hyperpolarizing the membrane. At these membrane sites one has to invoke active efflux of Cl^- to generate the necessary Cl^- gradient. At such loci, a high capacity Cl^-/HCO_3^- exchanger would be undesirable since, by allowing Cl^- influx, it could shunt the membrane to this ion.

Given this uncertainty with respect to the regulatory role played by the Cl^-/HCO_3^- exchanger, how can we explain the influence of pH_o and $[HCO_3^-]_o$ on the rate of H^+ extrusion? As discussed, $[H^+]_o$ would exert its effect by altering the chemical gradient for H^+ translocation. By the same token, $[HCO_3^-]_o$ would influence HCO_3^- flux, and it seems that it does not matter if the normal direction of Cl^-/HCO_3^- exchange is that suggested, with HCO_3^- leaving the cell. Thus, if this exchange provides a substantial H^+ leak it will reduce *net* H^+ translocation, and an increased $[HCO_3^-]_o$ would slow down this leak, allowing net H^+ translocation to approach the rate of H^+ extrusion via the Na^+/H^+ antiporter.

It seems natural to assume that the ion exchanges discussed provide the mechanisms of pH_i regulation in the intact brain. The question, though, is whether neurons and glial cells contain similar antiporters. Probably, Na^+/H^+ exchange driven by the Na^+ gradient, and thereby indirectly by ATP energy, is a universal mechanism of pH_i regulation. It has been known for some time that glial cells possess both a Na^+/H^+ and a Cl^-/HCO_3^- exchanger (Kimelberg and Bourke, 1982, 1984; Kimelberg, 1983) and regulation of pH_i in vertebrate neurons is probably similar to that previously demonstrated for invertebrates. There are no reasons to believe, therefore, that fundamental differences exist in the regulation of pH_i in various cell types, except perhaps in the capacity and the function of anion exchange systems (the "H^+ leak").

Changes in pH_i in pathological states

In this section, I wish to briefly summarize cerebral metabolic changes in ischemia, hypoglycemia, and epileptic seizures, discuss how these relate to transmembrane fluxes of the major ions, and review present information on changes in pH_i. For more detailed accounts of changes in energy state and of ionic fluxes, the reader is referred to recent review articles (Nicholson, 1980; Hansen and Zeuthen, 1981; Siesjö, 1981, 1984; Hossmann, 1982; Siesjö and Wieloch, 1985).

A previous review article (Siesjö, 1981) discusses and illustrates changes in cerebral cortical ATP concentration and calculated adenylate energy charge as well as in lactate concentrations. In ischemia, energy failure is rapid and extensive while tissue lactate contents are either markedly (starved animals) or excessively (fed animals) increased. Hypoglycemia also leads to marked deterioration of cerebral energy state, albeit less extensive than in ischemia. In contrast to ischemia, though, tissue lactate content is *decreased*, reflecting the cellular utilization of endogenous substrates. In status epilepticus, finally, energy failure is virtually absent and tissue lactate content only moderately increased.

As described in the review articles referred to above, ischemia leads to massive efflux of K^+ from cells, and to cellular uptake of Na^+, Cl^-, and Ca^{2+}. In hypoglycemia, the rise in K_e^+ concentration is somewhat less pronounced but cellular uptake of Ca^{2+} is as extensive as in ischemia (Harris et al., 1984). Probably, membrane fluxes of Na^+ and Cl^- are similar. In epileptic seizures, K^+ homeostasis is only moderately perturbed but considerable decreases in Ca_e^{2+} nevertheless occur (see Heinemann et al., 1977). We proceed to discuss cerebral acid-base events in the three conditions.

Hypoglycemia

Since hypoglycemia leads to consumption of endogenous carbohydrate and amino acid substrates, and since many of these are anions of metabolic acids, one would expect that their oxidation should increase intracellular buffer base concentration, i.e. raise pH_i. Calculations of pH_i from HCO_3^- distribution first suggested that pH_i was unchanged

(Lewis et al., 1974; Feise et al., 1976). However, when it was found that hypoglycemia raised CBF and reduced ECF volume it became clear that pH_i was significantly increased in both pre-coma and in coma (Pelligrino et al., 1981b). Obviously, hypoglycemia causes extensive energy failure and loss of ion homeostasis in the absence of cellular or extracellular acidosis.

The increase in pH_i during hypoglycemia is predictable. One can also predict that hypoglycemia, by reducing the concentrations of available metabolic acids and by preventing their production from glucose, should inhibit metabolic regulation of pH_i in hypercapnia and hypocapnia (Pelligrino and Siesjö, 1981). However, in the absence of information on transmembrane fluxes of H^+/HCO_3^- one cannot foresee how such inhibition will affect pH_i. Experiments showed that, in hypoglycemic coma, the pH_i changes were not those expected from the physiochemical buffer capacity and the "metabolic" buffer base changes (Pelligrino and Siesjö, 1981). In both hypocapnia and hypercapnia, pH_i was higher than values so predicted, suggesting that transmembrane ion fluxes had occurred (H^+ out, of HCO_3^- in). In hypocapnia, such fluxes caused pH_i to rise markedly. In fact, in four of the eight experiments, the ratio $[HCO_3^-]_i/[HCO_3^-]_e$ rose towards one and, at the low prevailing P_{CO_2}, pH_i approached 7.7. In hypercapnia, however, the fluxes of H^+/HCO_3^- must have achieved regulation of pH_i, i.e. these fluxes curtailed the fall in pH_i at the raised P_{CO_2}.

As stated, hypoglycemic coma markedly reduces cerebral energy state, but it leaves 20–30% of the ATP content unhydrolyzed. During marked hypocapnia, which caused moderate arterial hypotension in some of the animals, the adenylate energy charge was further reduced (Fig. 16). Furthermore, a direct correlation was found between energy charge and pH_i, suggesting that efflux of H^+/influx of HCO_3^- was enhanced by aggravation of cellular energy failure. The mechanisms for this uncontrolled accumulation of HCO_3^- in intracellular fluids are not known but seem related to the enhanced energy failure, and further depolarizations of membranes.

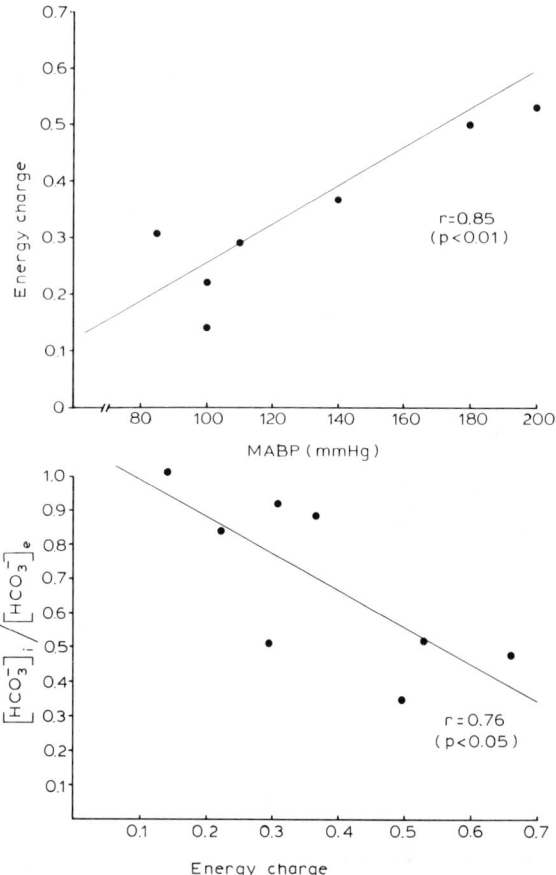

Fig. 16. Relationship between energy failure and intracellular alkalosis in hypoglycemic coma, induced in animals during respiratory alkalosis ($P_{a(CO_2)} \approx 15$ mmHg). The hypoglycemia gave rise to energy failure (normal energy charge about 0.94) and intracellular alkalosis. However, moderate reductions in blood pressure caused further reduction of energy charge, and enhanced alkalosis. At the low P_{CO_2} employed, pH_i rose to maximal values of about 7.7. (Reproduced with permission from Pelligrino and Siesjö, 1981.)

During hypercapnia, cerebral energy state was better maintained in the hypoglycemic animals (Pelligrino and Siesjö, 1981). This could be the reason why some regulation of pH_i was observed. Thus, one can envisage the persistence of ATP-driven Na^+ efflux, with Na^+ re-entering the cell in exchange for H^+. Whatever are the mechanisms, the results clearly show that even in severely hypoglycemic animals brain cells are protected against the acidifying effects of hypercapnia, but not against the alkalinizing effects of hypocapnia.

Epileptic seizures

Recordings of pH_e with surface or intracerebral electrodes, measurement of tissue lactic acid content, and calculation of changes in pH_i from the creatine kinase equilibrium have shown that seizures cause moderate lactic acidosis in the brain (for literature, see Howse et al., 1974; Siesjö et al., 1985a). Under standard conditions, i.e. when neither oxygen nor glucose supply becomes limiting, tissue lactate content increases to 8–10 μmol · g^{-1} during the first 3–5 min of seizure discharge, and remains unchanged thereafter (Duffy et al., 1975; Chapman et al., 1977). If oxygen supply is reduced by moderate lowering of arterial P_{O_2}, or of blood pressure, tissue lactate content can rise to 15–25 μmol · g^{-1} (Blennow et al., 1977) and if glucose supply becomes limiting as a result of moderate hypoglycemia, the lactate content of the tissue is reduced (Blennow et al., 1979; see also Folbergrová et al., 1981). Although such variations in steady-state lactate content must influence pH_i, values cannot be predicted as long as the contribution of H^+/HCO_3^- exchange between intra- and extracellular spaces has not been assessed.

Recently, changes in pH_e and pH_i were estimated for fluorothyl-induced seizures of 5–20 min duration, as well as for the immediate postepileptic period (Siesjö et al., 1985a). The main results are shown in Fig. 17. Changes in pH_e were dominated by an initial, fast acidification which sometimes exceeded 0.4 units (not shown in the Fig.), and by a sustained decrease in pH of about 0.35 units. Recovery was very slow. The change in pH_i was smaller, amounting to about 0.2 units after 5, and to 0.12 units after 20 min of seizures. Arrest of seizure activity led to a fast normalization of pH_i, with a subsequent increase above control values.

As discussed in the original article (Siesjö et al., 1985a) production of lactic acid during seizures is too slow and too small to explain the fast, initial acidification of ECF. Very probably, this initial shift of pH_e is due to fast Na^+/H^+ exchange. We recall that enhanced Na^+/H^+ exchange is a mechanism of pH_i regulation which is stimulated by a

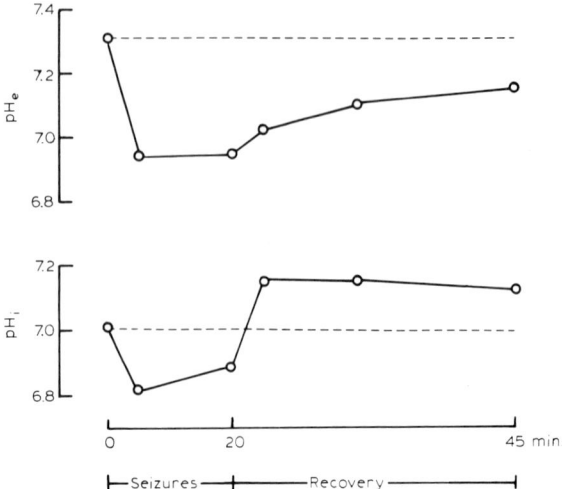

Fig. 17. Changes in pH_e and pH_i of cerebral cortex during and following 20 min of fluorothyl-induced seizures. The results demonstrate that pH_e decreases by about 0.35 unit during seizures, and is only slowly normalized during recovery. In contrast, pH_i changes less, seems subject to regulation during seizures, and shows postepileptic increase. (Data from Siesjö et al., 1985a.)

fall in pH_i. Thus, regulation of pH_i may be the reason for the suggested increase in pH_i during ongoing seizures. It is conceivable that the massive agonist-receptor interaction during seizures stimulates phospholipase C, and that the ensuing activation of C-kinase contributes to the increase in Na^+/H^+ exchange. A sustained activation of Na^+/H^+ exchange, and slow oxidation of lactate accumulated, can explain why pH_i increases above normal upon arrest of seizure activity (Siesjö et al., 1985a).

Under normal circumstances, therefore, seizure activity is accompanied by very moderate changes in pH_i. Furthermore, available results suggest that regulation of pH_i occurs during ongoing seizures. This would suggest that changes in pH_i during seizures do not become pronounced enough to trigger deleterious cellular reactions of the type discussed in subsequent sections. However, one brain region, the substantia nigra, seems to provide an exception. Experiments with fluorothyl-induced status epilepticus, and long-term recovery to allow assessment of the final neuronal damage, revealed a pancellular necrosis ("infarction") of the substantia nigra, pars reticulata, after seizure periods of 45 min or longer (Nevander et al., 1984, 1985). Preliminary autoradiographic estimates of tissue acid-base changes, with ^{14}C-DMO as the indicator, suggest that marked acidosis develops in the substantia nigra during ongoing seizures (Siesjö and Ingvar, 1985), and accumulation of lactate is marked (Ingvar et al., 1985). It is clear, therefore, that acidosis must be discussed as one mechanism underlying the development of infarction (see below).

Ischemia

It has been clearly documented that ischemia leads to extra- and intracellular acidosis. The evidence stems from studies in which pH_e was measured with ion-specific electrodes (Siemkowicz and Hansen, 1981; Kraig et al., 1983; Mutch and Hansen, 1984), or pH_i was estimated with pH indicators (Kogure et al., 1980a,b; Andersson and Sundt, 1983; Csiba et al., 1983). The results reported are variable, probably because acid production (which was not measured) varied with the type, density, and duration of the ischemia studied. The article by Kraig et al. (1985) is centered on quantitative relationships between lactic acidosis and changes in $P_{t(CO_2)}$ and pH_e. For that reason, the following discussion mainly concerns intracellular acid-base events, changes in pH_e being considered when (and if) they are essential for an understanding of alterations in pH_i.

The crucial acid-base events in ischemia are the deterioration of cerebral energy state, and the ensuing stimulation of anaerobic glycolysis, with conversion of glucose (and glycogen) to lactic acid. Some of the acid equivalents released stem from the hydrolysis of ATP which proceeds according to the reaction

$$\text{ATP} + \text{HOH} \rightarrow \text{ADP} + \text{P}_i + n\text{H}^+ \quad (18)$$

where n has been estimated to 0.7 (Wilkie, 1979; Alberti and Cuthbert, 1982). In severe ischemia, the ATP hydrolyzed is that contained in the ATP pool, and that formed from phosphocreatine (PCr) according to the reaction

$$\text{PCr} + \text{ADP} + n\text{H}^+ \rightarrow \text{ATP} + \text{Cr} \quad (19)$$

However, since n in this reaction is about 0.3 (Wilkie, 1979) the hydrolysis of all PCr (about 4 μmol · g^{-1}) and ATP (about 3 μmol · g^{-1}) should only release about 4 μmol · g^{-1} of acid.

Several other reactions in the cell will generate H$^+$ ions. However, all of them are of minor importance in comparison to anaerobic glycolysis, in which each mole of glucose is converted to two moles of lactic acid, the latter ionizing into H$^+$ and lactate ions. The amounts of lactic acid formed during ischemia are illustrated in Fig. 18. During complete ischemia, the lactate accumulated corresponds to the pre-ischemic stores of glucose and glycogen which vary with the plasma glucose concentration (Ljunggren et al., 1974). The same must be true in severe, incomplete ischemia; however, in that condition the remaining blood flow is a source of exogenous glucose. Accordingly, long periods of incomplete ischemia may cause excessive accumula-

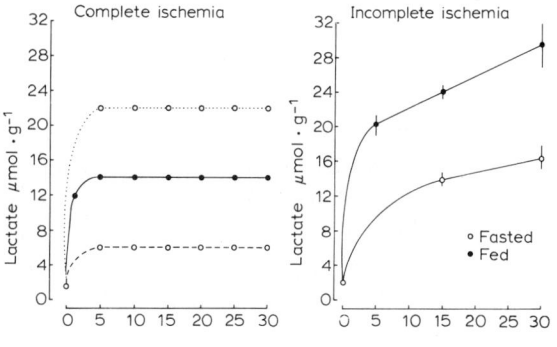

Fig. 18. Amounts of lactate accumulated during complete and during severe, incomplete ischemia. During complete ischemia, tissue lactate content can be lowered by induced hypoglycemia (lowermost curve) or increased by induced hyperglycemia (uppermost curve). During incomplete ischemia, the amount of lactate accumulated is different in fasted and fed rats. In the latter, which become hyperglycemic during the ischemia, lactate contents may in individual animals exceed 30 μmol · g^{-1}. (Reproduced with permission from Siesjö and Wieloch, 1985.)

tion of lactic acid in the tissue (Nordström et al., 1978; Welsh et al., 1980; Rehncrona et al., 1981).

In ischemia, the acidosis is due to changes in [BB] and P_{CO_2}, the two independent variables. Consider a situation of hypoxia in which CBF is not reduced, and $P_{t(CO_2)}$ remains constant. The H^+ ions released during ATP hydrolysis and anaerobic glycolysis react with HCO_3^- and with non-bicarbonate buffers, the change in $[H^+]$ at any given lowering of [BB] being functions of pH, $[HCO_3^-]$ and of the C and K_{Ha} values of non-bicarbonate buffers. In the course of this buffering, CO_2 is being blown off when H^+ combines with HCO_3^-. We have referred to the fact that when P_{CO_2} is held constant, the HCO_3^-/H_2CO_3 buffer system is uniquely efficient. However, in ischemia the reduction of CBF retards or prevents CO_2 from leaving the tissue, and P_{CO_2} rises. Thus, it is permissible to state that acidosis during ischemia is due to both a reduction of buffer base concentration, and a rise in P_{CO_2}. Our five-buffer theoretical system, whose behavior is assumed to mimic that of intracellular fluids, demonstrates the relative importance of changes in [BB] and P_{CO_2} (Fig. 19). Clearly, at low [BB] values changes in P_{CO_2} have only moderate effects on pH_i. In extracellular fluid, which contains no non-bicarbonate buffers, a rise in P_{CO_2} has a larger effect on pH (see below).

Complete ischemia converts the brain into a closed system. Given the lactate contents of the cerebral cortex in ischemic hypo-, normo- and hyperglycemic rats, and a constant total CO_2 content, Ljunggren et al. (1974) calculated expected changes in $P_{t(CO_2)}$ and pH_i. For Δ lactate values of 4, 14, and 21 $\mu mol \cdot g^{-1}$, the $P_{t(CO_2)}$ values were 65, 130, and 210 mmHg, and pH_i values were 6.8, 6.4, and 6.1, respectively.

Measurements have now been performed which allow a less speculative derivation of pH_i changes during and following severe, incomplete forebrain ischemia in the rat (von Hanwehr, Smith and Siesjö, submitted). Measurements were made of Pt_{CO_2}, pH_e, ECF volume, and T_{CO_2}, the values obtained allowing calculation of $[HCO_3^-]_e$, $[HCO_3^-]_i$, and pH_i. In the starved animals employed, lactate con-

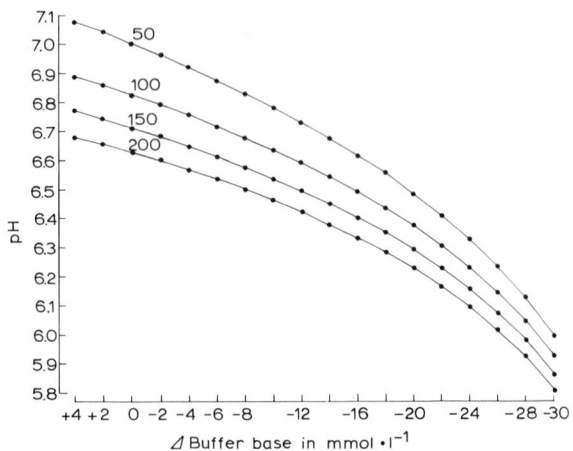

Fig. 19. Influence of changes in buffer base concentration, and in P_{CO2}, on pH in a system mimicking the buffer capacity of cerebral intracellular fluids. The curves were generated by using five buffer acids, each having $C = 0.010$ mol $\cdot l^{-1}$, with pK_{Ha} values in the range 7.6–6.4. P_{CO2} values in mmHg are shown as insets in each curve.

tents at the end of 15 min of ischemia varied but little (13–16 $\mu mol \cdot g^{-1}$). During ischemia, Pt_{CO_2} rose to a mean value of 150 mmHg, pH_e fell by an average of 0.7 unit, ECF volume decreased to 55% of control, and T_{CO_2} remained constant, or decreased moderately. Calculated pH_i fell from a value of 7.04 to 6.12 (range 5.9–6.4).

The values thus obtained, and those published previously (Mabe et al., 1983), give information on pH_i changes during and following severe, incomplete ischemia (Fig. 20). The values obtained by the HCO_3^-/H_2CO_3 method were validated by independent techniques. Thus, similar data during recovery were obtained by calculation from the creatine kinase equilibrium (see Fig. 20). Furthermore, values obtained during ischemia compared favourably to those calculated from our composite five-buffer system. At a pH_i of 7.05 and a $P_{t(CO_2)}$ of 45 mmHg, [BB] is 0.036 mol $\cdot l^{-1}$. Suppose that the increase in lactic acid concentration during ischemia (13 $\mu mol \cdot kg^{-1}$ of wet weight) is homogenously distributed in intra- and extracellular water (volume fraction 0.76), and that ATP hydrolysis contributes 0.005 mol $\cdot l^{-1}$ of acid. Then, Δ [BB] is 0.022 mol $\cdot l^{-1}$. We can now insert into our equation values for $P_{t(CO_2)}$ (150 mmHg) and pH_i (6.19) during ischemia, and calculate [BB]. This yields a Δ [BB] value of 0.023 mol · l^{-1}, i.e. virtually identical to that derived from acid production.

Inspection of Fig. 20 reveals that in spite of the marked acidosis during ischemia, pH_i normalizes after 15 min of recirculation and subsequently increases above control. The rapid normalization is not due to oxidation of lactate whose concentration is only moderately reduced in that period (Mabe et al., 1983). Probably, enhancement of Na$^+$/H$^+$ exchange leads to rapid extrusion of H$^+$ from cells. It also seems likely that the subsequent alkalosis is due to oxidation of lactate, with removal of a stoichiometrical amount of H$^+$ at a time when Na$^+$/H$^+$ exchange has brought pH_i back to normal. It cannot be excluded, though, that sustained activation of phospholipase C and of C-kinase leads to a long-lasting enhancement of Na$^+$/H$^+$ exchange.

Predictably, the severity of extra- and intracellular acidosis during ischemia must depend on the blood glucose concentration. A relationship between tissue lactate content and pH_e during complete ischemia has been demonstrated by Kraig et al. (1985). The influence of induced hypo- and hyperglycemia on tissue acid-base changes during and following incomplete forebrain ischemia is presently being studied in our laboratory (Smith, von Hanwehr, Rehncrona, and Siesjö, in preparation). The results have so far demonstrated that hyperglycemia exaggerates the extra- and intracellular acidosis, and that it prolongs the postischemic period during which net acidosis persists. In hyperglycemic animals, with tissue lactate contents of close to 20 μmol · g^{-1}, pH_i is reduced to just below 6.0. Obviously, at even higher lactate values, pH_i should fall well below 6.

Acidosis and molecular mechanisms of ischemic brain damage

Although it has long been suspected that acidosis adversely affects the viability of cerebral tissues, and that it promotes cell swelling (Friede and van Houten, 1961; Lindenberg, 1963), the hypothesis received strong support only recently when Myers observed that pre-ischemic feeding or glucose-infusion aggravated ischemic brain damage, apparently because these procedures enhanced lactic acid production in the ischemic brain (Myers and Yamaguchi, 1977; Myers, 1979). The results were soon confirmed and extended (Siemkowicz and Hansen, 1978; Ginsberg et al., 1980; Welsh et al., 1980; Rehncrona et al., 1981; Kalimo et al., 1981; Pulsinelli et al., 1982). Although the point has not been conclusively proven, we will assume that the adverse effects of hyperglycemia are mediated via an exaggerated lactic acidosis. In his studies, Myers noted that hyperglycemic animals developed gross tissue edema (Myers, 1979). Since extensive astrocytic swelling has been noted by others (Kalimo et al., 1981), it appears that loss of cell volume control is one cardinal feature in the acidosis-promoted brain injury.

In this last section, I will discuss cellular and molecular mechanisms which may provide the link between acidosis and ischemic brain injury. These are conveniently discussed under three headings: cell volume regulation, mitochondrial metabolism, and free radical injury to cell membranes.

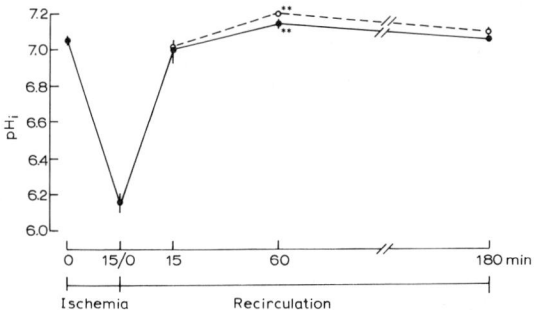

Fig. 20. Intracellular pH in the brain before, during, and following 15 min of incomplete ischemia in rats. Filled circles denote values derived with the CO_2/HCO_3^- method, unfilled circles those calculated from the creatine kinase equilibrium. (Data are from Mabe et al., 1983; and from unpublished work of von Hanwehr, Smith and Siesjö, submitted.)

Cell volume regulation

The most popular hypothesis for regulation of cell volume is the double Donnan pump-leak hypothesis (Tosteson and Hoffmann, 1960; MacKnight and Leaf, 1977). An elementary description is given in Fig. 21. The presence of impermeable anions in the cell favors swelling by Donnan forces, i.e. permeable ions tend to be concentrated on the inside of the membrane, with an associated flux of water. However, a double Donnan system is created by the Na^+/K^+ pump which maintains a high concentration of Na^+ on the outside of the membrane, thereby balancing the effect of the impermeable intracellular anions. In this new situation cell volume is determined by the balance between active Na^+ extrusion ("the pump") and passive Na^+ entry ("the leak").

Although it has been generally recognized that active Na^+ transport is essential to cell volume regulation, the nature of the Na^+ "leak" remained uncertain. It now seems established that, in a variety of cells, ion fluxes of importance for cell volume regulation occur via electroneutral ion exchange systems (antiporters). Some cells, notably nucleated erythrocytes, respond to osmotic swelling or shrinkage by regulatory volume decrease (RVD) and regulatory volume increase (RVI), respectively (see Cala, 1980, 1983). In RVD, K^+ and Cl^- are lost from the cell, with osmotically obliged water, via K^+/H^+ and Cl^-/HCO_3^- exchange (Fig. 22). During RVI, a corresponding ion exchange allows Na^+, Cl^-, and H_2O to enter the cell. In both cases, fluxes of H^+ and HCO_3^- are cyclic, and do not contribute to water movement.

In some cells, electroneutral ion fluxes are by cotransport, e.g. by the symport-coupled movement

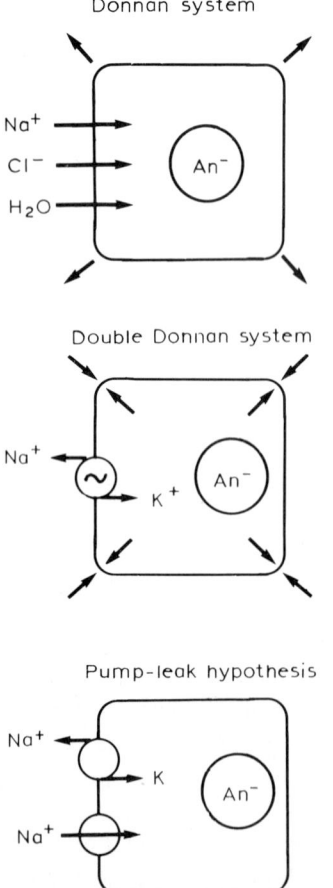

Fig. 21. Elementary description of double Donnan pump-leak hypothesis of cell volume regulation. Due to the presence of impermeant intracellular anions, permeant ions tend to accumulate in intracellular fluids, with osmotically obliged water. This swelling tendency is counteracted by a Na^+ pump which maintains this ion extracellularly ("effectively impermeant"). At steady state, cell volume is a function of the balance between Na^+ pump and Na^+ leak.

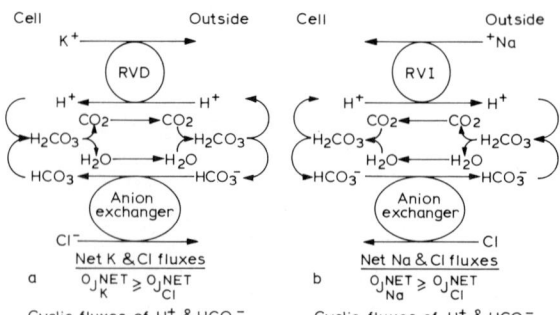

Fig. 22. Ionic and water fluxes during regulatory volume decrease (RVD) and regulatory volume increase (RVI), following osmotically induced cell swelling and shrinkage, respectively. RVD is shown to involve cellular loss of K^+ and Cl^-, with osmotically obliged water, and RVI gain of Na^+ and Cl^-, with osmotically obliged water. In both instances, cation and Cl^- fluxes occur via electroneutral ion exchanges with H^+ and HCO_3^- as the counterions. (Reproduced with permission from Cala, 1983.)

of Na^+, K^+, and Cl^- (Kregenow, 1981; Haas et al., 1982; Cala, 1983). However, coupled antiporters of the type shown in Fig. 22 probably exist in a majority of cells. Their existence in neurons and glial cells have been proven (e.g. Kimelberg, 1983; Kimelberg and Bourke, 1982). Since Na^+/H^+ exchange may be a general mechanism of pH_i regulation, and since Cl^-/HCO_3^- exchange may provide a pathway for back leakage of H^+ into the cell, the relationship between pH_i regulation and cell volume regulation is obvious (see Cala, 1983; Grinstein et al., 1983).

It seems likely, therefore, that the Na^+/H^+ antiporter provides the leak pathway predicted by the pump-leak hypothesis of cell volume control. However, since cell swelling requires influx of both Na^+ and Cl^- an increased Na^+/H^+ exchange must be accompanied by coupled exchange via the Cl^-/HCO_3^- antiporter. An intriguing situation then arises (Fig. 23). Thus, if H^+ is constantly pumped out in exchange for Na^+, and if back leakage occurs by Cl^-/HCO_3^- exchange, the cell would constantly gain Na^+, Cl^-, and osmotically obliged water. As pointed out previously (Siesjö, 1984), this swelling tendency could be counteracted by an electrogenic

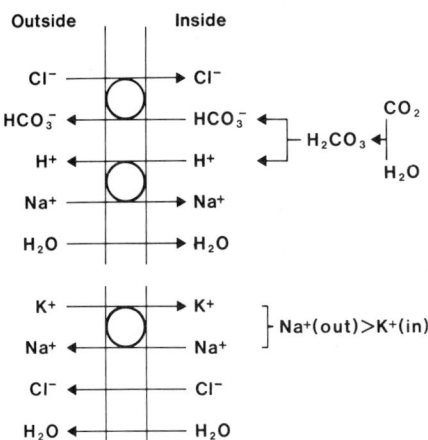

Fig. 23. Proposed model of ion and water fluxes in glial cells. Regulation of pH_i by Na^+/H^+ exchange and HCO_3^- outflux via a Cl^-/HCO_3^- antiporter favor accumulation of Na^+ and Cl^-, with osmotically obliged water (upper panel). This swelling tendency may be counteracted by an electrogenic Na^+ pump, which, by exporting positive charge, causes a balancing outflux of Cl^-. (Reproduced with permission from Siesjö, 1984.)

Na^+/K^+ pump which, by exporting Na^+ and, thereby, positive charge, would allow efflux of Cl^- via a conductive pathway.

The pump and leak relationships depicted in Fig. 23 are speculative. However, considerable evidence exists that the cation and the anion antiport systems are involved in glial swelling. It has been shown, for example, that swelling occurs after K^+-induced depolarization, or after addition of certain agonists (noradrenaline, adenosine and histamine), by mechanisms which are HCO_3^--dependent, which lead to uptake of Cl^-, and which are inhibited by diuretics acting on the Cl^-/HCO_3^- exchanger (Kimelberg, 1982; Kimelberg and Bourke, 1982, 1984). It seems very likely, therefore, that events which accelarate coupled Na^+/H^+ and Cl^-/HCO_3^- exchange will promote glial swelling. As discussed earlier in this article, Na^+/H^+ exchange can be accelerated by intracellular acidosis. It is my proposal that acidosis disrupts volume regulation in glial cells by leading to grossly enhanced Na^+/H^+ exchange. Clearly, marked swelling can only occur if the Na^+ gradient is maintained by continued ATPase activity. This could explain why astrocytic swelling develops first when circulation is restored after ischemia, or in "penumbra" regions with a higher blood flow rate than the ischemic core in stroke. In both instances we have to assume that oxygen supply and mitochondrial function are sufficient to maintain glial ATPase activity, but insufficient to prevent gross stimulation of aerobic glycolysis.

If the initiating event in cell swelling is enhancement of Na^+/H^+ exchange, how is Cl^- influx via the Cl^-/HCO_3^- antiporter maintained? Tentatively, Cl^- influx is driven by the HCO_3^- gradient, this in turn being maintained by the Na^+/H^+ exchanger which, by extruding H^+, increases intracellular and decreases extracellular HCO_3^-. We recall that the force driving Cl^- into the cell is the difference between the Cl^- and the HCO_3^- gradients (i.e. $RT \ln [Cl^-]_i/[Cl^-]_o - RT \ln [HCO_3^-]_i/[HCO_3^-]_o$). Thus, as long as H^+ efflux maintains this gradient there is no energy barrier to continued outward translocation of HCO_3^-. Since $[HCO_3^-]_o$ is bound to be very low in a situation of severe acidosis one can envisage the therapeutic advantage of promoting HCO_3^- flux from blood to ECF.

I wish to emphasize that the Na^+ and Cl^- contained in the ECF cannot sustain glial swelling of the magnitude discussed. Such swelling requires that a delivery line is established for Na^+ and Cl^- in the direction blood → ECF → ICF. For K^+, the overall flux is in the reverse direction. Under normal circumstances, any influx of Cl^- via the anion exchanger must be balanced by a corresponding efflux, either occurring as an electrophoretic drag created by an electrogenic Na^+ pump, or as conductive flux along the electrochemical gradient. It remains to be shown if this back flux is curtailed by a reduction of the electrogenic component of the pump, or by a reduction of membrane potential.

So far, I have laid the emphasis on glial cell swelling, assuming that these cells contain the coupled cation and anion antiporters. As observed in fixed tissue samples, neurons behave more erratic since some swell, some remain unchanged, and some show pronounced shrinkage (e.g. Kalimo et al., 1977; Jenkins et al., 1979, 1981). We do not know why these differences exist. It has been emphasized that whereas an increase in the "Na^+ leak" will cause cell swelling, a selective increase in K^+ permeability can lead to cell shrinkage (MacKnight and Leaf, 1977; see also Cala, 1983; and Fig. 22). Since an increase in K^+ "permeability" can be triggered by Ca^{2+} influx it is tempting to relate cell shrinkage to Ca^{2+} influx. However, any such link would at present be highly speculative, and we cannot exclude that some cells lack tightly coupled Na^+/H^+ and Cl^-/HCO_3^- exchanges. Until further information is available, we must conclude that cells differ with respect to the "leak" pathways which are established in adverse conditions.

Mitochondrial respiration

During complete or near-complete ischemia mitochondrial respiratory functions have ceased, or are severely depressed. If some oxygen supply persists it will depend on the circumstances whether or not useful mitochondrial functions persist. The same holds true for mitochondrial function in the recirculation period following complete or near-complete ischemia. What are those circumstances? In discussing one of them, cytosolic pH, we recall that mitochondria can be functionally depressed, or show structural injury. In the first case, they would be expected to respire normally when incubated under optimal conditions in vitro. In the latter, such in vitro incubation reveals the structural damage which may be transient or permanent.

When rats are subjected to 30 min of ischemia under conditions which cause excessive tissue lactic acidosis, isolated mitochondria show deficient respiratory functions (decreased State 3 respiration) which persist in the recirculation period (Rehncrona et al., 1979; Hillered et al., 1984a). During recirculation, tissue ATP levels are not adequately restored and excessive amounts of lactate accumulate (Nordström et al., 1978; Welsh et al., 1980). These results demonstrate deranged mitochondrial functions in vitro and in vivo. However, mitochondrial functions are restored after 30 min (Rehncrona et al., 1979, 1981), and even after 60 min of ischemia (Hossmann and Kleihues, 1973; Hossmann et al., 1977; Hossmann, 1982) provided that conditions are optimal. Notably, one requirement is that hyperglycemia does not induce excessive tissue acidosis (Rehncrona et al., 1981).

The results raise the question of how acidosis influences mitochondrial function and structural integrity. When normal brain mitochondria are incubated in vitro, State 3 respiration decreases with pH of the incubation medium, complete inhibition being observed at pH < 6.0 (Fig. 24). These results suggest that mitochondrial ATP formation is severely depressed in ischemic tissue with very low pH. The question arises: can the delay in restoration of pH_i following ischemia in hyperglycemic animals prevent adequate resumption of mitochondrial function? After 15 min of ischemia mitochondrial function, as studied in vitro, was quickly restored, demonstrating the absence of a persisting structural defect (Hillered et al., 1984a). Furthermore, in spite of the pronounced acidosis during

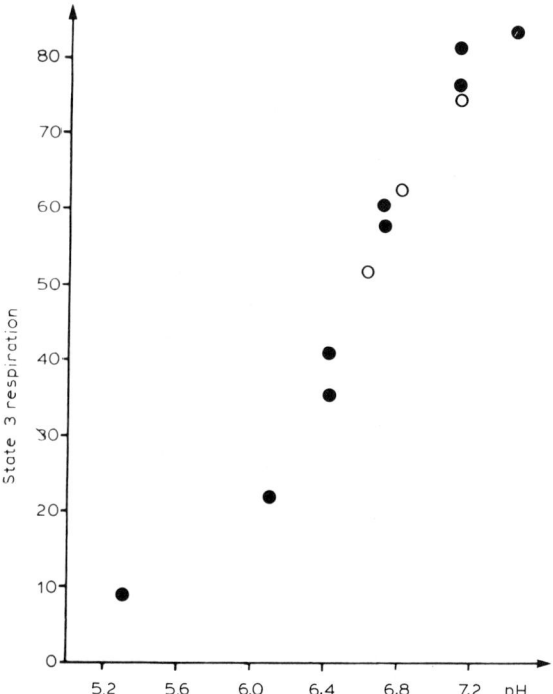

Fig. 24. The effects of in vitro lactic acidosis (●) and of hypercapnia (○) on the oxygen consumption rate (nmol O_2 min^{-1} · mg^{-1} protein) in State 3 (substrate-phosphate-, and ADP-stimulated) respiration in isolated rat brain mitochondria. (Slightly modified after Hillered et al., 1984b.)

ischemia cerebral energy state was quickly restored, demonstrating adequacy of mitochondrial function in vivo. We have to conclude, therefore, that the detrimental influence of excessive acidosis on the final outcome of a 15-min ischemic insult does not seem to be caused by a deficient mitochondrial function in the immediate recovery period.

Following a longer ischemic insult (e.g. 30 min in the rat) the situation is obviously different. Starved and fed animals show similar cerebral metabolic changes save for the lactic acidosis. It seems highly likely, therefore, that exaggeration of the acidosis triggers a derangement in mitochondrial function which outlasts the ischemic period and prevents adequate restoration of cellular energy state.

Lipid peroxidation

We obviously have to define the molecular mechanisms by which acidosis can aggravate the final cell damage after short periods of ischemia, and precipitate immediate mitochondrial failure after long periods of ischemia. One such mechanism, albeit of speculative nature, is peroxidative membrane damage caused by free radicals.

Free radical damage, if occurring, is likely to primarily involve the formation of superoxide radicals ($\cdot O_2^-$), a product of autoxidation of many compounds and of several enzymatic reactions (e.g. Fridovich, 1978). In the presence of hydrogen peroxide (H_2O_2) the reaction described by Haber and Weiss (1934) can then lead to the formation of hydroxyl radicals ($\cdot OH$), a likely initiator of deleterious reactions such as those leading to lipid peroxidation and crosslinking of proteins. It is now known that the uncatalyzed Haber-Weiss reaction is too slow to be of any importance; however iron catalysis can overcome this hindrance (see Freeman and Crapo, 1982; Halliwell and Gutteridge, 1984) and initiate the following reactions

$$Fe^{3+} + \cdot O_2^- \rightarrow Fe^{2+} + O_2 \qquad (20)$$

$$\underline{Fe^{2+} + H_2O_2 \rightarrow Fe^{3+} + \cdot OH + OH^- \qquad (21)}$$

$$\cdot O_2^- + H_2O \rightarrow O_2 + \cdot OH + OH^- \qquad (22)$$

These are not the only reactions by which iron catalysis of free radical reactions can occur. Whatever are the reactions, though, the participation of decompartmentalized iron seems likely.

When studying free radical formation in vitro by the thiobarbituric acid (TBA) method for malondialdehyde, Barber and Bernheim (1967) found that reduced pH enhanced formation of TBA reactive material. Since the TBA method does not unequivocally reflect rate of formation of free radicals, and extent of lipid peroxidation, our own laboratory studied the influence of lowered pH, measuring malondialdehyde formation, water- and lipid-soluble scavengers, and phospholipid-bound free fatty acids (Siesjö et al., 1985b). It could be shown that a lowering of pH from 7.0 to 6.5 markedly enhanced malondialdehyde formation, reduced the content of α-tocopherol, and caused part of the pool of phospholipid-bound polyenoic fatty acids to disappear (Fig. 25). Thus, it appears established that, at least in vitro, a lowering of pH to values encountered during ischemia markedly enhances initiation and propagation of free radical reactions.

Barber and Bernheim (1967) postulated that the effect of low pH was to cause decompartmentalization of iron bound to tissue constituents. In view of the pro-oxidant effect of free iron, such binding is mandatory. In the cell, iron in the ferrous form is chelated to transferrin, ferritin and other macromolecules (Aisen, 1979). At least in transferrin (TFn), the reversible binding of iron involves the formation of a bicarbonate (or carbonate) bridge according to the reaction

$$Fe^{3+} + HCO_3^- + H_3TFn \rightleftharpoons FeTFnHCO_3^- + 3H^+ \quad (23)$$

Thus, protonic attack on this bridge can lead to release of the iron.

Although the reactions outlined form a plausible series of events, mediating the effects of acidosis, other possibilities exist. Gebicki and Bielski (1981) have emphasized that the superoxide radical ($\cdot O_2^-$) is the anion of an acid ($HO_2^\cdot$) whose pK' is close to 4.7. Since the acid is both more lipid-soluble and a stronger pro-oxidant than $\cdot O_2^-$, a lowering of pH could cause lipid peroxidation by shifting the equilibrium towards formation of the acid form.

It should be emphasized that free radical induced damage is a likely but still speculative mechanism of ischemic brain damage (Kogure et al., 1985).

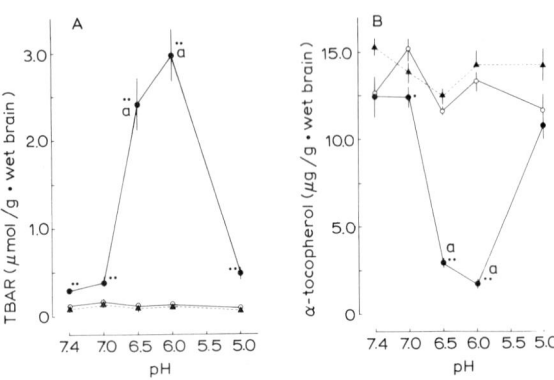

Fig. 25. The effect of lactic acidosis on free radical formation in brain homogenates fortified with ferrous sulfate and ascorbic acid. Reduction of pH to 6.5 (or 6.0) markedly enhanced the formation of thiobarbituric acid reactive material (TBAR) and the reduction of α-tocopherol content. Filled circles denote values obtained with 5–15% O_2, unfilled circles those with N_2. (Slightly modified from Siesjö et al., 1985b.)

Possibly, free radical damage only becomes important when iron is deposited in the tissue, e.g. due to gross intracerebral bleeding or trauma. However, we should not ignore the possibility that the adverse effects of acidosis on mitochondrial or other cellular membranes in ischemia involves enhancement of free radical reactions, e.g. triggered by release of compartmentalized iron.

Acknowledgements

This study was supported by grants from the Swedish Medical Research Council (No. 14X-263), and from U.S. Public Health Service (NIH grant No. 2 RO1 NS07838). The author is grateful to Erna Björkengren and Yvonne Hansson for skilful secretarial help.

References

Ahmad, H.R. and Loeschcke, H.H. (1982) Fast bicarbonate-chloride exchange between brain cells and brain extracellular fluid in respiratory acidosis. *Pflügers Arch.*, 395: 293–299.

Aisen, P. (1979) Some physicochemical aspects of iron metabolism. In: *Iron Metabolism* (CIBA Foundation Symposium 51). Elsevier, Amsterdam, pp. 1–17.

Alberti, K.G.M.M. and Cuthbert, C. (1982) The hydrogen ion in normal metabolism: a review. In: *Metabolic Acidosis* (CIBA Foundation Symposium 87). Pitman Books Ltd., London, pp. 1–19.

Ammann, D., Lanter, F., Steiner, R.A., Schulthess, P., Shijo, Y. and Simon, W. (1981) Neutral carrier based hydrogen ion selective microelectrode for extra- and intracellular studies. *Anal. Chem.*, 53: 2267–2269.

Andersson, R.E. and Sundt, T.M. (1983) Brain pH in focal cerebral ischemia and the protective effects of barbiturate anesthesia. *J. Cereb. Blood Flow Metabol.*, 3: 493–497.

Arieff, A.I., Kerian, A., Massry, S.G. and DeLima, J. (1976) Intracellular pH of brain: alterations in acute respiratory acidosis and alkalosis. *Am. J. Physiol.*, 230(3): 804–813.

Barber, A.A. and Bernheim, F. (1976) Lipid peroxidation: its measurement, occurrence, and significance in animal tissues. *Adv. Gerontol. Res.*, 2: 355–403.

Benos, D.J. (1982) Amiloride: a molecular probe of sodium transport in tissues and cells. *Am. J. Physiol.*, 242: C131–C145.

Berridge, M.J. (1984) Inositol triphosphate and diacylglycerol as second messengers. *Biochem. J.*, 220: 345–360.

Blennow, G., Nilsson, B. and Siesjö, B.K. (1977) Sustained epileptic seizures complicated by hypoxia, arterial hypotension or hyperthermia: effects on cerebral energy state. *Acta Physiol. Scand.*, 100: 126–128.

Blennow, G., Folbergrová, J., Nilsson, B. and Siesjö, B.K. (1979) Effects of bicuculline-induced seizures on cerebral metabolism and circulation of rats rendered hypoglycemic by starvation. *Ann. Neurol.*, 5: 139–151.

Boron, W.F. and de Weer, P. (1976a) Intracellular pH transients in squid giant axons caused by CO_2, NH_3, and metabolic inhibitors. *J. Gen. Physiol.*, 67: 91–112.

Boron, W.F. and de Weer, P. (1976b) Active proton transport stimulated by CO_2/HCO_3^-, blocked by cyanide. *Nature*, 259: 240–241.

Boron, W.F. and Boulpaep, E.L. (1983) Intracellular pH regulation in the renal proximal tubule of the salamander. Na-H exchange. *J. Gen. Physiol.*, 81: 29–52.

Boron, W.F., McCormick, W.C. and Roos, A. (1979) pH regulation in barnacle muscle fibers: dependence on intracellular and extracellular pH. *Am. J. Physiol.*, 237(3): C185–C193.

Brooks, D.J., Lammertsma, A.A., Beaney, R.P., Leenders, K.L., Buckingham, P.D., Marshall, J. and Jones, T. (1984) Measurement of regional cerebral pH in human subjects using continuous inhalation of $^{11}CO_2$ and positron emission tomography. *J. Cereb. Blood Flow Metabol.*, 4: 458–465.

Buxton, R.B., Wechsler, I.R., Alpert, N.M., Ackerman, R.H., Elmaleh, D.R. and Correia, J.A. (1984) Measurement of brain pH using $^{11}CO_2$ and positron emission tomography. *J. Cereb. Blood Flow Metabol.*, 4: 8–16.

Cala, P.M. (1980) Volume regulation by amphiuma red blood cells. The membrane potential and its implications regarding the nature of the ion-flux pathways. *J. Gen. Physiol.*, 76: 683–708.

Cala, P.M. (1983) Volume regulation by red blood cells. Mechanisms of ion transport. *Molec. Physiol.*, 4: 33–52.

Carter, N.W., Rector, F.C., Champion, R.T. and Seldin, D.W. (1976) Measurement of intracellular pH of skeletal muscle with pH-sensitive glass micro-electrodes. *J. Clin. Invest.*, 46: 920–933.

Chapman, A.G., Meldrum, B.S. and Siesjö, B.K. (1977) Cerebral metabolic changes during prolonged epileptic seizures in rats. *J. Neurochem.*, 28: 1025–1035.

Conway, E.J. and Fearon, P.J. (1944) The acid-labile CO_2 in mammalian muscle and the pH of the muscle fibre. *J. Physiol. (Lond.)*, 103: 274–289.

Csiba, L., Paschen, W. and Hossmann, K.-A. (1983) A topographic quantitative method for measuring brain tissue pH under physiological and pathophysiological conditions. *Brain Res.*, 289: 334–337.

Davies, D.G., Fitzgerald, R.S. and Gurtner, G.H. (1973) Acid-base relationships between CSF and blood during acute metabolic acidosis. *J. Appl. Physiol.*, 34(2): 243–248.

Davis, R.P. (1967) Logland: a gibbsian view of acid-base balance. *Am. J. Med.*, 42: 159–162.

Duffy, T.E., Howse, D.C. and Plum, F. (1975) Cerebral energy metabolism during experimental status epilepticus. *J. Neurochem.*, 24: 925–934.

Edsall, J.T. and Wyman, J. (1958) *Biophysical Chemistry*, Vol. 1. Academic Press, New York, pp. 699–753.

Feise, G., Kogure, K., Busto, R., Scheinberg, P. and Reinmuth, O.M. (1976) Effect of insulin hypoglycemia upon cerebral energy metabolism and EEG activity in the rat. *Brain Res.*, 126: 263–280.

Fencl, V. (1985) Acid-base balance in cerebral extracellular fluids. In: *Handbook of Physiology*. Am. Physiol. Soc. In press.

Fencl, V., Miller, T.B. and Pappenheimer, J.R. (1966) Studies on the respiratory response to disturbances of acid-base balance, with deductions concerning the ionic composition of cerebral interstitial fluid. *Am. J. Physiol.*, 210(3): 459–472.

Fenn, W.O. and Maurer, F.W. (1936) The pH of muscle. *Protoplasma*, 24: 337–345.

Folbergrová, J., Norberg, K., Quistorff, B. and Siesjö, B.K. (1975) Carbohydrate and amino acid metabolism in rat cerebral cortex in moderate and extreme hypercapnia. *J. Neurochem.*, 25: 457–462.

Folbergrová, J., Ingvar, M. and Siesjö, B.K. (1981) Metabolic changes in cerebral cortex, hippocampus, and cerebellum during sustained bicuculline-induced seizures. *J. Neurochem.*, 37(5): 1228–1238.

Freeman, B.A. and Crapo, J.D. (1982) Biology of disease. Free radicals and tissue injury. *Lab. Invest.*, 47(5): 412–426.

Fridovich, L. (1978) The biology of oxygen radicals. The superoxide radical is an agent of oxygen toxicity; superoxide dismutases provide an important defense. *Science*, 201: 875–880.

Friede, R.L. and van Houten, W.H. (1961) Relations between post-mortem alterations and glycolytic metabolism in the brain. *Exp. Neurol.*, 4: 197–204.

Gardiner, A., Smith, M.L., Kågström, E., Shohami, E. and Siesjö, B.K. (1982) Influence of blood glucose concentration on brain lactate accumulation during severe hypoxia and subsequent recovery of brain energy metabolism. *J. Cereb. Blood Flow Metabol.*, 2: 429–438.

Gebicki, J.M. and Bielski, B.H.J. (1981) Comparison of the

capacities of the perhydroxyl and the superoxide radicals to initiate chain oxidation of linoleic acid. *J. Am. Chem. Soc.*, 103: 7020–7022.

Ginsberg, M.D., Frank, A.W. and Budd, W.W. (1980) Deleterious effect of glucose pretreatment on recovery from diffuse cerebral ischemia in the cat. *Stroke*, 11(4): 347–354.

Grinstein, S., Clarke, C.A. and Rothstein, A. (1983) Activation of Na^+/H^+ exchange in lymphocytes by osmotically induced volume changes and by cytoplasmic acidification. *J. Gen. Physiol.*, 82: 619–638.

Grinstein, S., Cohen, S. and Rothstein, A. (1984) Cytoplasmic pH regulation in thymic lymphocytes by an amiloride-sensitive Na^+/H^+ antiport. *J. Gen. Physiol.*, 83: 341–369.

Haas, M., Schmidt, III W.F. and McManus, T.J. (1982) Catecholamine-stimulated ion transport in duck red cells. Gradient effects in electrically neutral Na + K + 2Cl co-transport. *J. Gen. Physiol.*, 80: 125–147.

Haber, F. and Weiss, J. (1934) The catalytic decomposition of hydrogen peroxide by iron salts. *Proc. Roy. Soc. London*, A147: 332–351.

Halliwell, B. and Gutteridge, J.M.C. (1984) Oxygen toxicity, oxygen radicals, transition metals and disease. *Biochem. J.*, 219: 1–14.

Hansen, A.J. and Zeuthen, T. (1981) Extracellular ion concentrations during spreading depression and ischemia in the rat brain cortex. *Acta Physiol. Scand.*, 113: 437–445.

Harris, R.J., Wieloch, T., Symon, L. and Siesjö, B.K. (1984) Cerebral extracellular calcium activity in severe hypoglycemia: relation to extracellular potassium and energy state. *J. Cereb. Blood Flow Metabol.*, 4: 187–193.

Heinemann, U., Lux, H.D. and Gutnick, M.J. (1977) Extracellular free calcium and potassium during paroxysmal activity in the cerebral cortex of the cat. *Exp. Brain Res.*, 27: 237–243.

Hilberman, M, Subramanian, V.H., Haselgrove, J., Cone, J.B., Egan, J.W., Gyulai, L. and Chance, B. (1984) In vivo time-resolved brain phosphorus nuclear magnetic resonance. *J. Cereb. Blood Flow Metabol.*, 4: 334–342.

Hillered, L., Siesjö, B.K. and Arfors, K.E. (1984a) Mitochondrial response to transient forebrain ischemia and recirculation in the rat. *J. Cereb. Blood Flow Metabol.*, 4: 438–446.

Hillered, L., Ernster, L. and Siesjö, B.K. (1984b) Influence of in vitro lactic acidosis and hypercapnia on respiratory activity of isolated rat brain mitochondria. *J. Cereb. Blood Flow Metabol.*, 4: 430–437.

Hindfelt, B. and Siesjö, B.K. (1971) Cerebral effects of acute ammonia intoxication. I. The influence on intracellular and extracellular acid-base parameters. *Scand. J. Clin. Lab. Invest.*, 28: 353–364.

Hossmann, K.A. (1982) Treatment of experimental cerebral ischemia. *J. Cereb. Blood Flow Metabol.*, 2: 275–297.

Hossmann, K.A. and Kleihues, P. (1973) Reversibility of ischemic brain damage. *Arch. Neurol.*, 29: 375–384.

Hossmann, K.A., Sakaki, S. and Zimmermann, V. (1977) Cation activities in reversible ischemia of the cat brain. *Stroke*, 8: 77–81.

Howse, D.C., Caronna, J.J., Duffy, T.E. and Plum, F. (1974) Cerebral energy metabolism, pH, and blood flow during seizures in the cat. *Am. J. Physiol.*, 227: 1444–1451.

Ingvar, M., Folbergrová, J. and Siesjö, B.K. (1985) The development of hypermetabolic infarction in the substantia nigra in status epilepticus. 1. Energy metabolism. Submitted for publication.

Jenkins, L.W., Povlishock, J.T., Becker, D.P., Miller, J.D. and Sullivan, H.G. (1979) Complete cerebral ischemia. An ultrastructural study. *Acta Neuropathol. (Berl.)*, 48: 113–125.

Jenkins, L.W., Povlishock, J.T., Lewelt, W., Miller, J.D. and Becker, D.P. (1981) The role of postischemic recirculation in the development of ischemic neuronal injury following complete cerebral ischemia. *Acta Neuropathol. (Berl.)*, 55: 205–220.

Kalimo, H., Garcia, J.H., Kamijyo, Y., Tanaka, J. and Trump, B.F. (1977) The ultrastructure of "brain death". II. Electron microscopy of feline cortex after complete ischemia. *Virchows Arch. B Cell. Pathol.*, 25: 207–220.

Kalimo, H., Rehncrona, S., Söderfeldt, B., Olsson, Y. and Siesjö, B.K. (1981) Brain lactic acidosis and ischemic cell damage. 2. Histopathology. *J. Cereb. Blood Flow Metabol.*, 1: 313–327.

Karmann, U. and Held, D.R. (1972) Equations treating the pH and (HCO_3^-) of buffered media as functions of PCO_2. *Respir. Physiol.*, 15: 343–349.

Kimelberg, H.K. (1983) Primary astrocyte cultures — a key to astrocyte function. *Cell Molec. Neurobiol.*, 3(1): 1–16.

Kimelberg, H.K. and Bourke, R.S. (1982) Anion transport in the nervous system. In: A. Lajtha (Ed.), *Handbook of Neurochemistry*, 2nd Ed., Vol. 1, *Chemical and Cellular Architecture*. Plenum Press, New York, pp. 31–67.

Kimelberg, H.K. and Bourke, R.S. (1984) Mechanisms of astrocytic swelling. In: A. Bes, P. Braquet, R. Paoletti and B.K. Siesjö (Eds.), *Cerebral Ischemia, ICS 654*. Excerpta Medica, Amsterdam-New York-Oxford, pp. 131–146.

Kjällquist, Å., Nardini, M. and Siesjö, B.K. (1969) The regulation of extra- and intracellular acid-base parameters in the rat brain during hyper- and hypocapnia. *Acta Physiol. Scand.*, 76: 485–494.

Kogure, K., Arai, H., Abe, K. and Nakano, M. (1985) Free radical damage of the brain following ischemia. *This volume*, pp. 237–259.

Kogure, K., Bust, R., Schwartzman, R.J. and Scheinberg, P. (1980a) The dissociation of cerebral blood flow, metabolism, and function in the early stages of developing cerebral infarction. *Ann. Neurol.*, 8: 278–290.

Kogure, K., Alonso, O.F. and Martinez, E. (1980b) A topographic measurement of brain pH. *Brain Res.*, 195: 95–109.

Koppel, M. and Spiro, K. (1919) Über die Wirkung von Moderatoren (Puffern) bei der Verschiebung des Säure-Basengleichgewichtes in biologischen Flüssigheiten. *Biochem. Z.*, 65: 409–439.

Kraig, R.P., Ferreira-Filho, C.R. and Nicholson, C. (1983) Alkaline and acid transients in cerebellar microenvironment. *J. Neurophysiol.*, 49(3): 831–850.

Kraig, R.P., Pulsinelli, W.A. and Plum, F. (1985) Heterogeneous distribution of hydrogen and bicarbonate ions during complete brain ischemia. *This volume*, pp. 155–166.

Kregenow, F.M. (1981) Osmoregulatory salt transporting mechanisms: control of cell volume in anisotonic media. *Ann. Rev. Physiol.*, 43: 493–505.

Lewis, L.D., Ljungren, B., Norberg, K. and Siesjö, B.K. (1974) Changes in carbohydrate substrates, amino acids and ammonia in the brain during insulin-induced hypoglycemia. *J. Neurochem.*, 23: 659–671.

Lindenberg, R. (1963) Patterns of CNS vulnerability in acute hypoxemia including anesthesia accidents. In: J. Schade and W. McMenemy (Eds.), *Selective Vulnerability of the Brain in Hypoxemia*. F.A. Davis, Philadelphia, pp. 189–210.

Ljunggren, B., Norberg, K. and Siesjö, B.K. (1974) Influence of tissue acidosis upon restitution of brain energy metabolism following total ischemia. *Brain Res.*, 77: 173–186.

Mabe, H., Blomqvist, P. and Siesjö, B.K. (1983) Intracellular pH in the brain following transient ischemia. *J. Cereb. Blood Flow Metabol.*, 3: 109–114.

MacKnight, A.D.C. and Leaf, A. (1977) Regulation of cellular volume. *Physiol. Rev.*, 57(3): 510–573.

MacMillan, V. and Siesjö, B.K. (1973) The influence of hypocapnia upon intracellular pH and upon some carbohydrate substrates, amino acids and organic phosphates in the brain. *J. Neurochem.*, 21: 1283–1299.

Messeter, K. and Siesjö, B.K. (1971a) Regulation of the CSF pH in acute and sustained respiratory acidosis. *Acta Physiol. Scand.*, 83: 21–30.

Messeter, K. and Siesjö, B.K. (1971b) The intracellular pH in the brain in acute and sustained hypercapnia. *Acta Physiol. Scand.*, 83: 210–219.

Miller, A.L., Hawkins, R.A. and Veech, R.L. (1975) Decreased rate of glucose utilization by rat brain in vivo after exposures to atmospheres containing high concentrations of CO_2. *J. Neurochem.*, 25: 553–558.

Moody, Jr., W.J. (1981) The ionic mechanism of intracellular pH regulation in crayfish neurones. *J. Physiol.*, 316: 293–308.

Moore, R.D. (1983) Effects of insulin upon ion transport. *Biochim. Biophys. Acta*, 737: 1–49.

Mutch, W.A.C. and Hansen, A.J. (1984) Extracellular pH changes during spreading depression and cerebral ischemia: mechanisms of brain pH regulation. *J. Cereb. Blood Flow Metabol.*, 4: 17–27.

Myers, R.E. (1979) Lactic acid accumulation as cause of brain edema and cerebral necrosis resulting from oxygen deprivation. In: R. Korobkin and G. Guilleminault (Eds.), *Advances in Perinatal Neurology*. Spectrum, New York, pp. 85–114.

Myers, R.E. and Yamaguchi, S. (1977) Nervous system effects of cardiac arrest in monkeys. *Arch. Neurol.*, 34: 65–74.

Nahas, G.G. (Ed.) (1966) Current concepts of acid-base measurement. *Ann. NY Acad. Sci.*, 133: 1–274.

Nevander, G., Ingvar, M., Auer, R. and Siesjö, B.K. (1984) Irreversible neuronal damage after short periods of status epilepticus. *Acta Physiol. Scand.*, 120: 155–157.

Nevander, G., Ingvar, M., Auer, R. and Siesjö, B.K. (1985) Status epilepticus in well oxygenated rats causes neuronal necrosis. *Ann. Neurol.*, in press.

Nicholson, C. (1980) Measurement of extracellular ions in the brain. *Trends Neurosci.*, 3: 216–218.

Norberg, K. (1976) Changes in the cerebral metabolism induced by hyperventilation at different blood glucose levels. *J. Neurochem.*, 26: 353–359.

Nordström, C.H., Rehncrona, S. and Siesjö, B.K. (1978) Effects of phenobarbital in cerebral ischemia. Part II. Restitution of cerebral energy state, as well as of glycolytic metabolites, citric acid cycle intermediates and associated amino acids after pronounced incomplete ischemia. *Stroke*, 9: 335–343.

Pelligrino, D. and Siesjö, B.K. (1981) Regulation of extra- and intracellular pH in the brain in severe hypoglycemia. *J. Cereb. Blood Flow Metabol.*, 1: 85–96.

Pelligrino, D.A., Musch, T.I. and Dempsey, J.A. (1981a) Interregional differences in brain intracellular pH and water compartmentation during acute normoxic and hypoxic hypocapnia in the anesthetized dog. *Brain Res.*, 214: 387–404.

Pelligrino, D., Almquist, L.-O. and Siesjö, B.K. (1981b) Effects of insulin-induced hypoglycemia on intracellular pH and impedance in the cerebral cortex of the rat. *Brain Res.*, 221: 129–147.

Pontén, U. and Siesjö, B.K. (1966) Gradients of CO_2 tension in the brain. *Acta Physiol. Scand.*, 67: 129–140.

Prichard, J.W., Alger, J.R., Behar, K.L., Petroff, O.A.C. and Shulman, R.G. (1983) Cerebral metabolic studies in vivo by ^{31}P NMR. *Proc. Natl. Acad. Sci. USA*, 80: 2748–2751.

Pulsinelli, W.A., Waldman, S., Rawlinson, D. and Plum, F. (1982) Moderate hyperglycemia augments ischemic brain damage: a neuropathologic study in the rat. *Neurology (NY)*, 32: 1239–1246.

Rehncrona, S., Mela, L. and Siesjö, B.K. (1979) Recovery of brain mitochondrial function in the rat after complete and incomplete cerebral ischemia. *Stroke*, 10: 437–446.

Rehncrona, S., Rosén, I. and Siesjö, B.K. (1981) Brain lactic acidosis and ischemic cell damage. 1. Biochemistry and neurophysiology. *J. Cereb. Blood Flow Metabol.*, 1: 297–311.

Rink, T.J., Esien, R.Y. and Pozzan, T. (1982) Cytoplasmic pH and free Mg^{2+} in lymphocytes. *J. Cell Biol.*, 95: 189–196.

Roos, A. (1965) Intracellular pH and intracellular buffering power of the cat brain. *Am. J. Physiol.*, 209: 1233–1246.

Roos, A. (1971) Intracellular pH and buffering power of rat brain. *Am. J. Physiol.*, 221(1): 176–188.

Roos, A. and Boron, W.F. (1981) Intracellular pH. *Physiol. Rev.*, 61(2): 296–434.

Siemkowicz, E. and Hansen, A. (1978) Clinical restitution following cerebral ischema in hypo-, normo-, and hyperglycemic rats. *Acta Neurol. Scand.*, 58: 1–8.

Siemkowicz, E. and Hansen, A.J. (1981) Brain extracellular ion composition and EEG activity following 10 minutes ischemia in normo- and hyperglycemic rats. *Stroke*, 12(2): 236–240.

Siesjö, B.K. (1971) Quantification of pH regulation in hypercapnia and hypocapnia. *Scand. J. Clin. Lab. Invest.*, 28: 113–119.

Siesjö, B.K. (1972) The regulation of cerebrospinal fluid pH. *Kidney Int.*, 1: 360–374.

Siesjö, B.K. (1973) Metabolic control of intracellular pH. *Scand. J. Clin. Lab. Invest.*, 32: 97–104.

Siesjö, B.K. (1981) Cell damage in the brain: a speculative synthesis. *J. Cereb. Blood Flow Metabol.*, 1: 155–185.

Siesjö, B.K. (1984) Cerebral circulation and metabolism. *J. Neurosurg.*, 60: 883–908.

Siesjö, B.K. and Messeter, K. (1971) Factors determining intracellular pH. In: B.K. Siesjö and S.C. Sørensen (Eds.), *Ion Homeostasis of the Brain* (Alfred Benzon Symposium III). Munksgaard, Copenhagen, pp. 244–262.

Siesjö, B.K. and Wieloch, T. (1985) Cerebral metabolism in ischemia: neurochemical basis for therapy. *Br. J. Anaesthesiol.*, 57: 47–62.

Siesjö, B.K., Ingvar, M. and Wieloch, T. (1985) Cellular and molecular events underlying epileptic brain damage. To be published by *Ann. NY Acad. Sci.*

Siesjö, B.K., Folbergrová, J. and MacMillan, V. (1972) The effect of hypercapnia upon intracellular pH in the brain, evaluated by the bicarbonate-carbonic acid method and from the creatine phosphokinase equilibrium. *J. Neurochem.*, 19: 2483–2495.

Siesjö, B.K., von Hanwehr, R., Nergelius, G., Nevander, G. and Ingvar, M. (1985a) Extra- and intracellular pH in the brain during seizures and in the recovery period following arrest of seizure activity. *J. Cereb. Blood Flow Metabol.*, in press.

Siesjö, B.K., Bendek, G., Koide, T., Westerberg, E. and Wieloch, T. (1985b) Influence of acidosis on lipid peroxidation in brain tissues in vitro. *J. Cereb. Blood Flow Metabol.*, Submitted.

Siggaard-Andersen, O. (1966) Titratable acid or base of body fluids. *Ann. NY Acad. Sci.*, 133: 41–58.

Stewart, P.A. (1981) *How to understand acid-base*. Edward Arnold, London, pp. 1–186.

Syrota, A., Castaing, M., Rougemont, D., Berridge, M., Baron, J.C., Bousser, M.G. and Pocidala, J.J. (1983) Tissue acid-base balance and oxygen metabolism in human cerebral infarction studied with positron emission tomography. *Ann. Neurol.*, 14: 419–428.

Thomas, R.C. (1974) Intracellular pH of snail neurones measured with a new pH-sensitive glass micro-electrode. *J. Physiol.*, 238: 159–180.

Thomas, R.C. (1976) The effect of carbon dioxide on the intracellular pH and buffering power of snail neurones. *J. Physiol.*, 255: 715–735.

Thomas, R.C. (1977) The role of bicarbonate, chloride and sodium ions in the regulation of intracellular pH in snail neurones. *J. Physiol.*, 273: 317–338.

Thulborn, K.R., du Boulay, G.H., Duchen, L.W. and Radda, G. (1982) A ^{31}P nuclear magnetic resonance in vivo study of cerebral ischaemia in the gerbil. *J. Cereb. Blood Flow Metabol.*, 2: 299–306.

Tosteson, D.C. and Hoffman, J.F. (1960) Regulation of cell volume by active cation transport in high and low potassium sheep red cells. *J. Gen. Physiol.*, 44: 169–194.

Van Slyke, D.D. (1922) On the measurement of buffer values and on the relationship of buffer value to the dissociation constant of the buffer and the concentration and reaction of the buffer solution. *J. Biol. Chem.*, 52: 525–570.

Vaughan-Jones, R.D. (1979) Regulation of chloride in quiescent sheepheart Purkinje fibres studied using intracellular chloride and pH-sensitive micro-electrodes. *J. Physiol.*, 295: 111–137.

Vigne, P., Frelin, C. and Lazdunski, M. (1982) The amiloride-sensitive Na^+/H^+ exchange system in skeletal muscle cells in culture. *J. Biol. Chem.*, 257(16): 9394–9400.

Wallace, W.M. and Hastings, A.B. (1942) The distribution of the bicarbonate ion in mammalian muscle. *J. Biol. Chem.*, 144: 637–649.

Welsh, F.A., Ginsberg, M.D., Rieder, W. and Budd, W.W. (1980) Deleterious effect of glucose pretreatment on recovery from diffuse cerebral ischemia in the cat. II. Regional metabolite levels. *Stroke*, 11(4): 355–363.

Weyne, J., Demeester, G. and Leusen, J. (1968) Brain and blood lactate during acute and prolonged respiratory acidosis and alkalosis. *Arch. Int. Physiol.*, 76: 157–159.

Wilkie, D.R. (1979) Generation of protons by metabolic processes other than glycolysis in muscle cells: a critical view. *J. Molec. Cell. Cardiol.*, 11: 325–330.

Woodbury, J.W. (1965) Regulation of pH. In: T.C. Ruch and H.D. Patton (Eds.), *Physiology and Biophysics*. Saunders, Philadelphia, pp. 899–934.

Heterogeneous distribution of hydrogen and bicarbonate ions during complete brain ischemia

Richard P. Kraig, William A. Pulsinelli and Fred Plum

Cerebrovascular Disease Research Center, Department of Neurology, Cornell University Medical College, 1300 York Avenue, New York, New York 10021, USA

Introduction

Heterogeneous distribution of H^+ in brain

H^+ exist in a non-equilibrium distribution between cells and the interstitial space in a number of tissues under normal conditions (Roos and Boron, 1981). Several methods have been used to calculate intracellular $[H^+]$ ($[H^+]_i$) including the distribution of weak acids and bases; colorimetry or fluorometry with H^+-sensitive dyes; ^{31}P nuclear magnetic resonance. In addition H^+-selective microelectrodes have been used to measure cytoplasmic $[H^+]$ (cytoplasmic is taken to mean intracellular). All of these techniques, except the use of H^+-selective microelectrodes, derive a tissue average $[H^+]_i$. Thus in tissues which consist of multiple cell types such as brain, where neurons, glia, and capillary endothelial cells are present, only an average $[H^+]_i$ for all cell types can be computed. Under normal steady-state conditions the histological heterogeneity of the brain may be unimportant since the $[H^+]_i$ is probably around pH 7 in all cells (Roos and Boron, 1981; Cohen and Kassirer, 1982).

When brain is perturbed from a resting state, however, functional changes may induce a heterogeneity in $[H^+]_i$ among different cell types because of varying abilities to generate or remove excess H^+. Cell metabolic activity is associated with acidification of biological fluids either through net production of acids or carbon dioxide (CO_2). Considerable disagreement exists in the literature with regard to the overall metabolic rate of brain. Neurons (Hertz and Schousboe, 1975; Quastel, 1975), astrocytes (Hertz and Schousboe, 1975; Hertz, 1981), or capillaries (Oldendorf et al., 1977) each have their champions as a major contributor to the brain total metabolic rate. Whichever type predominates, if the metabolic rate does vary from one brain cell type to another while the physicochemical H^+ buffer capacities are similar, $[H^+]_i$ might also vary during states of enhanced metabolic activity. Alternatively, $[H^+]_i$ could be equally heterogeneous if rates of H^+ production in individual brain cell types are similar but H^+ physicochemical buffer capacities differ. Furthermore, the ultimate extrusion of excess H^+ from brain cells via plasma membrane antiport systems (see below) may vary among neurons, glia, or endothelial cells. Such differences could arise because of differences in H^+-related counter transport or because of differences in the microenvironment to which these antiporters are exposed to during increased brain activity (Kraig et al., 1985a).

Local inhomogeneities in $[H^+]$ are known to occur in the brain interstitial space (Kraig et al., 1983; Nicholson et al., 1985). Repetitive surface electrical stimulation of rat cerebellar cortex produces rectilinear excitation of granule cell axons and Purkinje cell dendrites (Fig. 1A). Such activation results in a rise in $[H^+]_o$ directly proportional to the rate (Fig. 1B), duration (Fig. 1C), and density (Fig. 1D) of brain excitation. Spreading depression, a more intense activation of brain biochemical and physio-

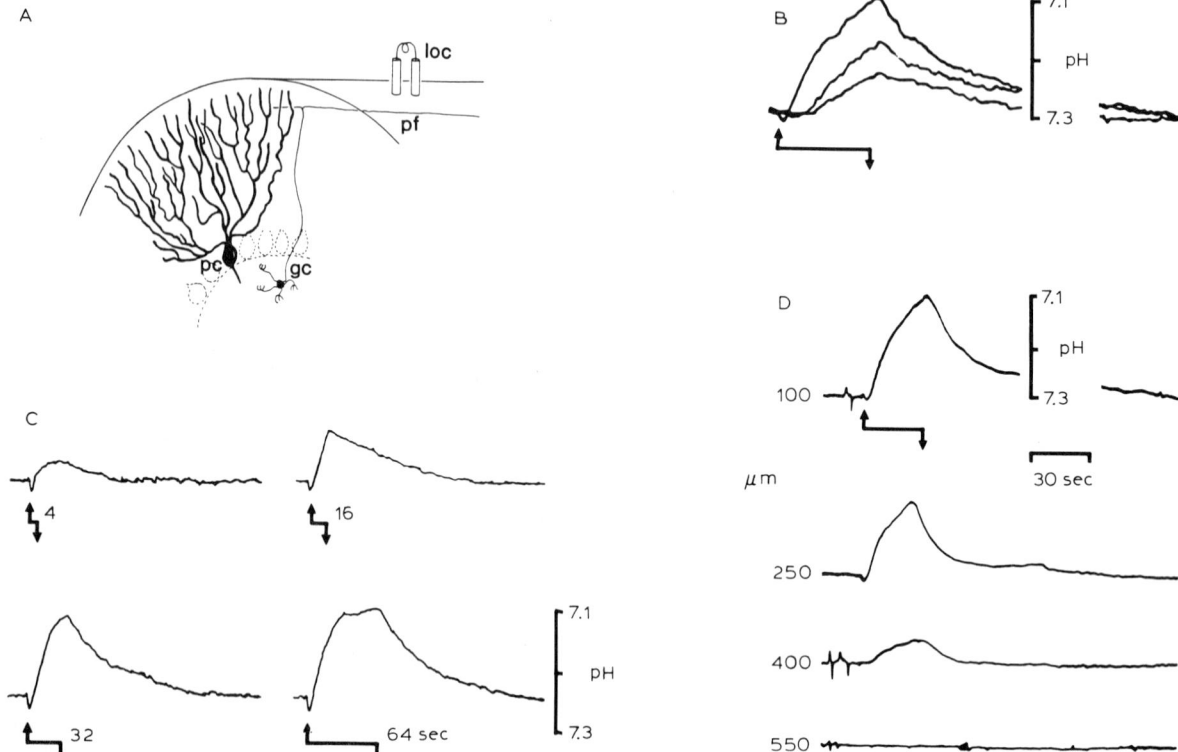

Fig. 1. Changes in pH_o associated with repetitive surface stimulation in the rat cerebellar cortex. The records show that heterogeneous levels of $[H^+]$ can be produced in the brain interstitial space which depend on the magnitude of brain excitation. (A) Local stimulation (loc) of the cerebellar surface excites a beam of parallel fibers (pf), which are axons of granule cells (gc), that in turn induce synaptic depolarization of Purkinje cell dendrites (pc) and interneurons. The cerebellar cortex is a highly ordered and well-defined laminar brain structure. Therefore, synchronous activation of a local population of parallel fibers and Purkinje cell dendrites produces well-defined changes in interstitial electrical potentials which can be used to accurately monitor microelectrode recording positions. Field potential analyses were used to determine pH_o recording depth in (B), (C), and (D). (B) Repetitive surface stimulation produced an alkaline then acid going response. Acidification of the interstitial space was proportional to the stimulus train rate. Records show pH_o transients 100 μm down in the cerebellar molecular layer in response to 5 Hz (lower record), 10 Hz (middle record), and 20 Hz (upper record) bipolar surface stimulation for 30 seconds. The stimulus began at the upward arrow and stopped at the downward arrow. The effect of increasing the duration of the stimulus train at 20 Hz is shown in (C). pH_o records again show an initial alkaline shift with initiation of the stimulus train (upward arrow). The subsequent acid shift increased in magnitude with the stimulus duration (4, 16, 32, and 64 seconds) until pH_o began to reach a steady-state after 64 seconds. (D) Acidification of the interstitial space was also directly proportional to the density of activated neural tissue. pH_o changes diminished in depth away from the beam of parallel fibers activated for 30 seconds at 20 Hz beginning at the upward arrow and stopping at the downward arrow. The H^+ selective microelectrode was advanced in increments of 150 μm vertically through a folium before each stimulus train (B), (C), and (D) are modified from Kraig et al., 1983.

logical processes (see Bureš et al., 1974; Nicholson and Kraig, 1981) than repetitive electrical stimulation, similarly acidifies the interstitial space in the cerebellum (Fig. 2) and the neocortex (Fig. 3). $[H^+]_o$ changes are directly proportional to the proximity of the H^+ selective microelectrode to brain involved in the wave of spreading depression (Fig. 2). Large changes in interstitial (and presumably intracellular) ion concentrations which occur during spreading depression (Kraig and Nicholson, 1978; Nicholson and Kraig, 1981) could differentially influence plasma membrane antiport mechanisms for $[H^+]_i$

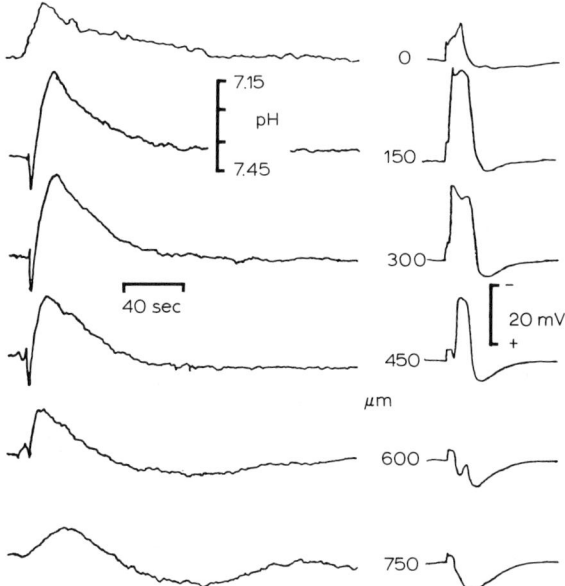

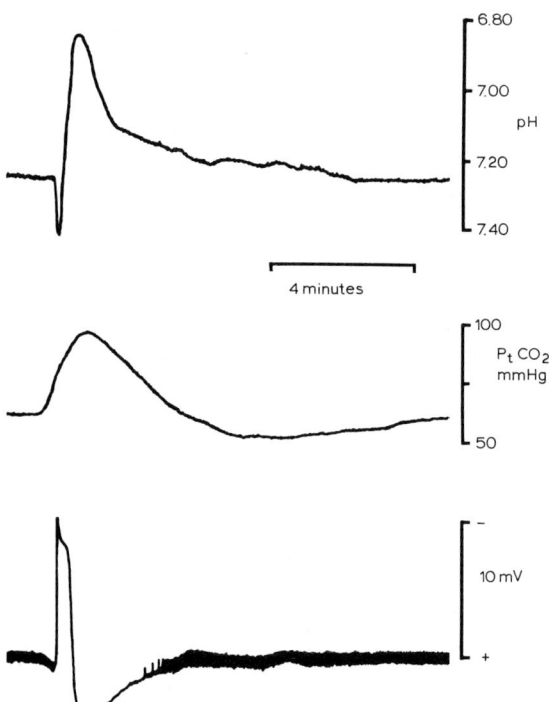

Fig. 2. Heterogeneous changes in pH$_o$ associated with spreading depression. Spreading depression is a pathological response of synaptically dense brain regions which consist of a cessation of spontaneous and evoked electrical activity, depolarization of brain cells, interstitial large negative d.c. signal, and massive deterioration of trans-membrane ion gradients which propagates through susceptible brain regions (see Nicholson and Kraig, 1981). pH$_o$ and slow d.c. potentials are shown from double barrelled H$^+$ selective microelectrodes. Spreading depression was evoked by 100 Hz surface stimulation for 1–5 seconds in cerebellum conditioned by exposure to proprionate Ringer solution (see Nicholson and Kraig, 1981). pH$_o$ shifted alkaline then acid during spreading depression and reached a higher peak acid level than during repetitive surface stimulation because of more intense metabolic stimulation during spreading depression. d.c. potential records show that spreading depression was localized to 150–300 μm below the pial surface. Maximum pH$_o$ changes occurred at this depth. Spreading depression did not propagate to 600 μm since the slow d.c. potential was positive there. Note that pH$_o$ changes at 600 and 750 μm swing acid first and then alkaline in a damped oscillation which may suggest that pH$_o$ changes at these depths occurred by diffusion from more superficially activated areas. (Results modified from Nicholson et al., 1985.)

Fig. 3. pH$_o$ and P$_{t(CO_2)}$ changes during spreading depression in rat neocortex. pH$_o$ (upper record) was recorded 500–600 μm below the pial surface in parietal neocortex with a double-barrelled H$^+$ selective microelectrode. pH$_o$ shifted initially alkaline and then acid as in the cerebellum. However, the peak acid shift reached 6.90 pH which may reflect enhanced lactic acidosis since blood glucose had been elevated to 17 mmol/l by previous intraperitoneal injection of dextrose. Spreading depression occurred spontaneously. Middle record shows simultaneous recording of P$_{t(CO_2)}$ from a surface carbon dioxide microelectrode. Since the time constant of the carbon dioxide microelectrode is greater than about 30 seconds, peak P$_{t(CO_2)}$ may be artifactually low. Nonetheless, these P$_{t(CO_2)}$ changes show that brain activity can crease local inhomogeneities in tissue CO$_2$ tension as well as [H$^+$]$_o$. Lower record shows the slow d.c. potential negative shift associated with spreading depression. Note that the thickness of the baseline reflects spontaneous electrical activity of the cortex which stops during spreading depression and then progressively returns. These data were recorded during experiments described in Kraig et al., 1984b, 1985c.

if intracellular ion concentration changes where dissimilar in neurons and glia. In addition, should the H$^+$ physicochemical buffer capacity of neurons differ from that of glia as suggested above, the rise in tissue carbon dioxide tension (P$_{t(CO_2)}$) which occurs during spreading depression (Fig. 3) would cause [H$^+$]$_i$ to rise further in the less buffered cell type.

H^+ homeostasis in brain

H^+ homeostasis in brain can be conceptually difficult to predict because [H^+] is subject to several simultaneously acting physicochemical constraints in a particular compartment. In addition to physicochemical H^+ buffers in a given brain compartment, ion transport across the compartment boundaries or metabolic production or consumption of acids and bases (Siesjö and Messeter, 1971; Siesjö, 1985) can influence [H^+]$_i$. We will deal with these issues separately.

Determinants of [H^+] in a single brain compartment

Stewart (1978, 1981, 1983) has recently presented a conceptual framework with which to solve problems of acid-base behavior in biological fluids. His approach employs the formalisms of solution chemistry to clearly define dependent and independent variables. Previously others, to varying degrees, have used a similar format (Edsall and Wyman, 1958; Siggaard-Andersen, 1963; Siesjö and Messeter, 1971).

Stewart begins by emphasizing the distinction between dependent and independent variables to an acid-base system (1978, 1981, 1983). Dependent variables are internal to a system. Furthermore, they are determined by equations relevant to a system (see Fig. 4) and by the values of externally imposed independent variables. Dependent variables include H^+, hydroxyl ions, carbonate ions, HCO_3^- ions, anions of weak acids (A^-) as well as undissociated weak acids (HA). Independent variables, on the other hand, are parameters whose values are imposed on a system from the outside. Independent variables do not influence one another but necessarily determine the values of dependent variables. Three independent variables are defined through Stewart's approach: the strong ion difference ([SID]), $P_{t(CO_2)}$, and total weak acid concentration ([A_{tot}]; where [A_{tot}] = [HA] + [A^-]). [SID] is the value of the strong base cations minus the strong acid anions. Important strong ions include sodium (Na^+), potassium (K^+), calcium, magnesium, chloride (Cl^-) and lactate. Weak acids (or bases) are represented by various ionizable groups on proteins.

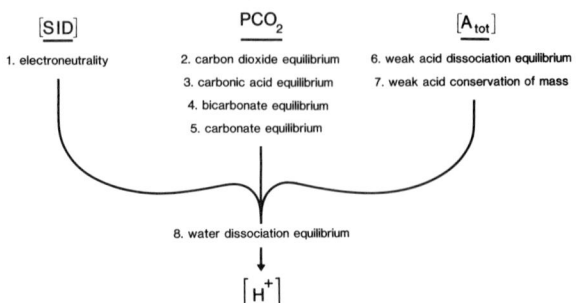

Fig. 4. Determinants of [H^+] in brain compartments. The putative pathogenesis of excessive acidosis during brain ischemia may be more readily defined if the [H^+] and how it is established can be understood in important brain compartments such as the interstitial space or glia and neuronal intracellular space. In biological fluids [H^+] is completely determined by the strong ion difference ([SID]), P_{CO_2}, and total weak acid concentration ([A_{tot}]) (Stewart, 1981, 1983). It is important to recognize that [SID], P_{CO_2}, and [A_{tot}] are three independent variables that completely define [H^+] and other dependent variables, [OH^-], [CO_3^{2-}], [A^-], [HA], and [HCO_3^-]. In brain trans-membrane ion fluxes influence [H^+] in a brain compartment through changes in [SID] while physicochemical H^+ buffers which are thought to remain confined to viable cells influence [H^+] through changes in [A_{tot}]. To accurately describe [H^+] in a given compartment, equations 1 through 8 must be solved simultaneously.

[H^+] in biological fluids is a function of the equilibria of, respectively, weak acids or bases, water dissociation, CO_2, carbonic acid, HCO_3^-, and carbonate solvation as well as the laws of electroneutrality and conservation of mass. Thus, to accurately describe [H^+] in any brain compartment, all relevant equations of ion species present in that compartment must be solved simultaneously (Fig. 4). For example, in brain intracellular fluid [H^+] is determined by [SID], $P_{t(CO_2)}$, and [A_{tot}] and requires simultaneous solutions for eight individual equations (Fig. 4). Siesjö (1984) has recently noted that the term buffer base (defined from the classical pH literature; Siggaard-Andersen, 1963) is equivalent to [SID]. In brain interstitial space, where weak acids are essentially absent, [H^+]$_o$ is determined solely by the [SID] and $P_{t(CO_2)}$ and can be approximated by the following equation:

$$[H^+] = \frac{K_1' \cdot S' \cdot P_{t(CO_2)}}{[SID]} \quad (1)$$

where K_1' is the first ionization constant for carbonic acid and S' is the solubility constant for CO_2 (Nicholson et al., 1985; Kraig et al., 1984b,e). Note that equation (1) is analogous to the classical Henderson equation (Henderson, 1908) since [SID] is essentially equivalent to the interstitial $[HCO_3^-]$ (Stewart, 1981).

Boundary characteristics for H^+ regulation of brain cells and interstitial space

Brain cells to survive must ultimately expel excess H^+, or their determinants, to the surrounding extracellular microenvironment (Kraig et al., 1985a). Primitive cells probably used a non-exclusive high energy phosphate such as adenosine triphosphate (ATP) directly to create a trans-membrane H^+ gradient which could also be employed to conduct other energy-requiring cell activities (Fig. 5) (Wilson and Maloney, 1976). Today bacteria and mitochondria continue to so use H^+ gradients while eukaryotic cells have evolved to employ the plasma membrane Na^+ gradient for similar cell requirements (Wilson and Maloney, 1976). In doing so, eukaryotic cells could regulate $[H^+]_i$ more accurately.

Electrically neutral Na^+/H^+ and Cl^-/HCO_3^- antiport in some combination are now known to remove excess H^+ from a number of different kinds of animal cells including mammalian astroglia (Kimelberg et al., 1978; 1979; 1982; Kimelberg and Bourke, 1982) and vertebrate neurons (Chesler and Nicholson, 1985). The trans-membrane Na^+ gradient, created by energy requiring Na^+ pumps and a selective membrane impermeability to Na^+, is thought to provide the energy needed for Na^+/H^+ antiport (Thomas, 1977; Roos and Boron, 1981; Thomas, 1984). The power source that drives Cl^-/HCO_3^- antiport remains unclear. In some cells Cl^-/HCO_3^- antiport may be an active process and require ATP (Boron and DeWeer, 1976). Alternatively, Cl^-/HCO_3^- may be driven by the Na^+ gradient (Thomas, 1977, 1984).

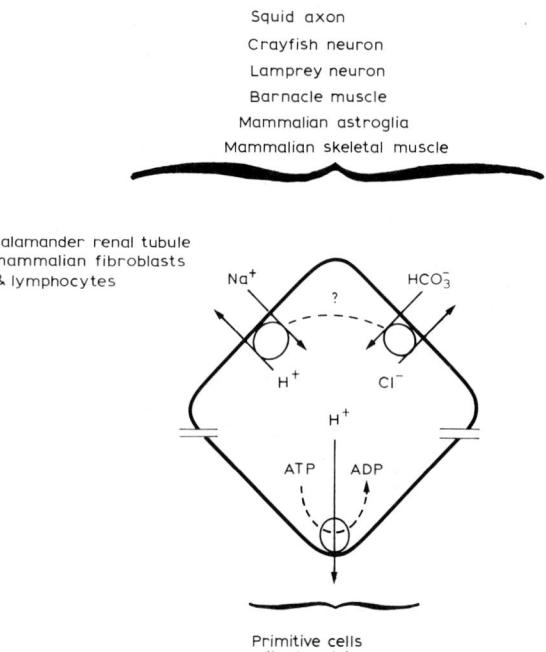

Fig. 5. $[H^+]$ homeostasis in animal cells. Primitive cells may have used a proton gradient as a power source to energize vital cell activities. Today bacteria and mitochondria continue to so use proton gradients while eukaryotic cells have evolved to substitute the plasma membrane Na^+ gradient for similar cell requirements (Wilson and Maloney, 1976). In so doing eukaryotic cells gained improved $[H^+]$ homeostasis which is likely to be more important to these latter cells because of their more numerous and complex enzyme systems and subcellular organelles. Today we know that excess intracellular H^+ are ultimately removed from a number of different animal cell types through two ion antiport systems, Na^+/H^+ and Cl^-/HCO_3^-. The plasma membrane Na^+ gradient drives Na^+H^+ antiport while the power source for Cl^-/HCO_3^- antiport remains unclear. In squid Cl^-/HCO_3^- antiport requires ATP. In barnacle muscle, squid axon, and snail or crayfish neurons Cl^-/HCO_3^- antiport may be driven by the Na^+ gradient through a variable coupling ratio (dotted line) (adapted from Thomas, 1984). For simplicity though one can regard plasma membrane H^+ regulation as some combination of Na^+/H^+ and Cl^-/HCO_3^- antiport.

In mammalian brain only astroglia are known to have Na^+/H^+ and Cl^-/HCO_3^- antiport mechanisms. However, the fact that these H^+ regulatory mechanisms have been conserved through a number of different cell types (Fig. 5) and have most recently been found in vertebrate (lamprey) neu-

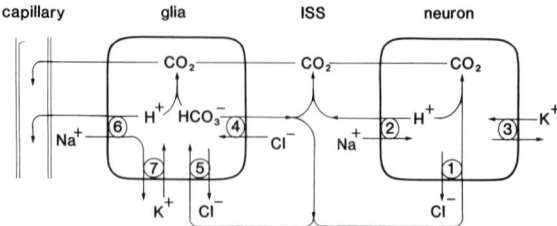

Fig. 6. Model of plasma membrane antiport systems for brain H^+ homeostasis under normal conditions. Excess neuronal H^+ could be neutralized to CO_2 by intracellular HCO_3^- or HCO_3^- that entered through Cl^-/HCO_3^- antiport (1). Otherwise, excess neuronal H^+ could be removed to the interstitial space (ISS) by Na^+/H^+ antiport (2) powered by the transmembrane Na^+ gradient created by Na^+/K^+ ATPase (3). Astroglia could manage excess H^+ similarly (adapted from Kimelberg et al., 1982). Na^+/H^+ antiport (6) would preferentially occur at the capillary-glia border so as to create a directional flux of H^+ toward blood while Cl^-/HCO_3^- antiport would be directed as needed to provide HCO_3^- to the ISS (4) and neurons (1) or buffer excess intraglial H^+ (5). Na^+/K^+ ATPase would maintain the glial Na^+ gradient (modified from Kraig et al., 1985a).

rons (Chesler and Nicholson, 1985) implies that they may be present in mammalian neurons as well. If so, H^+ regulation by plasma membrane antiport systems can be schematized as in Fig. 6 (Kraig et al., 1984b).

Results and discussion

Through the work of Myers (1979) and others it is now well recognized that carbohydrate stores in brain can greatly influence the severity of outcome after nearly complete ischemia in animals (Welsh et al., 1980; Siemkowicz and Hansen, 1978; Rehncrona et al., 1981; Kalimo et al., 1981; Pulsinelli et al., 1982) and man (Pulsinelli et al., 1983). Under normoglycemic conditions only selective neurons are lost after 30 minutes of nearly complete forebrain ischemia in rats created by occlusion of four cervical arteries (Pulsinelli and Duffy, 1983). On the other hand, equivalent ischemia under hyperglycemic conditions leads to brain infarction (Pulsinelli et al., 1982).

The above findings have led Myers (1979) and others to postulate that lactic acidosis may worsen ischemic brain injury. If so, the microphysiological mechanisms remain undefined. Nearly complete brain ischemia during normoglycemia results in selective neuronal destruction and lactate accumulation to a level up to 13 mmol/kg neocortex (Pulsinelli and Duffy, 1983). In contrast, equivalent ischemia under hyperglycemic conditions produces necrosis of all tissue elements and lactate accumulation to greater than 19 mmol/kg (Pulsinelli et al., 1982). Since H^+ is generated in a 1:1 stoichiometric relationship with lactate during complete ischemia (Krebs et al., 1975; Alberti and Cuthbert, 1982) one might expect to find a similar narrow range or threshold of $[H^+]$ beyond which all brain cells are destroyed. As a first approach to disclose such a threshold we measured $[H^+]$ in a single brain compartment, the interstitial space, as well as the total neocortical lactate content. Furthermore, to avoid the possible exchange of H^+ or its determinants across the blood brain barrier, we performed the experiments during complete ischemia, making the brain a closed system. If plasma membranes remain intact during complete ischemia, the brain can be considered as a three compartment system consisting of neurons, glia, and the interstitial space (Fig. 6). Pertinent aspects of the experimental paradigm are summarized in Fig. 7 and Kraig et al., 1984a,b, 1985a,b,c.

Complete ischemia

Animals had pre-ischemic blood glucose values that ranged from 3–7 mmol/l (normoglycemia) and 17–80 mmol/l (hyperglycemia). The groups were associated respectively with brain lactate contents that ranged from 8–13 mmol/kg and 16–31 mmol/kg (Kraig et al., 1984a,b, 1985a,b,c). High energy phosphates (measured by enzyme fluorometric techniques) deteriorated to similar levels in both groups, making energy in the form of ATP-related metabolites unavailable to either group for regulation of $[H^+]$. $[H^+]_o$ rose as soon as blood pressure fell in all animals. However, peak $[H^+]_o$ was bimodally distributed between the two groups. Although pre-ischemic blood glucoses in normogly-

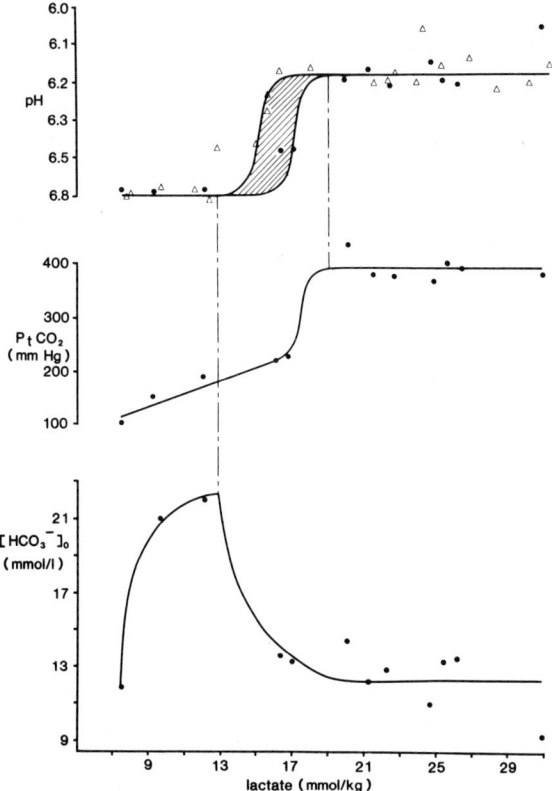

Fig. 7. Carbonic acid buffer peak changes after complete ischemia. pH_o recordings were made with double barrelled H^+ selective microelectrodes placed 800 μm down in parietal cortex of anesthetized rats. $P_{t(CO_2)}$ was measured with a surface microelectrode. Brain carbohydrate stores were modulated by pretreatment with intraperitoneal dextrose or intravenous insulin injections. Ischemia was induced by cardiac arrest caused by intravenous injection of KCl. When changes in pH_o and $P_{t(CO_2)}$ reached a peak, animals were decapitated and their heads frozen in liquid nitrogen for subsequent enzyme fluorometric analysis of neocortical lactate content. Upper graph shows peak pH_o compared to tissue lactate. Triangles show data from Kraig et al., 1985a and dots represent data from Kraig et al., 1984b, 1985c. The zone between 15–17 mmol/kg lactate is shaded with diagonal lines to reflect the variability in peak pH_o there. The constant peak level of pH_o between 8–13 and 16–31 mmol/kg lactate implies that $[H^+]_o$ is at a steady-state, but not equilibrium, with respect to $[H^+]$ in other brain compartments during complete ischemia. The middle graphs shows concomitant changes in $P_{t(CO_2)}$. $P_{t(CO_2)}$ initially rises linearly with increasing lactate up to about 17 mmol/kg. Then $P_{t(CO_2)}$ rises abruptly and remains constant at 389 ± 9 mmHg after 19 mmol/kg lactate. The constancy of peak $P_{t(CO_2)}$ above 19 mmol/kg lactate implies that HCO_3^- stores were exhausted from acid producing cells. If $[H^+]_o$ continues to be determined by [SID] and $P_{t(CO_2)}$ (see equation 1) during complete ischemia, then the lower graph shows the concomitant changes in $[HCO_3^-]_o$ which would be expected from the measured changes in pH_o and $P_{t(CO_2)}$. Notice that $[HCO_3^-]_o$ rises from 8–13 mmol/kg lactate, when pH_o is constant at 6.81 pH and then begins to fall when pH_o and $P_{t(CO_2)}$ change abruptly between 13–19 mmol/kg lactate. $[HCO_3^-]_o$ then remains constant at about 12.3 mmol/l above 19 mmol/kg lactate. Thus HCO_3^- and H^+ both remain heterogeneously distributed between the interstitial space and acid producing cells during complete ischemia.

cemic animals ranged from 3–7 mmol/l and brain lactates ranged from 8–13 mmol/kg, $[H^+]_o$ always rose by a constant amount from about 7.25 pH to a peak of 6.81 ± 0.02 pH ($n = 7$) (triangles in Fig. 7). Similarly, inspite of the fact that pre-ischemic blood glucoses in hyperglycemic animals ranged from 17–80 mmol/l and brain lactates ranged from 16–31 mmol/kg, $[H^+]_o$ again always rose by a constant, but larger amount, from 7.25 pH to a peak of 6.18 ± 0.02 pH ($n = 12$) (triangles in Fig. 7). In a second series of experiments where $[H^+]_o$ and $P_{t(CO_2)}$ were simultaneously monitored in a similar experimental paradigm (black dots in Fig. 7). $[H^+]_o$ reached peak levels of 6.79 ± 0.02 pH ($n = 3$) during normoglycemic ischemia and 6.19 ± 0.02 pH ($n = 7$) during hyperglycemic ischemia.

The constancy of peak $[H^+]_o$ levels for normoglycemic and hyperglycemic conditions suggests that $[H^+]_o$ arrives at a steady-state not in equilibrium with $[H^+]$ in other brain compartments. This inference stems from the conclusion that $[H^+]$ must be rising in some compartment other than the interstitial space because neocortical lactate content is rising (Krebs et al., 1975; Alberti and Cuthbert, 1982). Physicochemical H^+ buffers alone can not account for the constancy of peak $[H^+]_o$ levels since the presence of physicochemical H^+ buffers in any brain compartment would only reduce, but not abolish, the rate of rise and levels that $[H^+]$ otherwise would attain (Koppel and Spiro, 1914; Van Slyke, 1922; Bull, 1964; Stewart, 1981). Accordingly, one must invoke energy in the form of membrane barriers or residual ion gradients across plasma membranes to explain the steady-state constancy of peak $[H^+]_o$.

CO_2 is a highly diffusable gas in tissues (Krogh, 1919; Gleichman et al., 1962; Kaethner and Bangham, 1977). Hence, $P_{t(CO_2)}$ will rise when HCO_3^- is neutralized by H^+ in any brain compartment of a closed system. Therefore, by simultaneous measurements of $[H^+]_o$ and $P_{t(CO_2)}$ during complete ischemia one can: (1) calculate remaining $[HCO_3^-]_o$ according to equation 1; (2) calculate the amount of brain HCO_3^- neutralized by lactic acidosis (where $[HCO_3^-]$ lost is equal to the change in $P_{t(CO_2)}$ multiplied by S'). Our results show that peak $P_{t(CO_2)}$ increased linearly with lactate content until lactate reached about 17 mmol/kg. Peak $P_{t(CO_2)}$ then rose abruptly to 389 ± 9 mmHg (n = 7) and remained constant through 31 mmol/kg lactate (Fig. 7).

These changes in $P_{t(CO_2)}$ help to clarify how $[H^+]_o$ could remain constant between 8–13 and 16–31 mmol/kg lactate (Fig. 7) (Kraig et al., 1984b, 1985c). For $[H^+]_o$ to have remained constant up to 13 mmol/kg lactate while $P_{t(CO_2)}$ rose, $[HCO_3^-]_o$ must have increased (Fig. 7 lower graph). Subsequently since peak levels in $P_{t(CO_2)}$ did not change after lactate reached 19 mmol/kg, HCO_3^- stores must have been exhausted in acid producing cells. Consequently, if no changes occurred in $P_{t(CO_2)}$ or $[SID]_o$ (which is essentially equivalent to $[HCO_3^-]_o$ in the interstitial space), no change in $[H^+]_o$ could have occurred above 19 mmol/kg lactate. If these inferences are correct, then above 19 mmol/kg lactate, remaining brain HCO_3^- was segregated to the interstitial space and perhaps those cells which no longer produced lactic acid. On the other hand, excess H^+ remained in acid producing cells. This suggests that under non-physiological conditions such as ischemia, H^+ and HCO_3^- can remain unequally distributed between cells and the interstitial space, and perhaps even unequally distributed between different cell types.

The changes in $P_{t(CO_2)}$ and $[H^+]_o$ (Fig. 7) can be further interpreted with the model of brain H^+ homeostasis shown in Fig. 6. During complete ischemia it is known that $[Na^+]_o$ falls from about 154 mmol/l to about 48 mmol/l and $[Cl^-]_o$ declines from about 129 mmol/l to about 72 mmol/l (Hansen, 1981). The lowered $[Na^+]_o$ is presumably associated with a significant deterioration in the trans-membrane Na^+ gradient across intact cell membranes. If so, this would impede H^+ from leaving brain cells via Na^+/H^+ antiport. Instead, Cl^-/HCO_3^- antiport alone might remain operational and powered by remaining Cl^- or HCO_3^- gradients. CO_2 is most readily hydrated in neocortex by carbonic anhydrase containing glia (Sapirstein, 1983). Glia would, therefore, be the likely candidates to secrete HCO_3^- to the interstitial space during normoglycemic ischemia (lactate of 8–13 mmol/kg in Fig. 7). Above 13 mmol/kg lactate glia would stop secreting HCO_3^- and by 19 mmol/kg lactate brain HCO_3^- would remain only in the interstitial space and, perhaps, some hypothetical cells which no longer produced acid.

Severe incomplete ischemia and reperfusion

We have now begun to examine the behavior of $[H^+]_o$ during and after severe incomplete ischemia according to the modified (Pulsinelli and Duffy, 1983) model of Pulsinelli and Brierley (1979). Under severe hyperglycemic conditions (blood glucose 17–57 mmol/l) $[H^+]_o$ rose as soon as blood flow fell and reached a peak of 6.1–6.2 pH after 30 minutes of ischemia (Kraig et al., 1985b) (Fig. 8). This value is similar to those of 6.18 (Kraig et al., 1984a, 1985b) and 6.19 (Kraig et al., 1984b, 1985c) found after terminal ischemia under hyperglycemic conditions (Fig. 7). It appears that brain cell impermeability to H^+ or their ionized determinants can be maintained for at least 30 minutes of ischemia.

A transient second rise in $[H^+]_o$ occurred with reperfusion. This second peak in $[H^+]_o$ was directly proportional to the pre-ischemic blood glucose. For example, with a pre-ischemic blood glucose of 57 mmol/l, $[H^+]_o$, reached as high as 5.4–5.5 pH several minutes after reperfusion (Fig. 8). Brain is known to swell during reperfusion from severe incomplete ischemia (Kalimo et al., 1981) and membrane permeability of edematous, acid producing cells may increase. Under these circumstances, increased

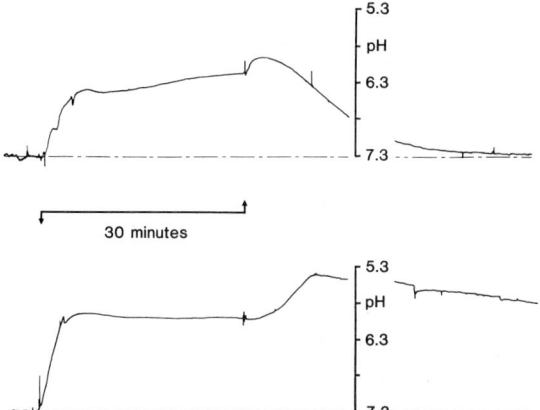

Fig. 8. pH_o changes with severe forebrain ischemia under hyperglycemic conditions. pH_o was recorded as described in Fig. 7. Ischemia was induced by occlusion of four cervical arteries as outlined in Pulsinelli and duffy (1983). Rats were pre-treated with intravenous dextrose to raise brain carbohydrate stores. Pre-ischemic blood glucose was 17 mmol/l (upper record) and 57 mmol/l (lower record) from two representative animals. pH_o rose as soon as carotid arteries were reversibly closed (upward arrow) and reached a peak between 6.1–6.2 pH under both conditions. With the release of the carotid artery clamps and reperfusion though, pH_o reached a secondary peak acid level which was directly proportional with pre-ischemic the pre-ischemic blood glucose level. When pre-ischemic blood glucose was as high as 57 mmol/l, pH_o fell as low as 5.4–5.5 pH during reperfusion. Astroglia swell and brain becomes edematous after reperfusion from severe incomplete ischemia under hyperglycemic conditions. Plasma membranes in general may increase their permeabilities to H^+ or their determinants under such conditions. If so, pH_o may accurately reflect brain H^+ content and suggest that maximum deterioration of brain H^+ buffering mechanisms occurs at this time after severe hyperglycemic ischemia (data from Kraig et al., 1985b).

cell membrane permeability to H^+ or their determinants ([SID]) could account for the further fall in $[HCO_3^-]_o$.

Previous investigations have shown that brain becomes acidotic during complete or nearly complete ischemia. Initially (Thorn and Heitmann, 1954; Crowell and Kaufman, 1961), surface H^+-selective glass semi-microelectrodes were used to show that $[H^+]_o$ shifted in the acid direction during ischemia. More recently H^+-selective glass microelectrodes have been used to show that $[H^+]_o$ rises to 6.80 pH after cardiac arrest (presumably under normoglycemic conditions) (Javaheri et al., 1984) or to about 6.1 pH during severe incomplete ischemia under hyperglycemic conditions (Siemkowicz and Hansen, 1981). Nemoto and Frinak (1981) recorded $[H^+]_o$ under similar ischemic conditions and also found that $[H^+]_o$ rose as high as about 6.1 pH. However, blood glucoses were not specified in these latter experiments. In addition, several indirect methods have been used to calculate ischemic $[H^+]_i$ including colorimetry (Kogure et al., 1980), fluorometry (Sundt et al., 1978; Welsh et al., 1982; Csiba et al., 1983), creatine kinase equilibrium and CO_2 distribution (Mabe et al., 1983), lactate content (Ljunggren et al., 1974), and ^{31}P nuclear magnetic resonance (Norwood et al., 1979). Such calculations, however, fail to account for inhomogeneities in $[H^+]_i$ such as those implied from our studies outlined above.

H^+-selective microelectrodes (Astrup et al., 1977; Gibson et al., 1983; Harris et al., 1984), ^{31}P nuclear magnetic resonance (Thulborn et al., 1982), and the distribution of 5,5-dimethyl-2,4-oxazolidinedione-^{14}C (Keitaro et al., 1984) have each been used to show brain acidosis during focal ischemia.

Conclusions

The enhancement by hyperglycemia of brain damage after severe incomplete ischemia is thought to result from excessive lactic acidosis in the tissue (Myers, 1979). Our results reveal an abrupt alteration in brain H^+-buffering mechanisms at levels of lactate accumulation which previously have correlated with the transition from ischemic neuronal damage to brain infarction. Furthermore, immediately after this transition zone, at 19 mmol/kg lactate, H^+ must remain unequally distributed between cells and the interstitial space. We propose that HCO_3^- stores are exhausted in those cellular compartments which continue to produce lactic acid.

An inability of excess H^+ to escape from brain cells may be a fundamental step in the genesis of irreversible ischemic brain injury. If HCO_3^- stores in acid producing cells are exhausted (i.e.

[HCO_3^-]$_i$ is at most 1 mmol/l and $P_{t(CO_2)}$ is 389 mmHg, then [H^+]$_i$ in that brain compartment will drop to a pH of about 5 during ischemia, according to the isohydric principle (Cohen and Kassirer, 1982) and the Henderson-Hasselbach equation (Hasselbach, 1916). This low value exceeds the peak [H^+]$_o$ occurring during reperfusion, when we speculate that acid producing brain cells become more permeable to H^+ or their determinants.

The molecular mechanisms by which such profound acidosis irreversibly damages brain cells remain unknown. However, we can now direct our attention to microphysiological processes which regulate the heterogeneous distribution of H^+ and their determinants among different brain cell types and the interstitial space during ischemia. These pathological processes must include conditions where [H^+]$_o$ reaches about 6.2 pH during ischemia or about 5 pH in acid producing cells and 5.4 pH afterwards in the interstitial space during reperfusion.

Acknowledgements

It is a pleasure to acknowledge the support of NINCDS Grants NS-19108 and NS-003346 as well as of a Teacher Investigator Development Award (NS-00767) to Richard P. Kraig. In addition we would like to thank Dr. C. Nicholson for reading this manuscript and for helpful discussions along with Dr. M. Chesler about hydrogen ion homeostasis in brain.

References

Alberti, K.G.M.M. and Cuthbert, C. (1982) The hydrogen ion in normal metabolism: a review. In: R. Porter and G. Lawrenson (Eds.), *Metabolic Acidosis*, Ciba Foundation Symposium 87. Pitman, London, pp. 1–15.

Astrup, J., Symon, L., Branston, N.M. and Lassen, N.A. (1977) Cortical evoked potential and extracellular K^+ and H^+ at critical levels of brain ischemia. *Stroke*, 8: 51–57.

Boron, W.F. and DeWeer, P. (1976) Active proton transport stimulated by CO_2/HCO_3^-, blocked by cyanide. *Nature (Lond.)*, 259: 240–241.

Bull, H.B. (1964) *An Introduction to Physical Biochemistry*. Davis, Philadelphia.

Bureš, J., Burešova, O. and Krivánek, J. (1974) *The Mechanism and Application of Leao's Spreading Depression of Electroencephalographic Activity*. Academic Press, New York.

Chesler, M. and Nicholson, C. (1985) Regulation of intracellular pH in vertebrate central neurons. *Brain Res.*, 325: 313–316.

Cohen, J.J. and Kassirer, J.P. (1982) *Acid Base*. Little, Brown, Co., Boston.

Crowell, J.W. and Kaufman, N. (1961) Changes in tissue pH after circulatory arrest. *Am. J. Physiol.*, 200: 743–745.

Csiba, L. Paschen, W. and Hossman, K.-A. (1983) A topographic quantitative method for measuring brain tissue pH under physiological and pathological conditions. *Brain Res.*, 289: 334–337.

Edsall, J.T. and Wyman, J. (1958) *Biophysical Chemistry*, Vol. 1. Academic Press, New York.

Gibson, G., Miller, S.A., Venalbes, G.S. and Strong, A.J. (1983) Evidence of acidosis in the ischemic penumbra. *J. Cereb. Blood Flow Metabol.*, 3, Suppl. 1: S401–S402.

Gleichman, U., Ingvar, D.H., Lübbers, D.W. and Siesjö, B.K. (1962) Tissue P_{O_2} and P_{CO_2} of the cerebral cotex related to blood gas tensions. *Acta Physiol. Scand.*, 55: 127–138.

Hansen, A.J. (1981) Extracellular ion concentrations during cerebral ischemia. In: T. Zeuthen (Ed.), *The Application of Ion-Selective Microelectrodes*. Elsevier/North-Holland, New York, pp. 239–254.

Harris, R. and Symon, L. (1984) Extracellular pH, potassium, and calcium activities in progressive ischaemia of rat cortex. *J. Cereb. Blood Flow Metabol.*, 4: 178–186.

Hasselbach, K.A. (1916) Die Berechnung der Wasserstoffzahl des Blutes aus der freien und gebundenen Kohlensäure desselben, und die Sauerstoffbindung des Blutes als Funktion der Wasserstoffzahl. *Biochem. Z.*, 78: 112–114.

Henderson, L.J. (1908) The theory of neutrality regulation in the animal organism. *Am. J. Physiol.*, 21: 427–448.

Hertz, L. (1981) Features of astrocytic function apparently involved in the response of central nervous tissue to ischemia-hypoxia. *J. Cereb. Blood Flow Metabol.*, 1: 143–153.

Hertz, L. and Schousboe, A. (1975) Ion and energy metabolism of the brain at the cellular level. In: C.C. Pfeiffer and J.R. Smythies (Eds.), *International Review of Neurobiology*, Vol. 10. Academic Press, New York, pp. 141–211.

Javaheri, S., Clendening, A., Papadakis, N. and Brody, J.S. (1984) pH changes on the surface of brain and in cisternal fluid in dogs in cardiac arrest. *Stroke*, 15: 553–557.

Kaethner, T.M. and Bangham, A.D. (1977) Selective compartmentation of the hydration products of carbon dioxide in liposomes, and its role in regulating water movement. *Biochim. Biophys. Acta*, 468: 157–161.

Kalimo, H., Rehncrona, S., Soderfeldt, B., Olsson, Y. and Siesjö, B.K. (1981) Brain lactic acidosis and ischemic cell damage.

2. Histopathology. *J. Cereb. Blood Flow Metabol.*, 1: 313–327.

Keitaro, K., Sako, K, Izawa, M., Yamamoto, Y.L. and Hakim, A.M. (1984) Autoradiographic determination of brain pH following middle cerebral artery occlusion in the rat. *Stroke*, 15: 540–547.

Kimelberg, H.K. and Bourke, R.S. (1982) Anion transport in the nervous system. In: A. Lajtha (Ed.), *Handbook of Neurochemistry*, 2nd Edn, Vol. 1, Chemical and Cellular Architecture. Plenum, New York, pp. 31–67.

Kimelberg, H.K., Biddlecome, S., Narumi, S. and Bourke, R.S. (1978) ATPase and carbonic anhydrase activities in bulk isolated neuron, glia, and synaptosome fractions from rat brain. *Brain Res.*, 141: 305–323.

Kimelberg, H.K., Bowman, C., Biddlecome, S. and Bourke, R.S. (1979) Cation transport and membrane potential properties of primary astroglial cultures from neonatal rat brains. *Brain Res.*, 177: 533–550.

Kimelberg, H.K., Bourke, R.S., Steig, P.E., Barron, K.D., Hirata, H., Pelton, E.W. and Nelson, L.R. (1982) Swelling of astroglia after injury to the central nervous system: mechanisms and consequences. In: R.G. Grossman and P.L. Gildenbery (Eds.), *Head Injury: Basic and Clinical Aspects*. Raven, New York, pp. 31–44.

Kogure, K., Alsonso, O.F. and Martinez, E. (1980) A topographic measurement of brain pH. *Brain Res.*, 195: 95–109.

Koppel, M. and Spiro, K. (1914) Über die Wirkung von Moderatoren (Puffern) bei der Verschiebung des Säure-Basengleichgewichtes in biologischen Flussigkeiten. *Biochem. Z.*, 65: 409–439.

Kraig, R.P. and Nicholson, C. (1978) Extracellular ionic variations during spreading depression. *Neuroscience*, 3: 1045–1059.

Kraig, R.P., Ferreira-Filho, C.R. and Nicholson, C. (1983) Alkaline and acid transients in the cerebellar microenvironment. *J. Neurophysiol.*, 49: 831–849.

Kraig, R.P., Pulsinelli, W.A. and Plum, F. (1984a) Proton buffering of the brain during complete ischemia. *Ann. Neurol.*, 16: 111 (abst.).

Kraig, R.P., Pulsinelli, W.A. and Plum, F. (1984b) Carbonic acid buffer behavior in brain during complete ischemia. *Soc. Neurosci.*, 10: 888 (abst.).

Kraig, R.P., Pulsinelli, W.A. and Plum, F. (1985a) Hydrogen ion buffering during complete ischemia. *Brain Res.*, 342: 281–290.

Kraig, R.P., Pulsinelli, W.A. and Plum, F. (1985b) Peak forebrain [H^+]$_o$ in severe hyperglycemic ischemia. *Stroke* (abst.), 16: 143.

Kraig, R.P., Pulsinelli, W.A. and Plum, F. (1985c) Carbonic acid buffer changes during complete brain ischemia (submitted for publication).

Krebs, H.A., Woods, H.F. and Alberti, K.G.M.M. (1975) Hyperlactemia and lactic acidosis. *Essays Med. Biochem.*, 1: 81–103.

Krogh, A. (1919) The rate of diffusion of gasses through animal tissues, with some remarks on the coefficient of invasion. *J. Physiol.*, 51: 391–408.

Ljunggren, B. and Siesjö, B.K. (1974) Influence of tissue acidosis upon restitution of brain energy metabolism following total ischemia. *Brain Res.*, 77: 173–186.

Mabe, H., Blomqvist, P. and Siesjö, Bo K. (1983) Intracellular pH in the brain following transient ischemia. *J. Cereb. Blood Flow Metabol.*, 3: 109–114.

Myers, R.E. (1979) Lactic acid accumulation as a cause of brain edema and cerebral necrosis resulting from oxygen deprivation. In: R. Korbkin and G. Guilleminault (Eds.), *Advances in Perinatal Neurology*. Spectrum Publ., New York, pp. 85–114.

Nemoto, E.M. and Frinak, S. (1981) Brain tissue pH after global brain ischemia and barbiturate loading in rats. *Stroke*, 12: 77–82.

Nicholson, C. and Kraig, R.P. (1981) The behavior of extracellular ions during spreading depression. In: T. Zeuthen (Ed.), *The Application of Ion-selective Microelectrodes*. Elsevier/North-Holland, New York, pp. 217–238.

Nicholson, C., Kraig, R.P., Ferreira-Filho, C.R. and Thompson, P. (1985) Hydrogen ion variations and their interpretation in the microenvironment of the vertebrate brain. In: M. Kessler, D.K. Harrison and J. Hoper (Eds.), *Recent Advances in the Theory and Application of Ion Selective Electrodes in Physiology and Medicine*. Springer-Verlag, New York, in press.

Norwood, W.I., Norwood, C.R., Ingwall, J.S., Castaneda, A.R. and Fossel, E.T. (1979) Hypothermic circulatory arrest. 31-Phosphorus nuclear magnetic resonance of isolated perfused neonatal rat brain. *J. Thorac. Cardiovasc. Surg.*, 78: 823–830.

Oldendorf, W.H., Cornford, E.M. and Brown, W.J. (1977) The large apparent work capacity of the blood-brain barrier: A study of the mitochondrial content of capillary endothelial cells in brain and other tissues of the rat. *Ann. Neurol.*, 1: 409–417.

Pulsinelli, W.A. and Brierley, J.B. (1979) A new model of bilateral hemispheric ischemia in the unanesthetized rat. *Stroke*, 10: 267–272.

Pulsinelli, W.A. and Duffy, T.E. (1983) Regional energy balance in rat brain after transient forebrain ischemia. *J. Neurochem.*, 40: 1500–1503.

Pulsinelli, W.A., Waldman, S., Rawlinson, D. and Plum, F. (1982) Moderate hyperglycemia augments ischemic brain damage: a neuropathologic study in the rat. *Neurology*, 32: 1239–1246.

Pulsinelli, W.A., Levy, D.E., Sigsbee, B., Scherer, P. and Plum F. (1983) Increased damage after ischemic stroke in patients with hyperglycemia with or without established diabetes mellitus. *Am. J. Med.*, 74: 540–544.

Quastel, J.H. (1975) Metabolic compartmentation in the brain and the effects of metabolic inhibitors. In: S. Berl, D.D. Clarke and D. Scheider (Eds.), *Metabolic Compartmentation and Neurotransmission*, Relation to Brain Structure and Function. Plenum, New York, pp. 337–361.

Rehncrona, S., Rosen, I. and Siesjö, B.K. (1981) Brain lactic acidosis and ischemic cell damage. I. Biochemistry and neurophysiology. *J. Cereb. Blood Flow Metabol.*, 1: 297–311.

Roos, A. and Boron, W.F. (1981) Intracellular pH. *Physiol. Rev.*, 61: 296–434.

Sapirstein, V.S. (1983) Carbonic anhydrase. In: A. Lajtha (Ed.), *Handbook of Neurochemistry*, 2nd Edn, Vol. 4. Plenum, New York, pp. 385–402.

Siemkowicz, E. and Hansen, A.J. (1978) Clinical restitution following cerebral ischemia in hypo-, normo-, and hyperglycemic rats. *Acta Neurol. Scand.*, 58: 1–8.

Siemkowicz, E. and Hansen, A.J. (1981) Brain extracellular ion composition and EEG activity following 10 minutes ischemia in normo- and hyperglycemic rats. *Stroke*, 12: 236–240.

Siesjö, B.K. (1984) Brain acid-base metabolism in health and disease. In: A. Bes, P. Braquet, R. Paoletti and B.K. Siesjö (Eds.), *Cerebral Ischemia, ICS 654*. Excerpta Medica, Amsterdam-New York-Oxford, pp. 157–165.

Siesjö, B.K. (1985) Acid-base homeostasis in the brain: physiology, chemistry, and neurochemical pathology. *This volume*, pp. 121–154.

Siesjö, B.K. and Messeter, K. (1971) Factors determining intracellular pH. In: B.K. Siesjö and S.C. Sorensen (Eds.), *Ion Homeostasis of the Brain*. Munksgaard, Copenhagen, pp. 244–262.

Siggaard-Andersen, O. (1963) The acid-base status of blood. *Scand. J. Clin. Lab. Invest.*, Suppl. 70: 1–134.

Stewart, P. (1978) Independent and dependent variables of acid-base control. *Respir. Physiol.*, 33: 9–26.

Stewart, P.A. (1981) *How to Understand Acid-Base*, Elsevier, New York.

Stewart, P.A. (1983) Modern quantitative acid-base chemistry. *Can. J. Physiol.*, 61: 1444–1461.

Sundt, Jr., T.F., Anderson, R.E. and Van Dyke, R.A. (1978) Brain pH measurements using a diffusable, lipid soluble pH sensitive fluorescent indicator. *J. Neurochem.*, 31: 627–635.

Thomas, R.C. (1977) The role of bicarbonate, chloride, and sodium ions in the regulation of intracellular pH in snail neurons. *J. Physiol.*, 273: 317–338.

Thomas, R.C. (1984) Experimental displacement of intracellular pH and the mechanism of its subsequent recovery. *J. Physiol.*, 354: 3P–22P.

Thorn, W. and Heitmann, R. (1954) pH der Gehirnrinde vom Kaninchen in Situ während perakuter, totaler Ischämie, reiner Anoxie und in der Erholung. *Pfluegers Arch.*, 258: 501–510.

Thulborn, K.R., du Boulay, G., Duchen, L.W. and Radda, G. (1982) A ^{31}P nuclear magnetic resonance in vivo study of cerebral ischaemia in the gerbul. *J. Cereb. Blood Flow Metabol.*, 2: 299–306.

Van Slyke, D.D. (1922) On the measurement of buffer values and on the relationship of buffer value to the dissociation constant of the buffer and the concentration and reaction of the buffer solution. *J. Biol. Chem.*, 52: 525–570.

Welsh, F., Ginsberg, M., Rieder, W. and Budd, W. (1980) Deleterious effect of glucose pretreatment on recovery from diffuse cerebral ischemia in the rat. II. Regional metabolite levels. *Stroke*, 353–363.

Welsh, F.A., O'Conner, M.J., Marcey, V.R., Spatacco, A.J. and Johns, R.L. (1982) Factors limiting regeneration of ATP following temporary ischemia in cat brain. *Stroke*, 13: 234–242.

Wilson, T.H. and Maloney, P.C. (1976) Speculations on the evolution of ion transport mechanisms. *Fed. Proc.*, 35: 2174–2179.

SECTION III

Alterations in Protein and Lipid Metabolism

Calmodulin and protein phosphorylation: implications in brain ischemia

Jerome H. Chin, Tom M. Buckholz and Robert J. DeLorenzo

Department of Neurology, Yale University School of Medicine, New Haven, CT 06510, USA

Introduction

Stroke is a major cause of mortality and physical disability in the later decades of life. More notable is the fact that despite numerous advances in other aspects of medical therapeutics, available modalities for the prevention of stroke and the preservation of neurological function after an ischemic insult are limited. It is critical therefore that a more detailed understanding of the etiology, pathophysiology, and biochemistry of ischemic brain damage be derived from both clinical studies and experimental stroke models.

It has become apparent in recent years that the brain may be more resistant to ischemia than previously suspected (Hossmann and Kleihues, 1973; Hossmann and Zimmerman, 1974; Plum, 1981). Hossmann and Zimmerman (1974) demonstrated that partial electrophysiological recovery of brain could occur after 60 min of total cerebral ischemia. These findings have raised the possibility of successfully intervening before the onset of irreversible cellular damage following ischemia. Towards this end, a molecular understanding of the crucial cytotoxic factors responsible for ischemic cell injury and the cascades they initiate which subsequently lead to cell death must be developed.

A considerable body of evidence has accumulated from studies in nerve and other tissues implicating calcium as a major initiator of ischemic cell injury (Farber et al., 1981; Nayler, 1981; Raichle, 1983). Although several molecular models have been proposed for calcium's mode of action in ischemia, it is still unclear which of the many biological systems responsive to calcium are directly involved in the morphological and functional alterations seen in ischemia-induced cell damage.

Research in our laboratory has been directed towards providing a molecular model for understanding the role of calcium in neuronal function and synaptic physiology. Calmodulin is now well-recognized as a ubiquitous calcium-dependent regulator protein that modulates the effects of calcium on a number of enzyme systems and cellular processes (Klee and Vanaman, 1982). Results from our studies have demonstrated that calmodulin regulates some of the effects of calcium on synaptic protein phosphorylation, neurotransmitter release, and cytoskeletal physiology (DeLorenzo, 1980, 1981, 1982; Burke and DeLorenzo, 1981, 1982a,b; Goldenring et al., 1983, 1984a,b; Larson et al., 1985). Because of the importance of calmodulin and calmodulin-dependent protein phosphorylation in many aspects of neuronal function (DeLorenzo et al., 1982; Klee and Vanaman, 1982; Nestler et al., 1984), it is appropriate that the involvement of calmodulin and protein phosphorylation in calcium-mediated ischemic cell damage be considered. In this presentation we will first review the evidence that calcium is involved in ischemic cell injury. Then we will discuss the role of calmodulin and calmodulin-dependent protein kinase in various aspects of brain metabolism and physiology. Finally, the possible effects of ischemia and a disordered calcium homeostasis on calmodulin-sensitive biochemical systems is discussed.

Calcium as an important mediator of ischemic cell injury

Several minutes following the cessation of blood flow to the brain major disruptions in normal ion homeostasis are observed. Using ion-sensitive microelectrodes (Hansen, 1981), a marked increase in potassium and a fall in sodium and calcium are observed in the extracellular space in brain. The movement of sodium and calcium into the cell as well as the release of calcium from intracellular storage sites results in a precipitous rise in cytoplasmic calcium concentrations. These events are in large part attributable to the ischemia-induced shortage of adenosine triphosphate (ATP) (Carvalho, 1982; Raichle, 1983).

Early studies by Nageotte (1910) and Cajal (1928) provided evidence for a damaging action of calcium on nerve tissue. They noted that fragments derived from peripheral nerves underwent in vitro myelin fragmentation when exposed to bivalent metals such as calcium. More recent studies by Schlaepfer and Bunge (1971a, 1973) have extended these original observations and demonstrated that calcium-mediated degenerative changes (such as the granular disruption of microtubules and neurofilaments) are dependent upon the concentration of calcium to which nerve preparations are exposed.

Studies in non-neuronal tissue have also supported a role for calcium in the pathogenesis of ischemic cell injury. Shen and Jennings (1972) demonstrated a dramatic 18-fold rise in total calcium accumulation by myocardial tissue after 40 min of ischemia followed by 10 min of reperfusion. Uptake of calcium was not observed in tissue not subjected to arterial reflow. Moreover, calcium accumulation was correlated with irreversible morphological cell damage and the appearance of intramitochondrial granules containing calcium phosphate. Subsequent studies have demonstrated a correlation between reperfusion-induced calcium accumulation and loss of functional myocardial recovery (Shine et al., 1978; Nayler, 1981). Most importantly, it was found that functional damage could be prevented by reperfusing ischemic tissue with low calcium solutions for 5 min before the introduction of normal calcium media. Presumably, this brief period of low calcium allowed the recovery of sufficient ATP stores to handle a large calcium influx and to repair other crucial cellular functions.

Farber and associates have provided evidence that calcium is intimately involved in destruction of liver cells by a variety of membrane-active toxins as well as ischemia-reperfusion (Chien et al., 1977; Schanne et al., 1979; Farber et al., 1981). Using primary cultures of adult rat hepatocytes, they demonstrated that the cytotoxic action of 10 different membrane-active toxins was absolutely dependent upon the presence or absence of calcium in the extracellular medium (Schanne et al., 1979). It was proposed that the functional consequence of each of these toxins was a disruption of the integrity of the plasma membrane leading to a massive accumulation of intracellular calcium upon exposure of the cells to calcium-containing medium. The rise in intracellular calcium then was responsible for the subsequent changes that characterize irreversible cell injury, namely permanent loss of mitochondrial function and further membrane damage. More recent studies by Farber and colleagues have focused on the role of calcium in ischemic liver damage (Farber et al., 1981). These studies have shown a correlation between reperfusion-induced mitochondrial calcium accumulation and permanent loss of mitochondrial function and cell viability. They hypothesize that ischemia induces a redistribution of intracellular calcium resulting in the activation of endogenous phospholipases and subsequent damage to cellular membranes. This damage in turn permits the influx of calcium during reperfusion.

It is apparent from the data presented above that calcium plays a pivotal role in ischemia-induced cell damage. The exact molecular mechanisms by which calcium's effects are manifest and their temporal importance in the development of irreversible ischemic cell injury however remain to be determined. It is the purpose of the remainder of this manuscript to examine the possible role of certain calcium-activated systems in brain that may mediate some of the functional alterations seen in ischemia.

Calmodulin is a major calcium regulator protein

The discovery of calmodulin and its subsequent recognition as a ubiquitous and versatile calcium-dependent regulator protein has dramatically altered our understanding of calcium's molecular mechanisms of action in various tissues and organisms (Cheung, 1980; Klee and Vanaman, 1982). Calmodulin is an abundant protein that is small, heat stable, and has an acidic pI. It contains four high-affinity binding domains for calcium ions. Interaction of calmodulin with its target proteins and their subsequent activation requires the presence of calcium. Trifluoperazine and other phenothiazine neuroleptics inhibit the interaction of calmodulin with its receptor proteins (Weiss et al., 1982), providing a pharmacological approach to the investigation of calmodulin's role in various cellular functions.

Calmodulin mediates the calcium-dependent activation of a variety of cellular processes and enzyme systems. The discovery of calmodulin resulted from its ability to activate calcium-dependent cyclic nucleotide phosphodiesterase activity in brain (Cheung, 1970; Kakiuchi and Yamazaki, 1970). Subsequently, calcium and calmodulin were also shown to regulate the synthesis of cAMP through the activation of adenylate cyclase in brain and cultured glial cells (Cheung et al., 1975; Ebersolt et al., 1981).

Calmodulin has been shown to play a role in various aspects of intermediary metabolism. Perhaps the most significant function discovered thus far is its role in mediating calcium-dependent regulation of the enzyme phosphorylase kinase. Cohen et al. (1978) demonstrated that calmodulin is an integral non-dissociable constituent of the enzyme complex, the δ-subunit. Recently, several calmodulin-dependent glycogen synthase kinase activities have been purified from rabbit liver and skeletal muscle that mediate the phosphorylation and inactivation of the enzyme (Woodget et al., 1982; Ahmad et al., 1982; Payne et al., 1983). Thus, calmodulin appears to have a dynamic integrative function in the control of glycogen metabolism.

Calmodulin is involved in the regulation of internal calcium concentrations via the activation of both plasma membrane and internal membrane calcium pump activities. Stimulation of both calcium ATPase activity and calcium uptake into sealed erythrocyte membrane vesicles by calmodulin has been described (Hinds et al., 1978). Moreover, calmodulin has been shown to stimulate calcium transport into vesicles prepared from cardiac sarcoplasmic reticulum (Katz and Remtulla, 1978), an effect which may involve calmodulin-dependent protein phosphorylation (Lepeuch et al., 1979; Plank et al., 1983).

A major function of calmodulin is in the transduction of the calcium signal to the contractile apparatus of smooth muscle and nonmuscle cells via the activation of myosin light chain kinases (Yagi et al., 1978; Dabrowska and Hartshorne, 1978). Phosphorylation of the light chain is mandatory for actomyosin ATPase activity. Calmodulin may also be involved in the action of calcium in flagellar systems through interaction with axonemal constituents such as the dynein ATPase. Blum et al. (1980) reported that the ciliary dynein ATPase of *Tetrahymena pyriformis* exhibits calcium-dependent activation by calmodulin.

Calmodulin plays an important role in the regulation of cytoskeletal dynamics. Immunocytochemical studies have localized calmodulin on microtubules (Wood et al., 1980; Derry et al., 1984). Moreover, calmodulin becomes associated during mitosis with the polar regions of the spindle fiber apparatus believed to contain microtubule-organizing centers (Welsh et al., 1978). In vitro (Marcum et al., 1978; Job et al., 1981) and in vivo studies (Keith et al., 1983) have demonstrated that calcium-calmodulin induces rapid depolymerization of microtubules. Calmodulin-dependent protein phosphorylation may also modulate tubulin dynamics by regulating the ability of certain proteins to confer cold-stability to microtubule preparations (Job et al., 1983) and by altering the ability of microtubule-associated proteins (MAPs) to induce microtubule assembly (Yamamoto et al., 1983; Yamauchi and Fujisawa, 1983a).

Calmodulin-dependent protein phosphorylation of endogenous substrates has now been observed in a number of tissues. Several calmodulin-dependent protein kinase activities have been isolated from brain tissue (Fukunaga et al., 1982; Goldenring et al., 1983; Bennett et al., 1983; McGuiness et al., 1983; Yamauchi and Fujisawa, 1983b; Schulman, 1984) that are distinct from the calmodulin-dependent kinases described in peripheral tissues, i.e. phosphorylase kinase, myosin light chain kinase, and glycogen synthase kinase. The brain enzymes are remarkably similar, if not identical, although different substrates were employed to monitor their distribution during the purification procedures. They have been designated type II calmodulin-dependent protein kinases. Our laboratory has described the purification and characterization of a calmodulin-dependent kinase from rat brain cytosol that phosphorylates tubulin and MAP-2 as major substrates (see below) (Goldenring et al., 1982, 1983).

The magnitude of cellular processes regulated by calmodulin indicate that any perturbance of normal calcium homeostasis is likely to affect calmodulin-modulated systems whether in a beneficial or detrimental fashion. Therefore, despite the absence of data on the possible role of calmodulin in calcium-induced cellular damage in ischemia, a role for calmodulin might be postulated. We now describe the results from our laboratory that suggest that calcium-calmodulin dependent protein phosphorylation provides an important mechanism for regulating neuronal activity in brain. The possible effects of ischemia on calmodulin kinase activity and the function and state of phosphorylation of its endogenous substrates is then discussed.

Calcium-calmodulin stimulated synaptic protein phosphorylation and neurotransmission

The role of calcium in synaptic function and neurotransmission is well established (Rubin, 1972; Rasmussen and Goodman, 1977). However, until recently little was known about the molecular mechanisms mediating the effects of calcium at the synapse. Evidence is accumulating to indicate that calcium-calmodulin regulated synaptic biochemical processes may mediate the actions of calcium on synaptic activity (DeLorenzo, 1980, 1981, 1982). Calmodulin is found in high concentrations in brain (Klee and Vanaman, 1982) and has been isolated from highly enriched brain synaptic vesicle preparations and nerve terminal synaptoplasm (DeLorenzo et al., 1979; DeLorenzo 1980, 1981).

Calcium's effects on endogenous protein phosphorylation were initially described in whole rat and human brain homogenates and synaptosome preparations (DeLorenzo, 1976, 1977; DeLorenzo and Glaser, 1976; DeLorenzo et al., 1977). These experiments revealed that calcium stimulated the phosphorylation of many brain proteins, especially proteins with molecular weights of 10 000–20 000, 50 000–54 000, 60 000–64 000, and 150 000–300 000. Two protein bands with molecular weights of 52 000–54 000 and 60 000–64 000 (protein bands DPH-M and DPH-L, respectively) were of particular interest since they were most dramatically stimulated by calcium and inhibited by phenytoin, an anticonvulsant that blocks several calcium-dependent processes including neurotransmitter release (DeLorenzo, 1981). From these results, the hypothesis was developed suggesting that calcium-dependent protein phosphorylation may regulate some of the effects of calcium on synaptic function and neurotransmitter release (DeLorenzo and Freedman, 1977, 1978).

The calcium-stimulated endogenous phosphorylation pattern described above was shown to be dependent on calmodulin in crude membrane preparations from brain (Schulman and Greengard, 1978). Calmodulin was also shown to mediate the effects of calcium on the phosphorylation of specific proteins in synaptic vesicle (DeLorenzo et al., 1979), enriched synaptic membrane (DeLorenzo, 1980), synaptic junctional complex (DeLorenzo, 1980), and postsynaptic density preparations (DeLorenzo, 1980; Grab et al., 1981b). Thus, considerable evidence has accumulated to indicate that calcium and calmodulin stimulate the endogenous phosphorylation of several synaptic proteins.

It was then demonstrated that the calcium-calmodulin dependent release of neurotransmitter substances from synaptic vesicles was also dependent on magnesium and ATP (DeLorenzo and Freedman, 1978; DeLorenzo et al., 1979; DeLorenzo, 1980), suggesting that utilization of ATP by synaptic protein kinases may involved in the release process. Experiments that simultaneously studied calcium-calmodulin stimulated neurotransmitter release and protein phosphorylation in isolated vesicles and intact synaptosomes supported the hypothesis that calmodulin-regulated synaptic protein phosphorylation may mediate some of the effects of calcium on neurotransmission (DeLorenzo, 1977, 1980, 1981, 1982). This evidence is summarized below.

Protein phosphorylation and neurotransmitter release in depleted synaptic vesicles was shown to be simultaneously stimulated by calcium and calmodulin (DeLorenzo et al., 1979; DeLorenzo 1980, 1981, 1982). In addition it was shown that vesicle protein phosphorylation and neurotransmitter release had the same requirements for magnesium, ATP, calcium, and calmodulin (DeLorenzo and Freedman, 1978; DeLorenzo, 1980). Phenytoin (DeLorenzo and Glaser, 1976; DeLorenzo et al., 1977) and diazepam (DeLorenzo et al., 1981) which specifically inhibit the vesicle calcium-calmodulin kinase system were also shown to significantly inhibit neurotransmitter release (DeLorenzo, 1980, 1981, 1982). Trifluoperazine also simultaneously inhibited vesicle protein phosphorylation and neurotransmitter release (DeLorenzo, 1980, 1981, 1982). Vesicles prepared under conditions that inactivated the labile calmodulin kinase system also showed no significant calcium-calmodulin stimulated release. These experiments demonstrated that protein phosphorylation and neurotransmitter release in isolated synaptic vesicles are simultaneously activated by calcium and calmodulin and that the release of neurotransmitter substances is directly dependent on the stimulation of vesicle protein phosphorylation.

In intact synaptosome preparations, depolarization of the synaptosome membrane in the presence of calcium stimulated the phosphorylation of an 80 000 dalton protein, designated protein I (Kreuger et al., 1977). Depolarization-dependent calcium uptake was also shown to simultaneously stimulate the phosphorylation of several proteins including DPH-L and DPH-M and neurotransmitter release in intact synaptosome preparations (DeLorenzo et al., 1979; DeLorenzo, 1980, 1981, 1982). Furthermore, the level of phosphorylation of protein DPH-M in synaptic vesicle, synaptic junction, and postsynaptic density fractions from intact synaptosomes was also shown to correlate with neurotransmitter release (DeLorenzo, 1980). Since the calcium-stimulated levels of phosphorylation of proteins DPH-L and DPH-M and several other proteins was shown to be dependent on calmodulin in vesicle, membrane, synaptic junction, and postsynaptic density preparations (DeLorenzo, 1980; Grab et al., 1981b), it is reasonable to conclude that the depolarization-dependent calcium uptake simultaneously stimulates calcium-calmodulin dependent protein phosphorylation and neurotransmitter release in intact synaptosome preparations.

Studies employing trifluoperazine, diazepam, and phenytoin provided evidence for a more direct relationship between phosphorylation and release (DeLorenzo, 1981, 1982). Trifluoperazine inhibited both synaptic protein phosphorylation and neurotransmitter release in intact synaptosome preparations. Trifluoperazine decreased phosphorylation by inhibiting depolarization-dependent calcium uptake induced by high K^+ and by directly inactivating the calmodulin kinase system, as seen in the presence of A23187. Phenytoin and diazepam also inhibited the activation of calmodulin kinase activity in intact synaptosomes while simultaneously diminishing neurotransmitter release. Thus, direct inactivation of calmodulin and the calmodulin kinase system correlates with inhibition of the calcium-dependent release process in intact synaptosomes. Combining the direct studies on the isolated vesicle system with the pharmacological data obtained in the intact synaptosome preparation, it is reasonable to suggest that synaptic calcium-calmodulin kinase activity may play a role in mediating some of the effects of calcium on synaptic transmission.

Calmodulin kinase and tubulin are major constituents of DPH-L and DPH-M

In order to further understand the role of calcium-calmodulin stimulated protein phosphorylation in mediating synaptic function, it was important to determine the identity and possible function of two of the major synaptic phosphoprotein bands, DPH-L and DPH-M. It was observed in our laboratory that these proteins had essentially the same molecular weight and comigrated with the α and β subunits of tubulin on SDS-polyacrylamide gel electrophoresis (PAGE) (Burke and DeLorenzo, 1981). Calcium plays a major role in the regulation of tubulin and microtubular assembly and function (Weisenberg, 1972; Olmsted and Borisy, 1975; Berkowitz and Wolff, 1981). Moreover, a number of studies have demonstrated that calmodulin may mediate some of the effects of calcium on microtubule dynamics and stability (Marcum et al., 1978; Job et al., 1981, 1983; Keith et al., 1983). These findings and the possible similarities between proteins DPH-L and DPH-M and the α and β subunits of tubulin stimulated our interest in studying the effects of calcium and calmodulin on the endogenous phosphorylation of tubulin.

Results from this laboratory have demonstrated that calcium stimulates the endogenous phosphorylation of neurotubulin isolated from rat brain and that a significant component (30–50%) of bands DPH-L and DPH-M are α- and β-tubulin (Burke and DeLorenzo, 1981, 1982,a,b). The calcium-stimulated phosphorylation of tubulin in synaptic cytosol (Burke and DeLorenzo, 1981), synaptic vesicle (Burke and DeLorenzo, 1982a), and intact synaptosome preparations (Burke and DeLorenzo, 1982b) is dependent upon the presence of calmodulin. Since tubulin is a major "structural" and "functional" protein in nerve cells, calcium and calmodulin-dependent phosphorylation of tubulin may have an important role in the control of certain aspects of neuronal and synaptic function.

With the purification of the calmodulin-dependent kinase from brain and the identification of its molecular subunit composition (see below), we have now determined that in addition to α- and β-tubulin, a major portion of phosphoprotein bands DPH-L and DPH-M represents the autophosphorylated subunits of the calmodulin kinase as revealed by two-dimensional gel electrophoresis, peptide mapping studies, and calmodulin-binding properties. These autophosphorylated kinase subunits co-migrate on one-dimensional SDS-PAGE with protein bands DPH-L and DPH-M with apparent molecular weights of 52 000 and 63 000 for the ρ and σ subunits respectively. Since the phosphorylation of protein bands DPH-L and DPH-M was shown to be particularly sensitive to calcium in a variety of brain subfractions (DeLorenzo, 1980), the identification of the subunits of calmodulin-dependent protein kinase as major components of these phosphoproteins bands suggests that the activation of this kinase is an important aspect of calcium's action in brain.

Purification and properties of calmodulin-dependent protein kinase from brain

Identification of tubulin as a major endogenous substrate for calcium-calmodulin dependent protein kinase activity provided a first step towards a molecular characterization of the role of calcium and protein phosphorylation in synaptic modulation. To further understand the function of this tubulin kinase system, we sought to purify the enzyme from brain. Initial attempts to purify the enzyme were unsuccessful due to the instability of the kinase activity post mortem and in crude enzyme preparations (Burke and DeLorenzo, 1981; Juskevich et al., 1982; Goldenring et al., 1983). However, we have now succeeded in stabilizing the tubulin kinase activity and have purified it to apparent homogeneity (Goldenring et al., 1982, 1983). The cytosolic kinase system was isolated from rat brain cytosol by sequential chromatography on phosphocellulose

TABLE 1

Purification of calmodulin-dependent protein kinase from brain

	Protein (mg)	Total activity (nmol/min)	Specific activity (nmol/min/mg)	Recovery (%)	-fold
Cytosol	1600	500	0.3	100	1
Phosphocellulose	13.8	186	13.5	37	45
Calmodulin affinity	1.5	98	65.0	20	216
Fractogel 55F	0.3	89	297.0	18	983

Calmodulin-dependent protein kinase was isolated from rat brain cytosol using tubulin as a phosphorylation substrate to monitor enzyme yield. (Data are reproduced from Goldenring et al., 1983.)

resin, calmodulin-affinity resin, Fractogel TSK HW-55 high resolution resin, and Sephacryl S-300 Superfine gel. Table 1 demonstrates that the Fractogel-purified enzyme preparation was over 980-fold purified compared to crude brain cytosol.

Chromatography of the Fractogel-purified enzyme on Sephacryl S-300 indicated that the kinase behaves as a homogenous complex of approximately 600 000 daltons (Fig. 1A). Silver staining of the Sephacryl kinase fraction subjected to SDS-PAGE revealed two polypeptide components of approximately 52 000 and 63 000 daltons, designated as enzyme subunits ρ and σ respectively (Fig. 1B). Both subunits bound ^{125}I-calmodulin on one-dimensional (Fig. 1B) and two-dimensional (Fig. 2A) denaturing gels. The ρ band routinely demonstrated higher affinity for calmodulin when corrected for protein concentration.

Both the ρ and σ subunits demonstrated autophosphorylation in the absence of added substrate as confirmed by one- and two-dimensional SDS-PAGE (Figs. 1B and 2B). Ahmad et al. (1982) reported that the subunits of liver glycogen synthase kinase demonstrate changes in mobility when phosphorylated in the absence of substrate. In a similar manner, autophosphorylation of the ρ and σ subunits of this calmodulin-dependent kinase over time generated lower mobility autophosphorylated species. Results of two-dimensional mapping of ^{125}I-labeled tyrosine-containing tryptic peptides suggested that the ρ and σ polypeptides are highly homologous yet distinct calmodulin-binding proteins.

Further characterization of the purified kinase activity was provided by subjecting phosphorylated proteins to phosphoamino acid analysis. While tubulin phosphorylation by endogenous magnesium-dependent kinase occurred primarily on serine residues, 60% of the phosphorylation of β-tubulin by calcium-calmodulin dependent kinase was found to occur on threonine residues.

α-Tubulin was primarily phosphorylated on serine residues as was myelin basic protein. MAP-2 and the autophosphorylation of the ρ and σ kinase subunits demonstrated mainly serine phosphorylation and a minimal amount of threonine phosphorylation. The kinase did not phosphorylate tyrosine residues on any of the substrates examined.

A number of kinetic parameters of the purified kinase were examined. Enzyme phosphorylation of β-tubulin reached a maximal level within several minutes and this was maintained for over 30 min of incubation, demonstrating that the final kinase preparation was essentially free of phosphatase activity. An apparent K_m for ATP of 7 μM was observed using β-tubulin as well as MAP-2 and α-tubulin as substrates. For all substrates and autophosphorylation, the kinase displayed half-maximal activity at 50 nM calmodulin and 1 mM MgCl$_2$. The apparent K_m for β-tubulin and α-tubulin were 0.13 μM and 0.11 μM. Finally, myelin basic protein displayed an apparent K_m of 1 μM, one order of mag-

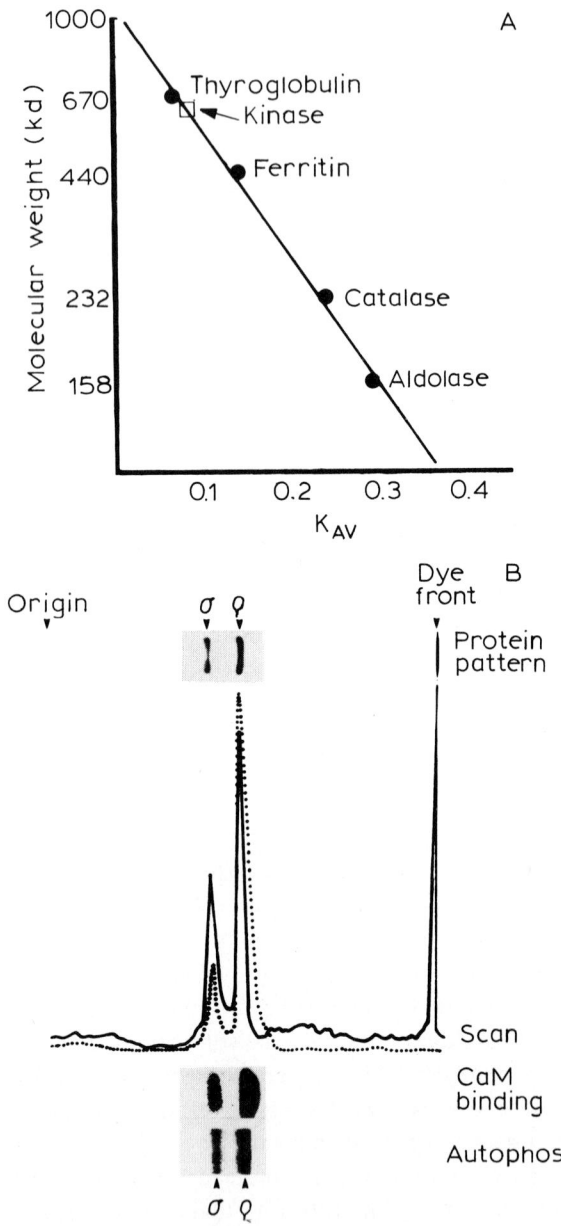

Fig. 1. Chromatography of brain calmodulin-dependent protein kinase on Sephacryl S-300 Superfine. (A) Fractogel-purified enzyme chromatographed on Sephacryl with an apparent molecular weight of approximately 600 000. (B) The kinase fraction obtained from chromatography on Sephacryl displayed only two silver-staining protein components of 52 000 (ρ) and 63 000 (σ) daltons, respectively, when resolved on one-dimensional SDS-PAGE. Both the ρ and σ subunits of the kinase bound calmodulin (CaM) in denaturing gels and displayed characteristic autophosphorylation. The densitometric scan demonstrates that the protein staining (......) and calmodulin binding (———) coincide. These patterns were identical to those seen for the Fractogel-purified enzyme (not shown). (Data are reproduced from Goldenring et al., 1983.)

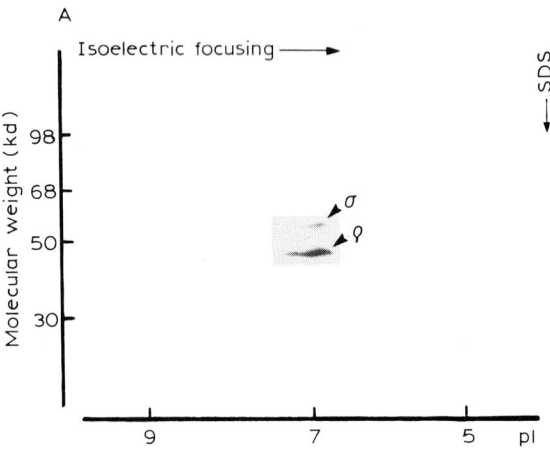

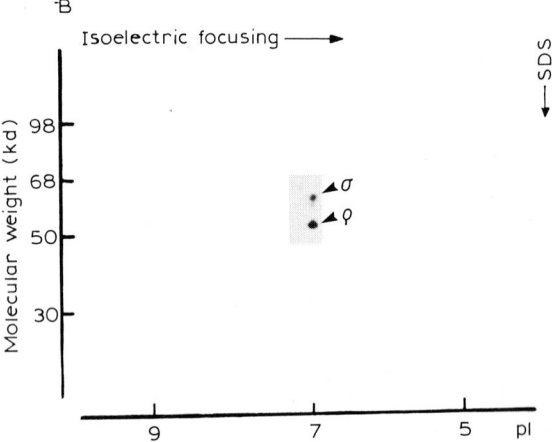

Fig. 2. ^{125}I-calmodulin binding and autophosphorylation of purified cytosolic calmodulin-dependent protein kinase. (A) Purified kinase was resolved on isoelectric focusing/SDS-PAGE and assayed for ^{125}I-calmodulin binding proteins as described (Goldenring et al., 1983). (B) Purified kinase was phosphorylated under standard conditions (Goldenring et al., 1983) in the presence of calcium and calmodulin and resolved on two-dimensional isoelectric focusing/SDS-PAGE. Gels were subsequently dried and exposed to X-ray film to produce the autoradiographs shown.

nitude higher than tubulin.

The properties of the brain cytosolic calmodulin-dependent protein kinase distinguish it from other calmodulin-dependent kinases including phosphorylase kinase, myosin light chain kinase, and glycogen synthase kinase (Cohen et al., 1978; Yagi et al., 1978; Ahmad et al., 1982; Payne et al., 1983). On the other hand, several laboratories have reported the purification of calmodulin-dependent kinase activities from brain which display many similar properties to the calmodulin kinase described above (Fukunaga et al., 1982; Bennett et al., 1983). All of these kinases phosphorylate a broad range of substrates. Previous confusion has centered around differences in the apparent substrate specificities of these kinases including their capacity to phosphorylate glycogen synthase, tubulin, and protein I. Recent evidence from several laboratories including ours suggests that the phosphorylation of these three substrates and others is dependent upon the procedures used for the preparation of the proteins. The presence of endogenous inhibitors or slight denaturation in the preparations apparently accounts for the variability in observed substrate specificities of the reported calmodulin-kinase activities. Current investigations in our laboratory and others indicate that the above proteins are indeed substrates for brain calmodulin-dependent protein kinase.

Calmodulin-dependent protein kinase and microtubule function

Calcium-calmodulin has significant effects on microtubule dynamics that involve both ATP-independent (Marcum et al., 1978; Job et al., 1981; Berkowitz and Wolff, 1981) and ATP-dependent mechanisms (Margolis and Rauch, 1981; Job et al., 1983; Yamamoto et al., 1983; Yamauchi and Fujisawa, 1983). The ATP-dependent mechanisms appear to involve the calcium-calmodulin dependent phosphorylation of several proteins that regulate microtubule polymerization and stability. For example, Margolis and associates (Pirollet et al., 1983) reported that cold-labile microtubules prepared from brain could be rendered cold-stable by the addition of a fraction containing a small number of polypeptides derived from cold-stable microtubules. In addition, cold-stable microtubules could be rendered cold-labile by the addition of MgATP (Margolis and Rauch, 1981). They subsequently demonstrated that the activity of these stabilizing proteins was abolished by calmodulin-dependent phosphorylation, a reaction blocked by trifluoperazine (Job et al., 1983). A number of high molecular weight microtubule-associated proteins (MAPs) have been shown to stimulate microtubule assembly under polymerizing conditions (Weingarten et al., 1975; Murphy and Borisy, 1975). Recently, the phosphorylation of MAPs by calcium-calmodulin-dependent protein kinases prepared from rat brain has been shown to inhibit the ability of MAPs to promote microtubule assembly (Yamamoto et al., 1983; Yamauchi and Fujisawa, 1983a). These results provide convincing evidence that calmodulin-dependent protein phosphorylation may play an important role in the physiological regulation of microtubule dynamics.

Recent results from our laboratory have provided additional evidence to support a role for calmodulin-dependent protein kinase in microtubule function. For example, we have demonstrated that the calmodulin-dependent protein kinase can be isolated in tight association with tubulin from brain cytosol (Goldenring et al., 1984b), suggesting a role for the enzyme as a tubulin-associated calmodulin-dependent kinase (TACK). Similarly, the calmodulin-dependent kinase has been identified as a major calmodulin binding enzyme system in cold-stable microtubule fractions prepared from rat brain (Larson et al., 1985). Table 2 demonstrates that a significant enrichment of calmodulin-dependent kinase activity was observed in cold-stable microtubule fractions. Significant calmodulin-dependent kinase activity was also present in twice-cycled microtubule fractions. Resolution of phosphorylated cold-stable microtubule protein in two-dimensions documented the phosphorylation (Fig. 3A) of α- and β-tubulin and MAP-2 as well as two phosphoproteins which focused near neutrality

TABLE 2

Calmodulin-dependent phosphorylation of MAP-2 in microtubule fractions

Fractions	MAP-2 phosphorylation	
	specific activity (cpm/μg)	relative activity
Cytosol	429	1
1st Cycle microtubules	2 402	5.6
Cold labile microtubules	4 464	10.4
Cold stable microtubules	9 047	21.1

Phosphorylation reactions (1 min) were performed in the presence of calcium and calmodulin as described (Larson et al., 1985). The amounts of MAP-2 were determined by densitometric scanning of Coomassie blue stained gels. Phosphorylation was quantified by excision of the specific protein bands (MAP-2) from the dried gels and scintillation counting. Specific activity is expressed as cpm/μg protein. Relative activity compared to cytosol is calculated in the right column.

and displayed apparent molecular weights of 52 000 and 63 000. These latter two phosphoproteins demonstrated identical mobilities to the autophosphorylated subunits of purified TACK subjected to two-dimensional electrophoresis (Fig. 3B).

The postsynaptic density (PSD) is a prominent structure of unknown function in central nervous system synapses. PSD fractions from brain have been found to contain significant amounts of α- and β-tubulin (Carlin et al., 1982), calmodulin (Grab et al., 1979), calmodulin-binding proteins (Carlin et al., 1981), and a number of enzymatic activities including a calmodulin-activatable protein kinase activity (DeLorenzo, 1980; Grab et al., 1981a,b). Our laboratory has recently demonstrated that the major 52 000 dalton postsynaptic density protein, which accounts for >50% of intrinsic PSD protein (Kelly and Cotman, 1977, 1978), is homologous to the major calmodulin binding ρ-subunit of TACK, suggesting that the major PSD protein may be a calmodulin-binding protein involved in kinase activity in the PSD (Goldenring et al., 1984). This was established by a number of criteria including identical autophosphorylation patterns and calmodulin binding properties on two-dimensional gels and homologous two-dimensional tryptic peptide maps. Taken together, the above findings strongly implicate the calmodulin-dependent protein kinase in

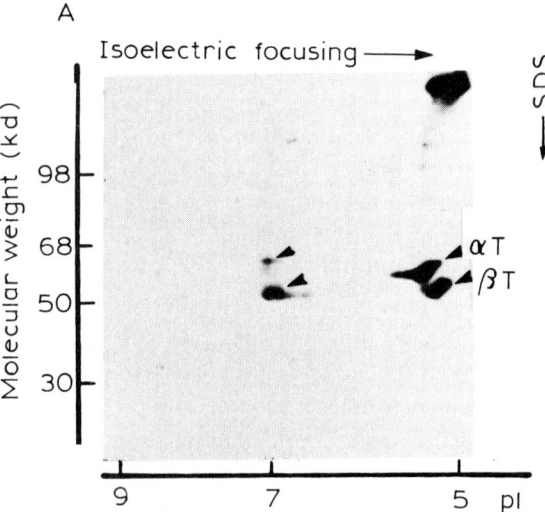

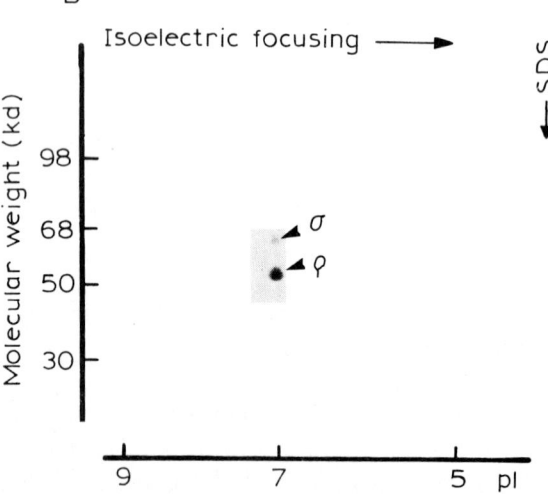

Fig. 3. Autoradiographs of two-dimensional gels of endogenous protein phosphorylation of cold-stable microtubule proteins (A) and purified calmodulin-dependent protein kinase (TACK) (B) from rat brain cytosol. The banding positions of α-tubulin (αT), and β-tubulin (βT) are indicated in A. The phosphoprotein spot at the top of the gel in A represents the endogenous phosphorylation of MAP-2. The arrowheads in A indicate the 63 000 dalton and 52 000 dalton phosphoproteins observed in cold stable microtubule fractions which focus near neutrality similar to the σ and ρ autophosphorylating subunits of TACK. (Data are reproduced from Larson et al., 1985.)

mediating some of the effects of calcium on microtubule and cytoskeletal function.

Calmodulin-dependent protein kinase, axonal transport, and brain ischemia

Axonal transport is essential for the maintenance of normal axonal and synaptic structure and function (Grafstein and Forman, 1980). Evidence from a number of sources indicate that microtubules are an integral component of the transport process (Kreutzberg, 1969; Banks et al., 1971; Schlaepfer et al., 1971; Brimijoin et al., 1979; Grafstein and Forman, 1980). Ochs and co-workers (Ochs et al., 1977; Chan et al., 1980; Ochs, 1981) have shown that axonal transport is sensitive to the axoplasmic calcium concentration and propose that calmodulin may modulate some of the effects of calcium on transport. Using desheathed peroneal nerves, they observed that axoplasmic transport could be arrested by placing desheathed nerves in a calcium-free media. Moreover, higher than normal levels of calcium in the incubation media resulted in the progressive failure of transport. This latter effect was correlated with a marked depletion of microtubules in the fibers (Ochs et al., 1977; Chan et al., 1979). It is probable that the loss of microtubules relates to the ability of calcium as well as calmodulin to induce the rapid disassembly of microtubules both in vitro and in vivo (Schlaepfer, 1971a; Weisenberg, 1972; Schlaepfer and Bunge, 1973; Marcum et al., 1978; Berkowitz and Wolff, 1981; Keith et al., 1983).

Disturbances in axoplasmic flow under the influence of anoxia-ischemia have been described (Ochs, 1972, 1974; Jacewicz and Levy, 1980). Moreover, disruption of microtubules is among the early changes observed following ischemic insults in the central nervous system (Jenkins et al., 1979). It is reasonable to speculate that ischemia-induced alterations in intracellular calcium homeostasis (Nayler et al., 1979; Raichle, 1982), resulting in a sustained elevation of internal calcium concentrations, may result in the progressive depolymerization of axonal microtubules through calmodulin-sensitive mechanisms. The disruption of microtubular integrity causes an interruption of normal axoplasmic flow that with time results in the compromise of the structural and functional integrity of the axon and nerve terminal. This may manifest itself in the loss of integrity of both plasma membranes and internal membranes (Fernando and Lau, 1978; Ekstrom von Lubitz and Diemer, 1982; Diemer and Ekstrom von Lubitz, 1983) and a further exacerbation of ion homeostasis within the nerve fiber. Thus, a degenerative cycle would ensue leading to the ultimate death of the neuron. Consistent with such a hypothesis is the observation that endoneurial injections of vincristine sulfate are accompanied by the complete disruption of microtubules, cessation of axonal transport, and the development of extensive Wallerian-type degenerative changes distal to the injection site (Schlaepfer, 1971).

Results from our laboratory and others (see above) indicate that the calcium-calmodulin-dependent protein kinase in brain is intimately involved in the regulation of microtubule dynamics and physiology. These findings suggest a role for the calmodulin-dependent kinase in mediating some of calcium's effects on axonal transport. If alterations in microtubular organization and axonal transport are involved in the initiation and propagation of irreversible cell damage in ischemia, it is possible that the calmodulin-dependent protein kinase may mediate some of these responses to ischemia. At this time, however, the role of the calmodulin kinase system in axonal transport and brain ischemia is merely speculative. More direct evidence from biochemical, physiological, and morphological studies will be necessary to support this hypothesis.

Lability of brain calmodulin-dependent kinase in ischemia

In our initial studies of endogenous calmodulin-dependent kinase activity in rat brain cytosol (Burke and DeLorenzo, 1981), we noted that maximal recovery of kinase activity was dependent on the rapid removal and homogenization of brain tissue following decapitation and the presence of protease

TABLE 3

Effect of prolonged preparation time, absence of PMSF, and type I kinase inhibitor in preparation media on endogenous activity of Ca^{2+}-calmodulin and cyclic AMP dependent protein kinases in tubulin-1 preparations

	Endogenous tubulin phosphorylation, %	
	Ca^{2+}-calmodulin kinase activity	cyclic AMP kinase activity
Control	100	100
Type I kinase inhibitor	99.2 ± 1.1	24.1 ± 3.2[a]
Prolonged preparation	11.3 ± 2.1[a]	92.4 ± 3.2
Absence of PMSF	24.2 ± 3.6[a]	98.3 ± 4.1

Crude tubulin preparations (T-1) partially depleted of calmodulin were prepared from brain cytosol by one cycle of microtubule polymerization (Burke and DeLorenzo, 1981) under control (standard) and various conditions. Endogenous phosphorylation of tubulin in these preparations was examined by incubation in the presence of Ca^{2+} and calmodulin (Ca^{2+}-calmodulin kinase activity) or cyclic AMP (cyclic AMP kinase activity) with or without type I protein kinase inhibitor. Data give the means ± SEM ($n = 10$) of endogenous kinase activity relative to maximally stimulated conditions (100%). For prolonged preparation conditions, rat brains were removed in 7–8 min instead of 20 s (control) after decapitation. For absence of PMSF (phenylmethylsulfonylfluoride) condition, PMSF was omitted from all media during preparation of T-1. (Data are reproduced from Burke and DeLorenzo, 1981.)

[a] $p < 0.001$ in comparison with maximally stimulated conditions.

inhibitors in the homogenization buffer (Table 3). Phosphorylation of tubulin by cAMP-dependent protein kinase activity in identical preparations was unaffected by the absence of protease inhibitors or prolonged preparation time (7–8 min), but was sensitive to inhibition by type I protein kinase inhibitor. These results indicated that the calmodulin-dependent protein kinase system in brain is particularly susceptible to inactivation post mortem.

Similar observations were reported by Wasterlain (1984) who found that in decapitation ischemia, the calcium-calmodulin stimulated phosphorylation of synaptic proteins in brain membranes was reduced within a few minutes, severely curtailed within 15 min, and vestigial after 30 min. Calmodulin kinase activity from synaptosomal cytosol and in partially-purified enzyme preparations also demonstrates marked lability upon storage (Juskevich et al., 1981; Goldenring et al., 1983), the loss of activity being greatly accelerated by the presence of calcium (Juskevich et al., 1982). It is possible that this represents an effect of endogenous calcium-protease activity.

The findings described above suggest that calmodulin-dependent protein kinase activity may be susceptible to inactivation *in vivo* during cerebral ischemia. Whether such inactivation would represent an initiating event in the pathogenesis of ischemic cell damage or an end result of irreversible ischemic injury is uncertain. Moreover, it is unclear if the loss of kinase activity observed *in vitro* is the result of the *in vivo* inactivation of the enzyme, or an increased susceptibility of the enzyme to (or increased activity of) endogenous inhibitors or proteases released during homogenization. Further studies will be necessary to characterize the effect of ischemia on endogenous calmodulin-dependent kinase activity and to determine the functional relationship of this kinase to the development of ischemic brain damage.

Conclusions

Considerable evidence indicates that calcium-calmodulin dependent protein phosphorylation plays a major role in mediating some of calcium's effects on neuronal function. Results from our laboratory have specifically implicated the brain calcium-calmodulin protein kinase system in regulating some of calcium's effects on synaptic function and microtubule dynamics. Although calcium has been shown to be intimately involved in the degenerative neuronal changes observed following anoxia-ischemia, its precise molecular actions are unknown. A number of findings suggest that calmodulin and calmodulin-dependent protein kinase may be involved in the calcium-induced ischemic changes. Further studies will be necessary however to determine the exact role of calmodulin-dependent kinase in ischemia. It is hoped that future studies of calcium's molecular actions in brain will provide insight into the pathogenesis of ischemic cell damage and lead to the development of effective modes of intervention for the preservation of nerve cell function in ischemia.

References

Ahmad, Z., DePaoli-Rauch, A.A. and Roach, P.J. (1982) Purification and characterization of a rabbit liver calmodulin-dependent protein kinase able to phosphorylate glycogen synthase. *J. Biol. Chem.*, 257: 8348–8355.

Banks, P., Mayor, D. and Tomlinson, D. (1971) Further evidence for the involvement of microtubules in the intra-axonal movement of noradrenaline storage vesicles. *J. Physiol.*, 219: 755–761.

Bennett, M.K., Erondu, N.E. and Kennedy, M.B. (1983) Purification and characterization of a calmodulin-dependent protein kinase that is highly concentrated in brain. *J. Biol. Chem.*, 258: 12735–12744.

Berkowitz, S.A. and Wolff, J. (1981) Intrinsic calcium sensitivity of tubulin polymerization. The contributions of temperature, tubulin concentration, and associated proteins. *J. Biol. Chem.*, 256: 11216–11223.

Blum, J.J., Haynes, A., Jamieson, G.A., Jr. and Vanaman, T.C. (1980) Calmodulin confers calcium sensitivity on ciliary dynein ATPase. *J. Cell Biol.*, 87: 533–538.

Brimijoin, S., Olsen, J. and Rosenson, R. (1979) Comparison of the temperature-dependence of rapid axonal transport and microtubules in nerves of the rabbit and bullfrog. *J. Physiol.*, 287: 303–314.

Burke, B. and DeLorenzo, R.J. (1981) Ca^{2+}- and calmodulin-stimulated endogenous phosphorylation of neurotubulin. *Proc. Natl. Acad. Sci. USA*, 78: 991–995.

Burke, B. and DeLorenzo, R.J. (1982a) Ca^{2+}- and calmodulin-dependent phosphorylation of endogenous synaptic vesicle tubulin by a vesicle-bound calmodulin kinase system. *J. Neurochem.*, 38: 1205–1218.

Burke, B. and DeLorenzo, R.J. (1982b) Ca^{2+}- and calmodulin-regulated endogenous tubulin kinase activity in presynaptic nerve terminal preparations. *Brain Res.*, 236: 393–415.

Cajal, S.R.Y. (1928) *Degeneration and Regeneration of the Nervous System*. Oxford University Press, London.

Carlin, R.K., Grab, D.J. and Siekevitz, P. (1981) Function of calmodulin in postsynaptic densities. III. Calmodulin-binding proteins of the postsynaptic density. *J. Cell Biol.*, 89: 449–455.

Carlin, R.K., Grab, D.J. and Siekevitz, P. (1982) Postmortem accumulation of tubulin in postsynaptic density preparations. *J. Neurochem.*, 38: 94–100.

Carvalho, A.G. (1982) Calcium in the nerve cell. In: A. Lajtha (Ed.), *Handbook of Neurochemistry*, 2nd Ed., Vol. 1. Plenum, New York, pp. 69–116.

Chan, S.Y., Ochs, S. and Jersild, R., Jr. (1979) Calcium localization in mammalian nerve fibers in relation to its regulation and axoplasmic transport. *Soc. Neurosci. Abstr.*, 5, 59.

Chan, S.Y., Ochs, S. and Worth, R.M. (1980) The requirement for calcium ions and the effect of other ions on axoplasmic transport in mammalian nerve. *J. Physiol.*, 301: 477–504.

Cheung, W.Y. (1970) Cyclic 3′,5′-nucleotide phosphodiesterase. Demonstration of an activator. *Biochem. Biophys. Res. Commun.*, 38: 533–538.

Cheung, W.Y. (1980) Calmodulin plays a pivotal role in cellular regulation. *Science*, 207: 19–27.

Cheung, W.Y., Bradham, L.S., Lynch, T.J., Lin, Y.M. and Tallant, E.A. (1975) Protein activator of cyclic 3′:5′-nucleotide phosphodiesterase of bovine or rat brain also activates its adenylate cyclase. *Biochem. Biophys. Res. Commun.*, 66: 1055–1062.

Chien, K.R., Abrams, J., Pfau, R.G. and Farber, J.L. (1977) Prevention by chlorpromazine of ischemic liver cell death. *Am. J. Pathol.*, 88: 539–558.

Cohen, P., Burchell, A., Foulkes, J.G., Cohen, P.T.W., Vanaman, T.C. and Nairn, A.C. (1978) Identification of the Ca^{2+}-dependent modulator protein as the fourth subunit of rabbit skeletal muscle phosphorylase kinase. *FEBS Lett.*, 92: 287–293.

Dabrowska, R. and Hartshorne, D.J. (1978) A Ca^{2+}- and modulator-dependent myosin light chain kinase from non-muscle cells. *Biochem. Biophys. Res. Commun.*, 85: 1352–1359.

Deery, W.J., Means, A.R. and Brinkley, B.R. (1984) Calmodulin-microtubule association in culture mammalian cells. *J. Cell Biol.*, 98: 904–910.

DeLorenzo, R.J. (1976) Calcium-dependent phosphorylation of specific synaptosomal fraction proteins: possible role of phosphoproteins in mediating neurotransmitter release. *Biochem. Biophys. Res. Commun.*, 71: 590–597.

DeLorenzo, R.J. (1977) Antagonistic action of diphenylhydantoin and calcium on the level of phosphorylation of particular rat and human brain proteins. *Brain Res.*, 134: 125–138.

DeLorenzo, R.J. (1980) Role of calmodulin in neurotransmitter release and synaptic function. *Ann. NY Acad. Sci.*, 356: 92–109.

DeLorenzo, R.J. (1981) The calmodulin hypothesis of neurotransmission. *Cell Calcium*, 2: 365–385.

DeLorenzo, R.J. (1982) Calmodulin in synaptic function and neurosecretion. In: W.Y. Cheung (Ed.), *Calcium and Cell Function*, Vol. III. Academic Press, New York, pp. 271–309.

DeLorenzo, R.J. and Glaser, G.H. (1976) Effect of diphenylhydantoin on the endogenous phosphorylation of brain protein. *Brain Res.*, 105: 381–386.

DeLorenzo, R.J. and Freedman, S.D. (1977) Calcium-dependent phosphorylation of synaptic vesicle proteins and its possible role in mediating neurotransmitter release and vesicle function. *Biochem. Biophys. Res. Commun.*, 77: 1036–1043.

DeLorenzo, R.J. and Freedman, S.D. (1978) Calcium dependent neurotransmitter release and protein phosphorylation in synaptic vesicles. *Biochem. Biophys. Res. Commun.*, 80: 183–192.

DeLorenzo, R.J., Emple, G.P. and Glaser, G.H. (1977) Regulation of the level of endogenous phosphorylation of specific brain proteins by diphenylhydantoin. *J. Neurochem.*, 28: 21–30.

DeLorenzo, R.J., Freedman, S.D., Yohe, W.B. and Maurer, S.C. (1979) Stimulation of Ca^{2+}-dependent neurotransmitter release and presynaptic nerve terminal phosphorylation by calmodulin and a calmodulin-like protein isolated from synaptic vesicles. *Proc. Natl. Acad. Sci. USA*, 76: 1838–1842.

DeLorenzo, R.J., Burdette, S. and Holderness, J. (1981) Benzodiazepine inhibition of the calcium-calmodulin protein kinase system in brain membrane. *Science*, 213: 546–549.

Diemer, N.H. and Ekstrom von Lubitz, D.K.J. (1983) Cerebral ischaemia in the rat: increased permeability of post-synaptic membranes to horseradish peroxidase in the early post-ischaemic period. *Neuropathol. Appl. Neurobiol.*, 9: 403–414.

Ebersolt, C., Perez, M. and Bockaert, J. (1981) Neuronal, glial and meningeal localizations of neurotransmitter-sensitive adenylate cyclase in cerebral cortex of mice. *Brain Res.*, 213: 139–150.

Ekstrom von Lubitz, D.K.J. and Diemer, N.H. (1982) Complete cerebral ischaemia in the rat: an ultrastructural and stereological analysis of the distal striatum in the hippocampal CA-1 region. *Neuropathol. Appl. Neurol.*, 8: 197–215.

Farber, J.L., Chien, K.R. and Mittnacht, S., Jr. (1981) The pathogenesis of irreversible cell injury in ischemia. *Am. J. Pathol.*, 102: 271–281.

Fukunaga, K., Yamamoto, H., Matsui, K., Higashi, K. and Miyamoto, E. (1982) Purification and characterization of a Ca^{2+}- and calmodulin-dependent protein kinase from rat brain. *J. Neurochem.*, 39: 1607–1617.

Goldenring, J.R., Gonzalez, B. and DeLorenzo, R.J. (1982) Isolation of brain Ca^{2+}-calmodulin tubulin kinase containing calmodulin binding proteins. *Biochem. Biophys. Res. Commun.*, 108: 421–428.

Goldenring, J.R., Gonzalez, B., McGuire, J.S. and DeLorenzo, R.J. (1983) Purification and characterization of a calmodulin-dependent kinase from rat brain cytosol able to phosphorylate tubulin and microtubule-associated proteins. *J. Biol. Chem.*, 258: 12632–12640.

Goldenring, J.R., McGuire, J.S. and DeLorenzo, R.J. (1984a) Identification of the major postsynaptic density protein as homologous with the major calmodulin-binding subunit of a calmodulin-dependent protein kinase. *J. Neurochem.*, 42: 1077–1084.

Goldenring, J.R., Casanova, J.E. and DeLorenzo, R.J. (1984b) Tubulin associated calmodulin-dependent kinase: evidence for an endogenous complex of tubulin with a Ca^{2+}-calmodulin-dependent kinase. *J. Neurochem.*, 43: 1669–1679.

Grab, D.J., Berzins, K., Cohen, R.S. and Siekevitz, P. (1979) Presence of calmodulin in postsynaptic densities isolated from the canine cerebral cortex. *J. Biol. Chem.*, 254: 8690–8696.

Grab, D.J., Carlin, R.K. and Siekevitz, P. (1981a) Function of calmodulin in postsynaptic densities. I. Presence of a calmodulin-activatable cyclic nucleotide phosphodiesterase activity. *J. Cell Biol.*, 89: 433–439.

Grab, D.J., Carlin, R.K. aand Siekevitz, P. (1981b) Function of calmodulin in postsynaptic densities. II. Presence of a calmodulin-activatable protein kinase activity. *J. Cell Biol.*, 89: 440–448.

Grafstein, B. and Forman, D.S. (1980) Intracellular transport in neurons. *Physiol. Rev.*, 60: 1167–1283.

Hansen, A.J. (1981) Extracellular ion concentrations in cerebral ischemia. In: T. Zeuthen (Ed.), *The Application of Ion-selective Microelectrodes*. Elsevier/North-Holland, Amsterdam, New York, pp. 239–254.

Hinds, T.R., Raess, B.U. and Vincenzi, F.F. (1981) Plasma membrane Ca^{2+} transport: antagonism by several potential inhibitors. *J. Membr. Biol.*, 58: 57–65.

Hossmann, K.-A. and Kleihues, P. (1973) Reversibility of ischemic brain damage. *Arch. Neurol.*, 29: 375–384.

Hossmann, K.-A. and Zimmerman, V. (1974) Resuscitation of brain after one hour of complete ischemia. I. Physiological and morphological observations. *Brain Res.*, 81: 59–74.

Jenkins, L.W., Povlishock, J.T., Becker, D.P., Miller, J.D. and Sullivan, H.G. (1979) Complete cerebral ischemia. *Acta Neuropathol. (Berlin)*, 48: 113–125.

Jacewicz, M. and Levy, D.E. (1980) Ischaemic effects on axonal transport in the CNS. *American Academy of Neurology*, 32nd Annual Meeting Abstract, p. 81.

Job, D., Fischer, E.H. and Margolis, R.L. (1981) Rapid disassembly of cold-stable microtubules by calmodulin. *Proc. Natl. Acad. Sci. USA*, 78: 4679–4682.

Job, D., Rauch, C.T., Fischer, E.H. and Margolis, R.L. (1983) Regulation of microtubule cold stability by calmodulin-dependent and -independent phosphorylation. *Proc. Natl. Acad. Sci. USA*, 80: 3894–3898.

Juskevich, J.C., Kuhn, D.M. and Lovenberg, W. (1982) Calcium enhanced inactivation of calmodulin-dependent protein kinase from synaptosomes. *Biochem. Biophys. Res. Commun.*, 108: 24–30.

Kakiuchi, S. and Yamazaki, R. (1970) Calcium dependent phosphodiesterase activity and its activating factor (PAF) from brain. Studies on cyclic 3′,5′-nucleotide phosphodiesterase(III). *Biochem. Biophys. Res. Commun.*, 41: 1104–1110.

Katz, S. and Remtulla, M.A. (1978) Phosphodiesterase protein activator stimulates calcium transport in cardiac microsomal preparations enriched in sarcoplasmic reticulum. *Biochem. Biophys. Res. Commun.*, 83: 1373–1379.

Keith, C., DiPaolo, M., Maxfield, F.R. and Shelanski, M.L. (1983) Microinjection of Ca^{2+}-calmodulin causes a localized depolymerization of microtubules. *J. Cell Biol.*, 97: 1918–1924.

Kelly, P.T. and Cotman, C.W. (1977) Identification of glycoproteins and proteins at synapses in the central nervous system. *J. Biol. Chem.*, 252: 786–793.

Kelly, P.T. and Cotman, C.W. (1978) Synaptic protein: characterization of tubulin and actin and identification of a distinct postsynaptic density polypeptide. *J. Cell biol.*, 79: 173–183.

Klee, C.B. and Vanaman, T.C. (1982) Calmodulin. In: C.B. Anfinsen, J.T. Edsall and F.M. Richards (Eds.), *Advances in Protein Chemistry*, Vol. 35, Academic Press, New York, pp. 213–321.

Kreuger, B.K., Forn, J. and Greengard, P. (1977) Depolarization-induced phosphorylation of specific proteins, mediated by calcium ion influx, in rat brain synaptosomes. *J. Biol. Chem.*, 252: 2764–2773.

Kreutzberg, G.W. (1969) Neuronal dynamics and axonal flow. IV. Blockade of intra-axonal enzyme transport by colchicine. *Proc. Natl. Acad. Sci. USA*, 62: 722–728.

Larson, R.E., Goldenring, J.R., Vallano, M.L. and DeLorenzo, R.J. (1985) Identification of endogenous calmodulin-dependent kinase and calmodulin binding proteins in cold-stable microtubule preparations from rat brain. *J. Neurochem.*, 44: 1566–1574.

LePeuch, C.J., Haiech, J. and Demaille, J.G. (1979) Concerted regulation of cardiac sarcoplasmic reticulum transport by cyclic adenosine monophosphate dependent and calcium-calmodulin-dependent phosphorylations. *Biochemistry*, 213: 139–150.

Marcum, J.M., Dedman, J.R., Brinklet, B.R. and Means, A.R. (1978) Control of microtubule assembly-disassembly by calcium-dependent regulator protein. *Proc. Natl. Acad. Sci. USA*, 75: 3771–3775.

Margolis, R.L. and Rauch, C.T. (1981) Characterization of rat brain crude extract microtubule assembly: correlation of cold stability with the phosphorylation state of a microtubule-associated 64K protein. *Biochemistry*, 20: 4451–4458.

McGuiness, R.L., Lai, Y., Greengard, P., Woodget, J.R. and Cohen, P. (1983) A multifunctional calmodulin-dependent protein kinase. *FEBS Lett.*, 163: 329–334.

Murphy, D.B. and Borisy, G.G. (1975) Association of high-molecular-weight proteins with microtubules and their role in microtubule-assembly in vitro. *Proc. Natl. Acad. Sci. USA*, 72: 2696–2700.

Nageotte, J. (1910) Action des métaux et de divers autres facteurs sur la dégéneration des nerfs en survie. *C.R. Seances Soc. Biol. Fil.*, 69: 556.

Nayler, W.G. (1981) The role of calcium in the ischemic myocardium. *Am. J. Pathol.*, 102: 262–270.

Nayler, W.G., Poole-Wilson, P.A. and Williams, A. (1979) Hypoxia and calcium. *J. Mol. Cell. Cardiol.*, 11: 683–706.

Nestler, E.J., Walaas, S.I. and Greengard, P. (1984) Neuronal phosphoproteins: physiological and clinical implications. *Science*, 225: 1357–1364.

Ochs, S. (1972) The dependence of fast transport in mammalian nerve fibers on metabolism. *Acta Neuropathol. (Berlin) (Suppl.)*, 5: 86–96.

Ochs, S. (1974) Energy metabolism and supply of P to the fast axoplasmic transport mechanism in nerve. *Fed. Proc.*, 33: 1049–1058.

Ochs, S. (1981) Calcium and the mechanism of axoplasmic transport. *Fed. Proc.*, 41: 2301–2306.

Ochs, S., Worth, R.M. and Chan, S.-Y. (1977) Calcium requirement for axonal transport in mammalian nerve. *Nature*, 279: 748–750.

Olmsted, J.B. and Borisy, G.G. (1975) Ionic and nucleotide regulation for microtubule polymerization in vitro. *Biochemistry*, 14: 2996–3005.

Payne, M.E.M., Schworer, C.M. and Soderling, T.R. (1983) Purification and characterization of rabbit liver calmodulin-dependent glycogen synthase kinase. *J. Biol. Chem.*, 258: 2376–2382.

Pirollet, F., Job, D., Fischer, E.H. and Margolis, R.L. (1983) Purification and characterization of sheep brain cold-stable microtubules. *Proc. Natl. Acad. Sci. USA*, 80: 1560–1564.

Plank, B., Wyskovsky, W., Hellmann, G. and Suko, J. (1983) Calmodulin-dependent elevation of calcium transport associated with calmodulin-dependent phosphorylation in cardiac sarcoplasmic reticulum. *Biochim. Biophys. Acta*, 732: 99–109.

Plum, F. (1983) What causes infarction in ischemic brain? *Neurology*, 33: 222–233.

Raichle, M.E. (1982) The pathophysiology of brain ischemia. *Ann. Neurol.*, 13: 2–10.

Rasmussen, H. and Goodman, D.B.P. (1977) Relationships between calcium and cyclic nucleotides in cell activation. *Physiol. Rev.*, 57: 421–509.

Rubin, R.P. (1972) The role of calcium in the release of neurotransmitter substances and hormones. *Pharm. Rev.*, 22: 389–428.

Schanne, F.A.X., Kane, A.B., Young, E.E. and Farber, J.L. (1979) Calcium dependence of toxic cell death: a final common pathway. *Science*, 206: 700–702.

Schlaepfer, W.W. (1971a) Experimental alterations of neurofilaments and neurotubules by calcium and other ions. *Exp. Cell Res.*, 67: 73–80.

Schlaepfer, W.W. (1971b) Vincristine-induced axonal alterations in rat peripheral nerve. *J. Neuropathol. Exp. Neurol.*, 30: 488–505.

Schlaepfer, W.W. and Bunge, R.P. (1973) Effects of calcium ion concentration on the degeneration of amputated axons in tissue culture. *J. Cell Biol.*, 59: 456–470.

Schulman, H. (1984) Phosphorylation of microtubule-associated proteins by a calcium/calmodulin-dependent protein kinase. *J. Cell Biol.*, 99: 11–19.

Schulman, H. and Greengard, P. (1978) Stimulation of brain membrane protein phosphorylation by calcium and an endogenous heat-stable protein. *Nature*, 271: 478–479.

Shen, A.C. and Jennings, R.B. (1972) Kinetics of calcium accumulation in acute myocardial ischemic injury. *Am. J. Pathol.*, 67: 441–452.

Shine, K.I., Douglas, A.M. and Ricchiuti, N.V. (1978) Calcium, strontium, and barium movements during ischemia and reperfusion in rabbit ventricle. Implications for myocardial preservation. *Circ. Res.*, 43: 712–720.

Wasterlain, C.G. (1984) Calcium- and calmodulin-dependent phosphorylation in ischemic brain. *Soc. Neurosci. Abstr.*, 10: 1005.

Weingarten, M.D., Lockwood, A.H., Hwo, S.Y. and Kirschner, M.W. (1975) A protein factor essential for microtubule assembly. *Proc. Natl. Acad. Sci. USA*, 72: 1858–1862.

Weisenberg, R.C. (1972) Microtubule formation in vitro in solutions containing low calcium concentrations. *Science*, 177: 1104–1105.

Weiss, B., Prozialeck, W.C. and Wallace, T.L. (1982) Interaction of drugs with calmodulin. *Biochem. Pharmacol.*, 31: 2217–2226.

Welsh, M., Dedman, J.R., Brinkley, B.R. and Means, A.R. (1978) Calcium-dependent regulator protein: localization in mitotic apparatus of eucaryotic cells. *Proc. Natl. Acad. Sci. USA*, 75: 1867–1871.

Wood, J.G., Wallace, R.W., Whitaker, J.N. and Cheung, W.Y. (1980) Immunocytochemical localization of calmodulin and a heat labile calmodulin-binding protein (CaM-BP$_{80}$) in basal ganglia of mouse brain. *J. Cell Biol.*, 84: 66–76.

Woodget, J.R., Tonks, N.K. and Cohen, P. (1982) Identification of a calmodulin-dependent glycogen synthase kinase in rabbit skeletal muscle distinct from phosphorylase kinase. *FEBS Lett.*, 148: 5–11.

Yagi, K., Yazawa, M., Kakiuchi, S., Oshima, M. and Uenishi, K. (1978) Identification of an activator protein for myosin light chain kinase as the Ca^{2+}-dependent-modulator protein. *J. Biol. Chem.*, 253: 1338–1340.

Yamamoto, H., Fukunaga, K., Tanaka, E. and Miyamoto, E. (1983) Ca^{2+}- and calmodulin-dependent phosphorylation of microtubule-associated protein 2 and factor, and inhibition of microtubule assembly. *J. Neurochem.*, 41: 1119–1125.

Yamauchi, T. and Fujisawa, H. (1983a) Disassembly of microtubules by the action of calmodulin-dependent protein kinase (kinase II) which occurs only in the brain tissues. *Biochem. Biophys. Res. Commun.*, 110: 287–291.

Yamauchi, T. and Fujisawa, H. (1983b) Purification and characterization of the brain calmodulin-dependent protein kinase (kinase II), which is involved in the activation of tryptophan-5-monooxygenase. *Eur. J. Biochem.*, 132: 15–21.

Mechanisms underlying the neuronal response to ischemic injury. Calcium-activated proteolysis of neurofilaments

William W. Schlaepfer and Un-Jin P. Zimmerman

Division of Neuropathology, Department of Pathology and Laboratory Medicine, University of Pennsylvania Medical School, Philadelphia, PA 19104, USA

Introduction

Neurofilaments (NF) are the predominant component of the neuronal cytoskeleton and function as a major determinant in the formation and maintenance of the markedly asymmetrical shape of the neuron. They occur in abundance throughout neuronal cytoplasm, especially within the axons and dendrites of large nerve cells. Moreover, NF are highly specific for neurons and are readily differentiated biochemically and immunochemically from other intermediate filaments which occur in astroglia and in mesenchymal elements of the nervous system. NF and their subunits have been well characterized so that they can be easily recognized and studied by morphological, biochemical and immunochemical methods. Thus NF can serve as a very useful set of neuronal marker proteins which can be examined and monitored under various experimental and pathological conditions.

Studies of NF in different systems indicate that they are highly susceptible to proteolysis by calcium-activated neutral protease (CANP). The presence of CANP in neuronal cytoplasm with no apparent barrier between the enzyme and NF substrate suggests that CANP is maintained in an inactive form within the cell, either due to the presence of an endogenous enzyme inhibitor or to insufficient levels of calcium to activate the enzyme. In either case, experimental influxes of calcium into the neuron lead to progressive proteolysis of NF by CANP. Furthermore, calcium-mediated degradation of NF is a natural consequence of pathological states, suggesting that activation of CANP may represent an important mechanism mediating neuronal reaction to injury. The present chapter reviews the topic of calcium-activated proteolysis of NF by describing the substrate and its relationship to the neuronal cytoskeleton, by describing the reaction whereby NF are degraded by calcium and by characterizing the enzyme which mediates the reaction.

Neurofilaments and the neuronal cytoskeleton

The neuron is a markedly asymmetrical cell with numerous processes (i.e., dendrites and axon) extending for variable distances away from the perikaryon. Patterns of neuritic arborization vary considerably among different groups of neurons. Yet, all neurons share the same cytoskeletal components, including NF proteins. Differences in neuritic arborization are reflected in varying admixtures of cytoskeletal components. For example, dendrites contain a higher density of microtubules (Wuerker and Kirkpatrick, 1972) and more of the MAPs 2 form of microtubule-associated proteins (MAP) (Huber and Matus, 1984) than do axons. Likewise, NF are more prevalent in axons, especially those of large size (Friede and Samorajski, 1970; Berthold, 1978). More recently, it has been proposed that NF are the major determinant of axonal calibre (Hoffman et al., 1984).

Quantitative differences of NF content are present within different parts of the neuron (e.g., perikaryon vs. neurite) as well as among different sets of neurons (e.g., large vs. small neurons). Variations in the relative amounts of individual NF subunits are also known to occur within the same neuronal population during development (Shaw and Weber, 1982; Willard and Simon, 1983; Pachter and Liem, 1984; Cochard and Paulin, 1984). More recently, immunochemical studies have shown that NF epitopes are differentially expressed within different parts of the same neuron as well as by different groups of neurons (Goldstein et al., 1983; Dahl, 1983; Bennett et al., 1984). Much of the regional variation in the immunohistochemical expression of NF may reflect post-translational modifications of NF protein subunits, such as their state of phosphorylation (Sternberger and Sternberger, 1984).

NF in situ appear as hollow cylindrical filaments of 8–11 nm diameter which are interconnected to themselves and microtubules by 4–6 nm strands (Wuerker and Kirkpatrick, 1972; Ellisman and Porter, 1980; Hirokawa, 1982). Crossbridges are unique to NF and may serve to maintain the minimal 30–40 nm circumferential spacings which occur around NF but not other intermediate filaments (Tohyama et al., 1983). Isolated NF reveal a cylindrical structure (Fig. 1) and are composed of 2–2.5 nm protofilaments (Schlaepfer, 1977; Krishnan et al., 1979) which can be disassembled by exposure to low ionic strength (Schlaepfer, 1971a and 1978a).

Mammalian NF are composed of three protein subunits: M_r 70 000 (NF70), M_r 150 000 (NF150) and M_r 200 000 (NF200). Subunits from different species reveal similar peptide maps but vary slightly in their electrophoretic mobilities (Thorpe et al., 1979; Dahl, 1979; Davison and Jones, 1980; Chiu et al., 1980). Each NF subunit possesses unique and shared epitopes (Liem et al., 1978; Anderton et al., 1980; Dahl, 1980; Yen and Fields, 1981) as well as epitopes which are shared by all intermediate filament proteins (Pruss et al., 1981). Intact NF are composed of all three NF subunits (Schlaepfer et al., 1981a; Willard and Simon, 1981) and sediment when centrifuged in non-ionic detergent solutions

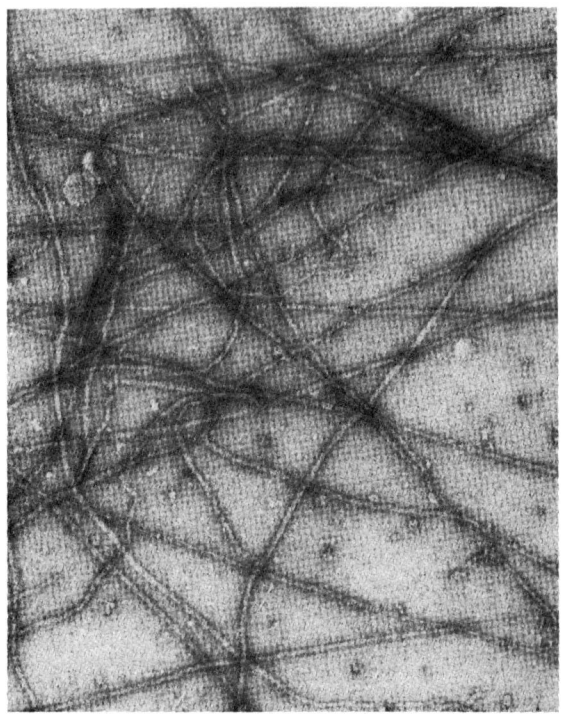

Fig. 1. Isolated neurofilaments from rat peripheral nerve appear as cylindrical structures with relatively smooth external surfaces (without apparent sidearms) when attached to a carbon-formvar film and viewed by negative imaging with an electron dense stain (1% uranyl acetate). Neurofilament profiles are 8–11 nm wide. × 100 000.

(e.g., 1% Triton X-100). Hypotonic disassembly of NF (Schlaepfer, 1971a and 1978a) leads to separation of protofilaments which are also composed of the triplet subunits but no longer sediment upon centrifugation (Carden and Eagles, 1983). NF subunits are solubilized in 8 M urea and can be separated chromatographically (Geisler and Weber, 1981; Chiu and Norton, 1982; Liem and Hutchison, 1982; Tokutake, 1984). Complete separation of subunits may be achieved by preparative electrophoresis (Hogue-Angeletti et al., 1982).

NF subunits contain domains which are similar to those described in other intermediate filament proteins, including a 10–12 000 dalton N-terminal portion rich in arginine residues, a 35–40 000 dalton rod segment of α-helical configuration and a C-terminal portion which comprises the bulk of NF150 and NF200 (Geisler et al., 1983). The N-terminus and rod segment are believed to anchor the subunits to the backbone of the filament while the C-terminus is felt to extend into the periphery of the filament. Mild chymotryptic digestion of intact NF separates large C-terminal portions of NF150 and NF200 (Julien and Mushynski, 1983). Digestion by trypsin can selectively degrade the C-termini of NF150 and NF200 without disrupting the filamentous structure of the NF (Chin et al., 1983). Intact NF can be reassembled most readily from isolated NF70 subunits (Geisler and Weber, 1981; Moon et al., 1981; Liem and Hutchison, 1982; Zackroff et al., 1982) but also from NF150 and, possibly NF200 as well (Gardner et al., 1984).

NF subunits are synthesized concomitantly as separate and independent events (Czosnek et al., 1980; Strocchi et al., 1982). Pulse-labeled NF subunits appear as insoluble proteins which move synchronously into and along the axon as the major component in the slowest phase (SCa) of axonal transport (Hoffman and Lasek, 1975). Movement of pulse-labeled NF in SCa retains a bell-shaped distribution (Lasek, 1982), suggesting that NF subunits are translocated as intact filaments or, at least, in very close association. Symmetrical enlargement of the bell-shaped wave of labeled NF subunits during axonal transit indicates that individual NF can move at slightly differing velocities. Rates of axonal transport of NF subunits differ in the central vs. peripheral branches of the primary sensory neuron (Mori et al., 1979), during development (Hoffman et al., 1983; Willard and Simon, 1983) and during nerve regeneration (Hoffman and Lasek, 1980), and may be accelerated (Monaco et al., 1983) or stopped (Griffin et al., 1978; Bizzi et al., 1984) in pathological states.

NF become phosphorylated (Julien and Mushynski, 1982; Honchar et al., 1982; Shecket and Lasek, 1982; Jones and Williams, 1982) either before or following their assembly into filaments and/or during their transit through the axon. Most phosphorylation sites are located on the large C-terminal fragments of NF150 and, especially, NF200 which are cleaved by mild chymotryptic digestion (Julien and Mushynski, 1983). Enzymes which mediate the phosphorylation of NF are associated with the neuronal cytoskeleton, including a cAMP-independent kinase that co-purifies with NF (Shecket and Lasek, 1982; Julien et al., 1983), a cAMP-dependent kinase associated with MAPs 2 (Runge et al., 1981; Letterrier et al., 1981) and cAMP-dependent and cAMP-independent kinases associated with neurofilament proteases (Zimmerman and Schlaepfer, 1984b). Phosphatases which dephosphorylate NF subunits have not as yet been characterized.

Most studies on NF metabolism have focused on the synthesis and transport of NF subunits through the axon. Very little attention has been directed at the fate of NF subunits after their transit through the axon. Lasek and Black (1977) showed that radiolabeled NF subunits are quickly degraded upon reaching axonal terminals and that this rapid turnover of NF subunits is dependent upon an intact and functioning synapse. They speculated that NF turnover may be regulated by calcium influxes associated with neurotransmission and that NF breakdown may be mediated by calcium-activated proteases at nerve endings. Experimental data from our laboratory in support of these hypotheses are reviewed in the following section.

Calcium-mediated breakdown of neurofilaments

Susceptibility of mammalian NF to degradation by calcium was initially noted during comparative studies of finely minced segments of rat peripheral nerve which had been incubated in solutions of different composition prior to fixation and examination by electron microscopy (Schlaepfer, 1971b). These studies showed that brief exposure to solutions containing free calcium led to a granular disintegration of axonal NF and microtubules whereas the same axonal cytoskeletal structures remained intact during prolonged incubations in phosphate buffer prior to fixation. Calcium-induced changes could be prevented by chelation of calcium and were not reproduced during parallel incubations with high levels of magnesium or during incubations with aluminum or lead.

The same granular disintegration of axonal NF

and microtubules occurred in long intact segments of rat peripheral nerve which had been excised and incubated in solutions containing free calcium (Schlaepfer, 1974a). The changes in excised nerves were identical to those of contralateral nerves which were transected and left to undergo Wallerian degeneration in situ (Fig. 2). Calcium-dependent changes in excised nerves were accelerated by increasing the calcium concentration and, especially, by permeating the axolemma by including detergents (e.g. Triton X-100) or calcium ionophore (e.g., A23187) in the incubation media (Schlaepfer, 1974b, 1978b). Degeneration of excised and transected nerves showed the same collapse and fragmentation of myelin sheaths, suggesting that calcium-induced disintegration of the axonal cytoskeleton caused liquifaction and collapse of the axonal compartment. Fragmentation of myelin sheaths into linear arrays of myelin ovoids is a characteristic feature of axonal degeneration.

Granular disintegration of NF of transected axons in vitro could be prevented by removal of calcium from the media (Schlaepfer and Bunge, 1973). Replacement of calcium to these cultures within a

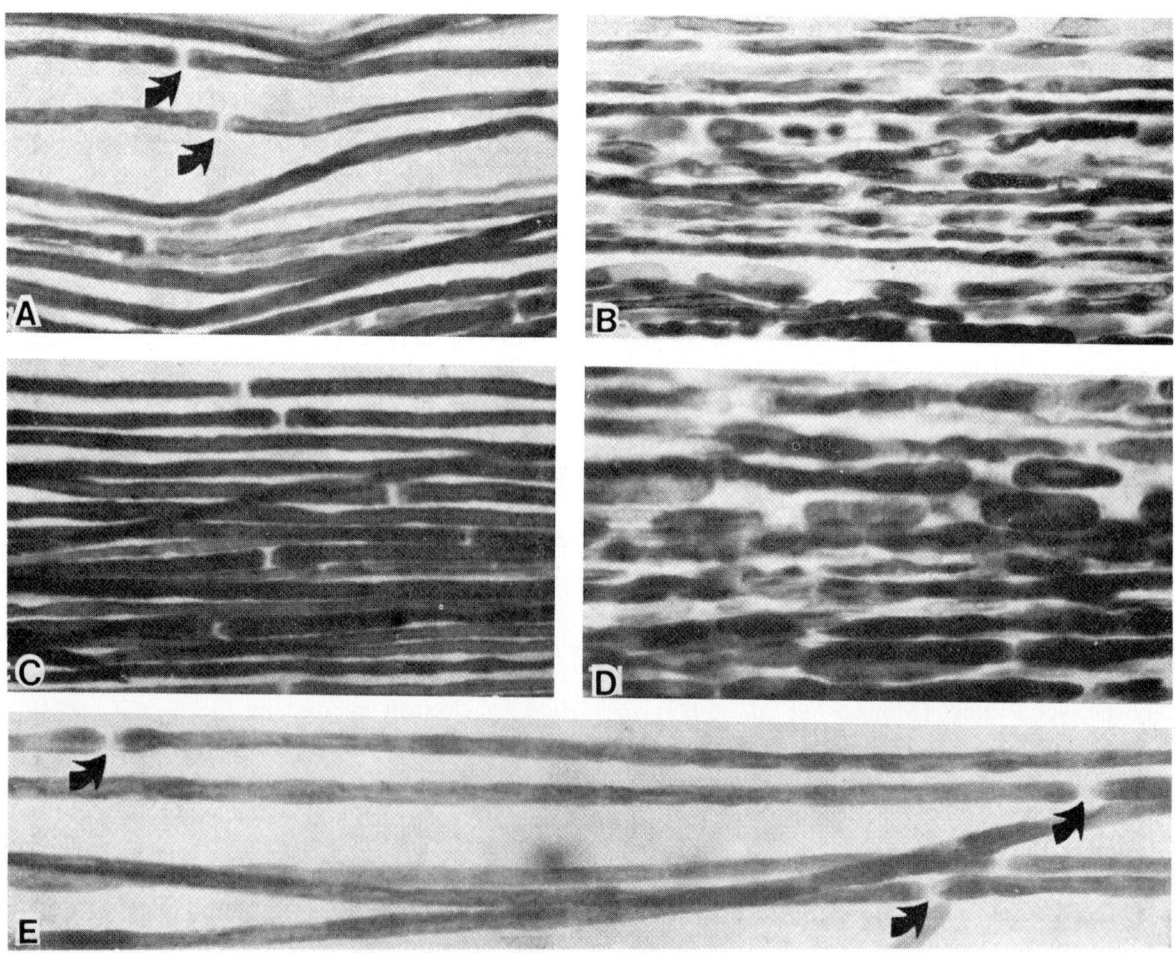

Fig. 2. Myelinated nerve fibers undergo fragmentation between the 24-hour (A and C) and 48-hour (B and D) intervals in transected rat sciatic nerves which are left to degenerate in vivo (A and B) or which are excised and placed in nutrient media at 37°C with calcium (C and D). Fragmentation of myelin does not occur in excised nerves which are placed in nutrient media lacking calcium (E). Fragmentation of myelin is due to the granular disintegration of the axonal cytoskeleton, especially the axonal neurofilaments and microtubules. Osmicated whole-mount preparations of nerve. × 175.

6-hour interval caused NF degradation. Similar granular disintegration of NF caused by incubation with calcium did not occur in transected neurites after 24- and 48-hour intervals in calcium-free media (Schlaepfer and Bunge, unpublished data), indicating that addtional factors were responsible for the calcium-dependent degradation of NF in vitro.

Studies of calcium-dependent disintegration of NF were facilitated by the use of transverse frozen sections of peripheral nerve which enhances the exposure and penetration of axoplasm to different solutes (Schlaepfer and Hasler, 1979a). These studies showed that calcium-dependent degradation of NF (1) occurred in all nerve fibers of rat peripheral nerve, but preferentially in small myelinated and unmyelinated fibers, (2) was inhibited by PCMB, a thiol protease inhibitor, (3) was prevented by prolonged preincubation of frozen sections in calcium-free media, and (4) did not continue in the absence of calcium. These findings were all consistent with the view that NF degradation is mediated by a soluble calcium-activated thiol protease.

Biochemical studies of peripheral nerves following experimental influxes of calcium showed that the calcium-dependent granular disintegration of NF is accompanied by a selective loss of the three NF protein subunits (Schlaepfer and Micko, 1979). Loss of NF70 and NF150 generally preceded loss of NF200. Tubulin was also degraded. Similar loss of NF subunits (Fig. 3) paralleled the granular disintegration of NF in transected rat peripheral nerve (Schlaepfer and Micko, 1978). Interestingly, some loss of NF subunits could be detected in nerves that were freeze-thawed in as little as 10 μM of free calcium (Schlaepfer et al., 1981b). Other studies showed that the NF protein subunits (as well as the protein subunits of glial filaments and vimentin filaments) in the rat spinal cord and optic nerve are also degraded following a calcium influx into these tissues (Schlaepfer and Zimmerman, 1981).

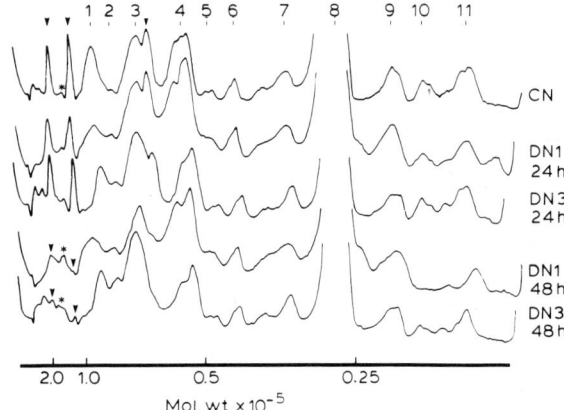

Fig. 3. Individual neurofilament proteins (arrowheads) are seen in densitometric tracings of proteins in whole nerve homogenates from control rat sciatic nerve (CN) and in proximal (DN1) and distal (DN3) portions of transected nerves at the 24-hour interval following transection. The three neurofilament proteins (200 000, 150 000 and 68 000 molecular weights) are lost from proximal and distal portions of transected nerves by the 48-hour interval following transection. Proteins were separated by electrophoresis in 12% SDS-acrylamide gels. Asterisk denotes a metachromatic staining collagen protein which served as an internal marker.

Isolation and characterization of calcium-activated protease that degrades neurofilaments

The identification and separation of a calcium-activated protease that degrades NF were advanced by studies which showed that NF isolated from rat spinal cord distintegrated in the presence of calcium and that this reaction was mediated by a separate tissue factor (Schlaepfer and Freeman, 1980). NF which were separated from the tissue factor remained unaltered in the presence of calcium but were rapidly degraded when the tissue factor was added back to the preparation (Fig. 4). This tissue factor was inactivated by heat, precipitated in ammonium sulfate and was inhibited by p-chloromercurobenzoate. It was active between pH 6.8–8.0 and at 4, 18 and 37°C.

Further purification of the calcium-activated neutral protease (CANP) from rat spinal cord was achieved by subjecting ammonium sulfate precipitates to anion exchange chromatography and gel filtration (Zimmerman and Schlaepfer, 1982, 1984a).

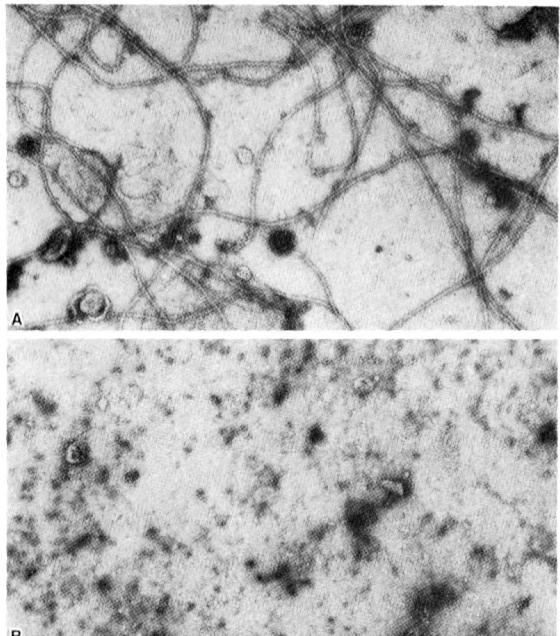

Fig. 4. Isolated neurofilaments which have been separated from soluble tissue factors remain intact during incubation with calcium (A) but undergo granular disintegration when tissue factors are added back to the incubation (B). Neurofilaments are from rat spinal cord and have been negatively stained with uranyl acetate. ×65000.

These procedures resulted in the separation of several forms of CANP which differ in their affinities for calcium as defined by the calcium concentration necessary for enzyme activation. The most active form of CANP has a low affinity for calcium and has been designated mCANP since it requires mM levels of calcium for activation. A high affinity enzyme form (μCANP) is activated at μM concentrations of calcium. μCANP elutes from DE52 at 0.08–0.12 M NaCl, whereas mCANP possesses greater charge and elutes from the same anion exchange column at 0.27–0.30 M NaCl. Multiple forms of CANP with high and low affinities for calcium have been isolated from many tissues (Zimmerman and Schlaepfer, 1984c).

The differing affinities of μCANP and mCANP for calcium can be utilized to separate as well as purify the different enzyme forms using substrate affinity chromatography (Zimmerman and Schlaepfer, 1984a). μCANP but not mCANP is retarded on a column containing casein or neurofilament proteins when the Ca/EGTA buffering system is adjusted to a calcium concentration of 10^{-5} M free calcium (Fig. 5A). Both μCANP and mCANP are retarded on the column at free calcium concentrations of 10^{-3} M, but only mCANP is eluted from the column when the calcium concentration is reduced to 10^{-5} M (Fig. 5B). Purified preparations of μCANP and mCANP from substrate affinity chromatography have M_r of 96 000 and 76 000 daltons, respectively, when examined by SDS acrylamide gel electrophoresis (Fig. 5). Furthermore, these enzyme forms differ markedly in their susceptibility to autoproteolysis in the presence of calcium.

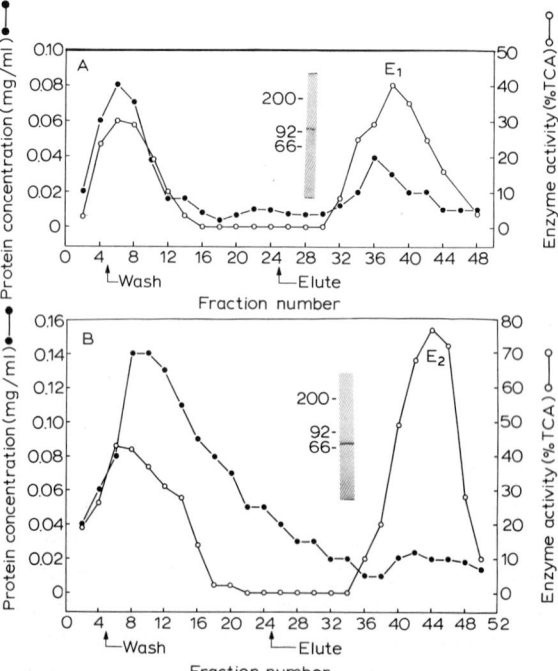

Fig. 5. Purification of μCANP (A) and mCANP (B) from rat brain by substrate affinity chromatography using a casein-conjugated Sepharose 4B column and adjusting calcium concentrations to activate and inactivate the enzyme. High affinity μCANP (E_1) remains bound to the column during application and washing of sample with 10^{-5} M calcium but is eluted when calcium is reduced to 10^{-7} M (A). Low affinity mCANP (E_2) remains bound to the column during application and washing of sample with 10^{-3} M calcium but is eluted when calcium is reduced to 10^{-5} M (B). μCANP and mCANP have molecular weights of 96 000 and 76 000 by SDS gel electrophoresis (inserts).

mCANP is rapidly inactivated when incubated in calcium (Fig. 6), a phenomenon accompanied by loss of the M_r 76 000 dalton band on SDS gels. μCANP is much more resistant to the presence of calcium.

It is not clear whether the various forms of CANP represent different gene products or whether they arise from modification of a larger protein with variable alterations of the calcium affinity site(s) on the enzyme. Enzyme forms with high and low affinities for calcium show considerable structural similarities (Yoshimura et al., 1983) and immunological cross-reactivity (Dayton et al., 1981; Wheelock, 1982) in non-neural tissues. Fig. 7 shows that affinity purified antisera to mCANP from rat muscle cross-reacts extensively with M_r 96 000 and M_r 76 000 protein bands of μCANP and mCANP purified by substrate affinity chromatography (Zimmerman and Schlaepfer, 1984a). Furthermore, this antiserum recognizes a larger enzyme form (M_r 154 000) with high affinity for calcium in crude preparations from rat brain. This large enzyme form could be the source from which both μCANP and mCANP are derived, with alteration of the calcium binding site(s) occurring in the mCANP form of the enzyme.

Phosphorylation may represent another regulatory feature associated with the different forms of CANP (Zimmerman and Schlaepfer, 1984b). Both μCANP and mCANP from rat muscle and rat brain co-purify with kinase activities which preferentially phosphorylate the different enzyme forms. Kinase activity associated with mCANP is cAMP-dependent, is inactivated by Walsh kinase inhibitor and is not altered by calmodulin. The kinase activity associated with μCANP is cAMP-independent and can still be detected after purification of the enzyme

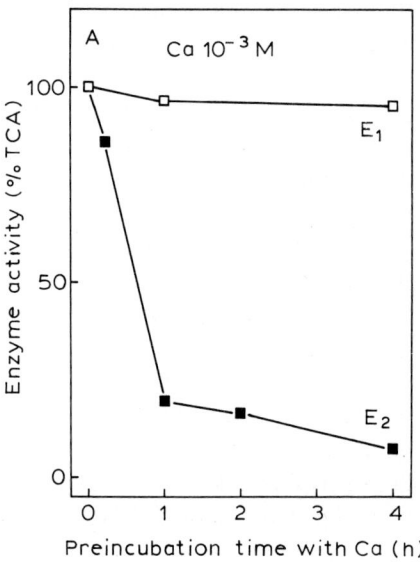

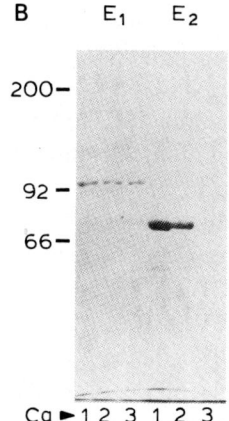

Fig. 6. mCANP (E_2) is inactivated during incubation with calcium (A) and disappears from electrophoretogram during the same 4-hour interval (B). μCANP (E_1) is less susceptible to inactivation by autoproteolysis.

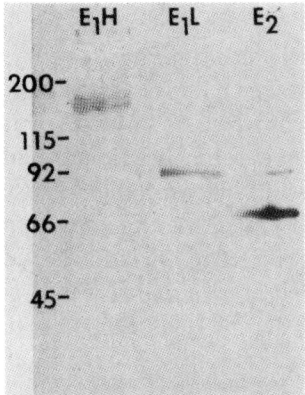

Fig. 7. Rabbit antisera to mCANP from rat brain immunoreacts with the 76 000 molecular weight protein band in mCANP preparation (E_2), with the 96 000 molecular weight protein band in μCANP preparation (E_1L) and with a 154 000 molecular weight protein in μCANP preparation (E_1H) which was separated from the smaller proteins in E_1L by gel filtration.

by substrate affinity chromatography. Phosphorylation reduces proteolytic activity of the enzyme but does not appear to alter the level of calcium required for activation of the different enzyme forms.

Proteolytic activity of CANP is also dependent upon an endogenous inhibitor which coexists with the enzyme in most tissues. The inhibitor tends to co-purify with μCANP and elutes from DE52 at low salt concentrations (Zimmerman and Schlaepfer, 1984a). Lower molecular weight forms of the enzyme are separated from the inhibitor by gel filtration; however, large enzyme forms (e.g., M_r 154000) with high affinity for calcium may be present but remain undetected due to close association with the endogenous inhibitor. The enzyme inhibitor is heat-stable and is believed to form an E-I complex, especially in the presence of calcium (Mellgren and Carr, 1983; Melloni et al., 1982).

Proteolysis of neurofilament proteins by calcium-activated protease

Very similar patterns of calcium-dependent degradation of NF proteins occurred under diverse experimental conditions, whether generated by crude or purified enzyme preparations at different temperature, pH and ionic composition (Zimmerman and Schlaepfer, 1982). NF subunit proteins were degraded with apparent K_m values of 3.9×10^{-8}, 4.4×10^{-8}, and 8.2×10^{-8} M from NF70, NF150 and NF200, respectively. The relatively greater K_m of NF200 is also apparent when NF proteolysis is induced in situ following experimental influxes of calcium into the tissues (Schlaepfer and Micko, 1979; Schlaepfer et al., 1981b). Conditions were not found which favored the selective breakdown of a single NF protein subunit as reported to occur in situ (Nixon et al., 1983) and to be associated with the cytoskeletal pellet from rat spinal cord (Ishizaka et al., 1983). Furthermore, a CANP specific for NF subunits has yet to be isolated.

The same patterns of NF breakdown also occur when isolated NF are degraded by different forms of purified CANP (Zimmerman and Schlaepfer, 1984a). For example, degradation of ^{125}I-NF proteins by μCANP and by mCANP generates identical radioactive peptide fragments. The same fragmentation of ^{125}I-NF proteins is brought about by μCANP and mCANP from rat brain and from rat muscle.

A more detailed analysis of NF fragmentation following calcium-activated proteolysis is provided by immunoblotting the peptide fragments which are generated during proteolysis (Schlaepfer et al., 1984b). Polyclonal and monoclonal antibodies to NF protein subunits enable the same broad or restricted set of epitopes to be studied among the parent NF proteins and the degraded fragments. Similarities in patterns of NF fragmentation by immunoblot are particularly strong indications of enzymatic homology since peptide fragments are compared by electrophoretic migration as well as their ability to retain specific NF immunoreactivities. Indeed, identical NF immunoblot patterns are generated when NF proteins are degraded by either μCANP or mCANP from muscle or from brain (Zimmerman and Schlaepfer, 1984a).

The immunoblot patterns generated by CANP proteolysis of NF are very similar to those which result following an influx of calcium into different rat tissues, such as peripheral nerve, spinal cord or spinal nerve roots (Schlaepfer et al., 1984b). Identical immunoreactive fragments of M_r 110000–120000 daltons are generated during the early stages of NF breakdown in each instance. Most immunoreactive products, however, have M_r between 40000–65000 daltons and appear as a series of closely spaced immunobands, following CANP proteolysis of NF and after calcium influx into the tissues. Furthermore, in both instances, the same immunoreactive products of M_r 57000 and 65000 persist. These products selectively react with a monoclonal antibody (2.2F3) to NF200.

Immunoblot studies have also shown that NF proteolysis by CANP mediates NF breakdown in transected nerve (Schlaepfer et al., 1984a). Most of the breakdown of NF occurs in the 24–48 hour interval following transection, corresponding to the period in which calcium influx into the axoplasmic compartment is believed to occur (Schlaepfer and

Micko, 1978). NF fragmentation in transected nerves generates the same peptide fragments as seen during an experimental calcium influx into the tissues as well as during NF proteolysis by CANP (Schlaepfer et al., 1984b).

Likewise in transected nerve, immunoblots revealed the presence of NF breakdown fragments of M_r 57 000 and 65 000 which appear relatively resistant to further breakdown, persisting in transected nerve for prolonged periods (Schlaepfer et al., 1984a). These NF fragments were detected by polyclonal antisera to NF proteins, but more selectively by the 2.2F3 monoclonal antibody to NF200. It is likely that these fragments are externalized following the collapse and disappearance of the axonal compartment (Schlaepfer and Hasler, 1979b). Interestingly, low levels of the same NF fragments are present in normal peripheral nerve as well as CNS tissues. It is uncertain whether these fragments reflect turnover of NF proteins within the tissues with persistence of the more protease-resistant domains of the NF protein subunits.

Conclusion

NF represent a major component of the neuronal cytoskeleton, thereby serving to establish and maintain the asymmetrical shape of the neuron. In fact, the synthesis and transport of NF tend to stabilize the axon since NF comprise the structural foundation of the axon. Much of the turnover of NF proteins appears to occur at the distal end of the axon, mediated by a CANP which can be isolated from neural and non-neural tissues. Activation of CANP at nerve endings may well be coupled to calcium influxes associated with neurotransmission. The enzyme, however, is not limited to synaptic endings but is also present throughout the neuronal cytoplasm. Like other neuronal proteins, it is undoubtedly synthesized in the perikarya and transported to distal sites. It is unclear whether the extremely low level of intracellular calcium is the only mechanism which maintains CANP in an inactive form. It is possible that the phosphorylation state of the enzyme or its close association with an endogenous inhibitor may also serve to limit the activation of the enzyme.

The presence of CANP, albeit in an inactive state, throughout the cytoplasm of the neuron represents a potential risk for the neuron. The enzyme can readily be activated by experimental influxes of calcium into neural tissues, a phenomenon which is a major determinant of the axonal degeneration which ensues following nerve transection. Similar influxes of calcium into the neuron could easily arise under a variety of metabolic conditions, including ischemia, which compromise the natural impermeability of the neuronal surface membrane to calcium. Alternatively, excessive calcium-activated proteolysis could arise in disease conditions which lead to inherent alterations in permeability of the neuronal surface membrane. It is also possible that other mechanisms could intervene in the activation of CANP, such as the selective degradation of enzyme inhibitor, the disruption of an E-I complex or altered states of phosphorylation of the enzyme. In any case, the degradation and loss of NF proteins represent changes in an important system with definitive cellular markers by which neuronal injury may be detected and monitored.

Acknowledgement

This work was supported by Grant NS 15722 from the National Institutes of Health.

References

Anderton, B.H., Thorpe, R., Cohen, J., Selvendran, S. and Woodhams, P. (1980) Specific neuronal localization by immunofluorescence of 10 nm filament polypeptides. *J. Neurocytol.*, 9: 835–844.

Bennett, G.S., Tapscott, S.J., DiLullo, C. and Holtzer, H. (1984) Differential binding of antibodies against the neurofilament triplet proteins in different avian neurons. *Brain Res.*, 304: 291–302.

Berthold, C.-H. (1978) Morphology of normal peripheral axons. In: S.G. Waxman (Ed.), *Physiology and Pathobiology of Axons*. Raven Press, New York, pp. 3–63.

Bizzi, A., Crane, R.C., Autilio-Gambetti, L. and Gambetti, P.

(1984) Aluminum effect on slow axonal transport: a novel impairment of neurofilament transport. *J. Neurosci.*, 4: 722–731.

Carden, M.J. and Eagles, P.A.M. (1983) Neurofilaments from ox spinal nerves. Isolation, disassembly, reassembly and cross-linking properties. *Biochem. J.*, 215: 227–237.

Chin, T.K., Eagles, P.A.M. and Maggs, A. (1983) The proteolytic digestion of ox neurofilaments with trypsin and a-chymotrypsin. *Biochem. J.*, 215: 239–252.

Chiu, F.-C. and Norton, W.T. (1982) Bulk preparation of CNS cytoskeleton and the separation of individual neurofilament proteins by gel filtration: dye-binding characteristics and amino acid composition. *J. Neurochem.*, 39: 1252–1260.

Chiu, F.-C., Korey, B. and Norton, W.T. (1980) Intermediate filaments from bovine, rat, and human CNS: mapping analysis of the major proteins. *J. Neurochem.*, 34: 1149–1159.

Cochard, P. and Paulin, D. (1984) Initial expression of neurofilaments and vimentin in the central and peripheral nervous system of the mouse embryo in vivo. *J. Neurosci.*, 4: 2080–2094.

Czosnek, H., Soifer, D. and Wisniewski, H.M. (1980) Studies on the biosynthesis of neurofilament proteins. *J. Cell Biol.*, 85: 726–734.

Dahl, D. (1979) The cyanogen bromide peptide maps of neurofilament polypeptides in axonal preparations isolated from bovine brain are different. *FEBS Lett.*, 103: 144–147.

Dahl, D. (1980) Study on the immunological cross-reactivity of neurofilament polypeptides in axonal preparations of bovine brain. *FEBS Lett.*, 111: 152–156.

Dahl, D. (1983) Immunohistochemical differences between neurofilaments in perikarya, dendrites and axons. *Exp. Cell Res.*, 149: 397–408.

Davison, P.F. and Jones, R.N. (1980) Neurofilament proteins of mammals compared by peptide mapping. *Brain Res.*, 182: 470–473.

Dayton, W.R., Schollmeyer, J.V., Lepley, R.A. and Cortes, L.R. (1981) A calcium-activated protease possibly involved in myofibrillary protein turnover. Isolation of a low calcium-requiring form of the protease. *Biochim. Biophys. Acta*, 659: 48–61.

Ellisman, M.H. and Porter, K.R. (1980) Microtrabecular structure of the axoplasmic matrix: visualization of cross-linking structures and their distribution. *J. Cell Biol.*, 87: 464–479.

Friede, R.L. and Samorajski, T. (1970) Axon caliber related to neurofilaments and microtubules in sciatic nerve fibers of rats and mice. *Anat. Rec.*, 167: 379–388.

Gardner, E.E., Dahl, D. and Bignami, A. (1984) Formation of 10-nanometer filaments from the 150K-dalton neurofilament protein in vitro. *J. Neurosci. Res.*, 11: 145–155.

Geisler, N. and Weber, K. (1981) Self-assembly in vitro of the 68 000 molecular weight component of the mammalian neurofilament triplet proteins into intermediate-sized filaments. *J. Mol. Biol.*, 151: 565–571.

Geisler, N., Kaufman, E., Fischer, S., Plessmann, U. and Weber, K. (1983) Neurofilament architecture combines structural principles of intermediate filaments with carboxy-terminal extensions increasing in size between triplet proteins. *EMBO J.*, 2: 1295–1302.

Goldstein, M.E., Sternberger, L.A. and Sternberger, N.H. (1983) Microheterogeneity ("neurotypy") of neurofilament proteins. *Proc. Natl. Acad. Sci. USA*, 80: 3101–3105.

Griffin, J.W., Hoffman, P.N., Clark, A.W., Carroll, P.T. and Price, D.L. (1978) Slow axonal transport of neurofilament proteins: impairment by β,β'-iminodipropionitrile administration. *Science*, 202: 633–635.

Hirokawa, N. (1982) Cross-linker system between neurofilaments, microtubules and membrane organelles in frog axons revealed by the quick-freeze, deep-etching method. *J. Cell Biol.*, 94: 129–142.

Hoffman, P.N. and Lasek, R.J. (1975) The slow component of axonal transport: identification of major structural polypeptides of the axon and their generality among mammalian neurons. *J. Cell Biol.*, 66: 351–366.

Hoffman, P.N. and Lasek, R.J. (1980) Axonal transport of MT-NF network during regeneration: constancy and change. *Brain Res.*, 202: 317–334.

Hoffman, P.N., Lasek, R.J., Griffin, J.W. and Price, D.L. (1983) Slowing of the axonal transport of neurofilament proteins during development. *J. Neurosci.*, 8: 1694–1700.

Hoffman, P.N., Griffin, J.W. and Price, D.L. (1984) Control of axonal caliber by neurofilament transport. *J. Cell Biol.*, 99: 705–714.

Hogue-Angeletti, R.A., Wu, H.-L. and Schlaepfer, W.W. (1982) Preparative separation and amino acid composition of neurofilament triplet proteins. *J. Neurochem.*, 38: 116–120.

Honchar, M.P., Bunge, M.B. and Agrawal, H.C. (1982) In vivo phosphorylation of neurofilament proteins in the central nervous system of immature rat and rabbit. *Neurochem. Res.*, 7: 365–372.

Huber, G. and Matus, A. (1984) Differences in the cellular distributions of two microtubule-associated proteins, MAPs 1 and MAPs 2, in rat brain. *J. Neurosci.*, 4: 151–160.

Ishizaka, Y., Tashiro, T. and Kurakawa, M. (1983) A calcium-activated protease which preferentially degrades the 160-kDa component of the neurofilament triplet. *Eur. J. Biochem.*, 131: 41–45.

Jones, S.M. and Williams, R.C. (1982) Phosphate content of mammalian neurofilaments. *J. Biol. Chem.*, 257: 9902–9905.

Julien, J.-P. and Mushynski, W.E. (1982) Multiple phosphorylation sites in mammalian neurofilament polypeptides. *J. Biol. Chem.*, 257: 10467–10470.

Julien, J.-P. and Mushynski, W.E. (1983) The distribution of phosphorylation sites among identified proteolytic fragments of mammalian neurofilaments. *J. Biol. Chem.*, 258: 4019–4025.

Julien, J.-P., Smoluk, G.D. and Mushynski, W.E. (1983) Characteristics of the protein kinase activity associated with rat neurofilament preparations. *Biochim. Biophys. Acta*, 755: 25–31.

Krishnan, N., Kaiserman-Abramof, I.R. and Lasek, R.J. (1979) Helical substructure of neurofilaments from *Myxicola* and squid giant axons. *J. Cell Biol.*, 82: 323–335.

Lasek, R.J. (1982) Translocation of the neuronal cytoskeleton and axonal locomotion. *Philos. Trans. Roy. Soc. Lond. (Series B)*, 299; 313–327.

Lasek, R.J. and Black, M.M. (1977) How do axons stop growing? Some clues from the metabolism of the proteins in the slow component of axonal transport. In: S. Roberts, A. Lajtha, and W.H. Gispen (Eds.), *Mechanisms, Regulation and Special Functions of Protein Synthesis in the Brain*. Elsevier, Amsterdam, pp. 161–169.

Leterrier, J.-F., Liem, R.K.H. and Shelanski, M.L. (1981) Preferential phosphorylation of the 150 000 molecular weight component of neurofilaments by a cyclic-AMP dependent, microtubule-associated protein kinase. *J. Cell Biol.*, 90: 755–760.

Liem, R.K. and Hutchison, S.B. (1982) Purification of individual components of the neurofilament triplet: filament assembly from the 70 000-dalton subunit. *Biochemistry*, 21: 3221–3226.

Liem, R.K. Yen, S.-H., Salomon, D. and Shelanski, M.L. (1978) Intermediate filaments in nervous tissues. *J. Cell Biol.*, 79: 637–645.

Mellgren, R.L. and Carr, T.C. (1983) The protein inhibitor of calcium-dependent protease: purification from bovine heart and possible mechanisms of regulation. *Arch. Biochem. Biophys.*, 225: 779–786.

Melloni, E., Sparatore, B., Salamino, F., Michetti, M. and Pontremoli, S. (1982) Cytosolic calcium dependent proteinase of human erythrocytes: formation of an enzyme-natural inhibitor complex induced by Ca^{2+} ions. *Biochem. Biophys. Res. Comm.*, 106: 731–740.

Monaco, S., Crane, R., Autilio-Gambetti, L. and Gambetti, P. (1983) Transport of neurofilaments is accelerated in 2,5-hexanedione axonopathy. *J. Neuropathol. Exp. Neurol.*, 42: 330a.

Moon, H.M., Wisniewski, T., Merz, P., DeMartin, J. and Wisniewski, H.M. (1981) Partial purification of neurofilament subunits from bovine brains and studies on neurofilament assembly. *J. Cell Biol.*, 82: 174–184.

Mori, H., Komiya, Y. and Kurokawa, M. (1979) Slowly migrating axonal polypeptides. Inequalities in their rate and amount of transport between two branches of bifurcating axons. *J. Cell Biol.*, 92: 192–198.

Nixon, R.A., Brown, B.A. and Marotta, C.A. (1983) Limited proteolytic modification of a neurofilament protein involves a proteinase activated by endogenous levels of calcium. *Brain Res.*, 275: 384–388.

Pachter, J.S. and Liem, R.K.H. (1984) The differential appearance of neurofilament triplet polypeptides in the developing rat optic nerve. *Dev. Biol.*, 103: 200–210.

Pruss, R.M., Mirsky, R., Raff, M., Thorpe, R., Dowding, A. and Anderton, B.H. (1981) All classes of intermediate filaments share a common antigenic determinant defined by a monoclonal antibody. *Cell*, 27: 419–428.

Runge, M.S., El-Maghrabi, M.R., Claus, T.H., Pilkis, S.J. and Williams, R.C. (1981) A MAPs 2-stimulated protein kinase activity associated with neurofilaments. *Biochemistry*, 20: 175–180.

Schlaepfer, W.W. (1971a) Stabilization of neurofilaments by vincristine sulfate in low ionic strength media. *J. Ultrastruct. Res.*, 36: 367–374.

Schlaepfer, W.W. (1971b) Experimental alteration of neurofilaments and neurotubules by calcium and other ions. *Exp. Cell Res.*, 67: 73–80.

Schlaepfer, W.W. (1974a) Calcium-induced degeneration of axoplasm in isolated segments of rat peripheral nerve. *Brain Res.*, 69: 203–215.

Schlaepfer, W.W. (1974b) Effects of energy deprivation on Wallerian degeneration in isolated segments of rat peripheral nerve. *Brain Res.*, 78: 71–81.

Schlaepfer, W.W. (1977) Studies on the isolation and substructure of mammalian neurofilaments. *J. Ultrastruct. Res.*, 61: 149–157.

Schlaepfer, W.W. (1978a) Observations on the disassembly of isolated mammalian neurofilaments. *J. Cell Biol.*, 76: 50–56.

Schlaepfer, W.W. (1978b) Structural alterations of peripheral nerve induced by the calcium ionophore, A23187. *Brain Res.*, 136: 1–9.

Schlaepfer, W.W. and Bunge, R.P. (1973) The effects of calcium ion concentration on the degeneration of amputated axons in tissue culture. *J. Cell Biol.*, 59: 456–470.

Schlaepfer, W.W. and Micko, S. (1978) Chemical and structural changes of neurofilaments in transected rat sciatic nerve. *J. Cell Biol.*, 78: 369–378.

Schlaepfer, W.W. and Micko, S. (1979) Calcium-dependent alterations of neurofilament proteins of rat peripheral nerve. *J. Neurochem.*, 32: 211–219.

Schlaepfer, W.W. and Hasler, M.B. (1979a) Characterization of the calcium-induced disruption of neurofilaments in rat peripheral nerve. *Brain Res.*, 168: 299–309.

Schlaepfer, W.W. and Hasler, M.B. (1979b) The persistence and possible externalization of axonal debris during Wallerian degeneration. *J. Neuropathol. Exp. Neurol.*, 38: 242–252.

Schlaepfer, W.W. and Freeman, L.A. (1980) Calcium-dependent degradation of mammalian neurofilaments by soluble tissue factor(s) from rat spinal cord. *Neurosci.*, 5: 2305–2314.

Schlaepfer, W.W. and Zimmerman, U.-J.P. (1981) Calcium-mediated breakdown of glial filaments and neurofilaments in rat optic nerve and spinal cord. *Neurochem. Res.*, 6: 243–255.

Schlaepfer, W.W., Lee, V. and Wu, H.-L. (1981a) Assessment of immunological properties of neurofilament triplet proteins. *Brain Res.*, 226: 259–272.

Schlaepfer, W.W., Zimmerman, U.-J.P. and Micko, S. (1981b) Neurofilament proteolysis in rat peripheral nerve: homologies with calcium-activated proteolysis of other tissues. *Cell Calcium*, 2: 235–250.

Schlaepfer, W.W., Lee, C., Lee, V.M.-Y. and Zimmerman, U.-J.P. (1984a) Comparison of neurofilament degradation in situ and during calcium activated proteolysis: an immunoblot study. *J. Neurochem.* (in press).

Schlaepfer, W.W., Lee, C., Trojanowski, J.Q. and Lee, V.M.-Y. (1984b) Persistence of immunoreactive neurofilament protein breakdown products in transected rat sicatic nerve. *J. Neurochem.*, 43: 857–864.

Shaw, G. and Weber, K. (1982) Differential expression of neurofilament triplet proteins in brain development. *Nature*, 298: 277–279.

Shecket, G. and Lasek, R.J. (1982) Neurofilament protein phosphorylation. Species generality and reaction characteristics. *J. Biol. Chem.*, 257: 4788–4795.

Sternberger, L.A. and Sternberger, N.H. (1983) Monoclonal antibodies distinguish phosphorylated and nonphosphorylated forms of neurofilaments in situ. *Proc. Natl. Acad. Sci. USA*, 80: 6126–6130.

Strocchi, P., Dahl, D. and Gilbert, J.M. (1982) Studies on the biosynthesis of intermediate filament proteins in rat CNS. *J. Neurochem.*, 39: 1132–1141.

Thorpe, R., Delacourte, A. and Anderton, B.H. (1979) The polypeptides of isolated 10 nm filaments and their association with polymerized tubulin. *Biochem. J.*, 181: 275–284.

Tohyama, K., Ide, C., Nitatori, T. and Yokota, R. (1983) Nearest-neighbor distance of intermediate filaments in axons and Schwann cells. *Acta Neuropathol.*, 60: 194–198.

Tokutake, S. (1984) Complete separation of the triplet components of neurofilament by DE-52 column chromatography depends upon urea concentration. *Anal. Biochem.*, 140: 203–207.

Wheelock, M.J. (1982) Evidence for two structurally different forms of skeletal muscle Ca^{2+}-activated protease. *J. Biol. Chem.*, 257: 12471–12474.

Willard, M. and Simon, C. (1981) Antibody decoration of neurofilaments. *J. Cell Biol.*, 89: 198–205.

Willard, M. and Simon, C. (1983) Modulations of neurofilament axonal transport during the development of rabbit retinal ganglion cells. *Cell*, 35: 551–559.

Wuerker, R.B. and Kirkpatrick, J.B. (1972) Neuronal microtubules, neurofilaments and microfilaments. *Int. Rev. Cytol.*, 33: 45–75.

Yen, S.-H. and Fields, K.L. (1981) Antibodies to neurofilament, glial filament and fibroblast intermediate filament proteins bind to different cell types of the nervous system. *J. Cell Biol.*, 88: 115–126.

Yoshimura, N., Kikuchi, T., Sasaki, T., Ditahara, A., Hatanaka, M. and Murachi, M. (1983) Two distinct Ca^{2+} proteases (calpain I and calpain II) purified concurrently by the same method from rat kidney. *J. Biol. Chem.*, 258: 8883–8889.

Zackroff, R.V., Idler, W.W., Steinert, P.M. and Goldman, R.D. (1982) In vitro reconstitution of intermediate filaments from mammalian neurofilament triplet polypeptides. *Proc. Natl. Acad. Sci. USA*, 79: 754–757.

Zimmerman, U.-J.P. and Schlaepfer, W.W. (1982) Characterization of brain calcium-activated protease that degrades neurofilament proteins. *Biochemistry*, 21: 3977–3983.

Zimmerman, U.-J.P. and Schlaepfer, W.W. (1984a) Multiple forms of Ca-activated protease from rat brain and muscle. *J. Biol. Chem.*, 259: 3210–3218.

Zimmerman, U.-J.P. and Schlaepfer, W.W. (1984b) Kinase activities associated with calcium-activated neutral proteases. *Biochem. Biophys. Res. Comm.*, 120: 767–774.

Zimmerman, U.-J.P. and Schlaepfer, W.W. (1984c) Calcium-activated neutral protease (CANP) in brain and other tissues. *Prog. Neurobiol.*, (in press).

Cerebral protein synthesis and ischemia

W. Bodsch, K. Takahashi, A. Barbier, B. Grosse Ophoff and K.-A. Hossmann

Max-Planck-Institute for Neurological Research, Department of Experimental Neurology, Cologne, FRG

Introduction

One of the unique characteristics of neurons with respect to other cell types is their morphological and biochemical communication with other neurons. The rapid rates of protein turnover found in synaptic fractions (Cunningham, 1983) reflect these specialized functions of the brain. Enzymes and proteins involved in synthesis and storage of neuronal transmitters, and membrane proteins involved in release mechanisms at the synapse have to turn over rapidly enabling the organism to adapt readily to changes in its environment. The dynamics of protein synthesis provide important insights into the function of the central nervous system at the cellular level. Continuous renewal in all cell types and anatomical regions of brain depends on mechanisms by means of which the organism can respond and adapt to various stimuli. Changes in rates of synthesis as well as rates of degradation may be involved.

It is known from developmental studies that the rough endoplasmatic reticulum of neurons becomes more abundant during maturation (Rennyson and Mytilineous, 1979), and that the development of this organized protein synthesis machinery correlates with the appearance of enzymes associated with the synthesis of neurotransmitters. This correlation has led to an important conclusion: the presence of a target is essential not only for neuronal survival but also for structural and biochemical maturation. When the neurons are deprived of their target, the protein synthesis machinery never matures, and as a result, the neurons die in a relatively immature state (Chiappinelli et al., 1976). Therefore, the development of protein synthesis machinery is a basic metabolic requirement of brain tissue.

In view of the anatomical complexity of the central nervous system, the investigation of the protein synthesis machinery should consider regional differences of neuronal activity. An autoradiographic approach was therefore developed to determine the regional protein synthesis of the brain under physiological conditions. A combination of the data obtained from autoradiography (Bodsch and Hossmann, 1983b), from measurements of in vivo accumulated specific activities of precursor pools (Bodsch and Hossmann, 1983a) and from in vitro determinations were then used. Yanagihara (1973) ascertained in vitro amino acid incorporation by incubating brain slices in media containing defined amounts of a radioactive amino acid. The first attempts to illustrate amino acid incorporation autoradiographically in the brain were reported by Merei and Gallyas (1964) using tracer doses of ^{35}S-methionine in rats. Other amino acids, leucine (Hershkowitz et al., 1975), tyrosine (Kleihues and Hossmann, 1973), valine and phenylalanine (Dwyer et al., 1982) have been used as radioactive tracers as well, however, the route of injection was often reported to influence the outcome of results. Flooding doses of amino acids containing tracer quantities of the isotopic compound (Dienel et al., 1980) minimize variations in the precursor pools of the brain during incorporation. Although quantitative rates of protein synthesis have been obtained in the normal state and the various precursor pools equilibrated by a radioactive tracer during the observation period, a number of problems arise when this approach is transferred to pathophysiological conditions without additional assumptions. Also, one may seriously argue whether or not autoradiograms of amino acid incorporation actually illustrate protein synthesis. They may represent numerous other pathobiochemical events unrelated to protein biosynthesis because of differences in amino acid transport at the blood-brain barrier, extensive amino acid metabolism, amino acylation or combination of these events (Bodsch, 1983). To decide if any of these non-specific processes were involved, additional biochemical measurements in tissue samples were carried out in combination with the autoradiographic studies of cerebral protein synthesis. This is particularly true when investigating under pathophysiological conditions. These measurements involved the two major amino acid pathways in brain — metabolism and aminoacylation — to form the actual precursors for protein incorporation. The reaction constants for aminoacylation are determined from measurements of the aminoacyl-tRNA pool and the charging and releasing parameters of these tRNAs. The reaction constant for metabolism, however, is determined at the end of the experiment from the amount of radioactive amino acids metabolized and the enzymatic activity of the enzyme responsible for the first metabolic reaction. Although cerebral protein synthesis rates (CPSR) have been elaborated in detail for the normal rat and gerbil brains in our laboratory, application of these techniques to other experimental animal models is still under investigation in order to confirm the validity of in vitro data. The in vitro results are used as a supplement to correct the end-point measurements of specific activities in the absence of knowledge about their time course during the 45 minutes of incorporation.

We have applied this approach to the study of regional cerebral protein synthesis in two models of cerebral ischemia. Functional and morphological investigations have revealed that irreversible neuronal damage may develop after as little as 5 minutes' ischemia in selectively vulnerable areas (Kirino, 1982), whereas recovery from ischemia seems to be possible in other regions of the brain after ischemia as long as 1 hour (Kleihues and Hossmann, 1971; Hossmann and Zimmermann, 1974). However, reinitiation of protein synthesis does not allow the conclusion that the correct proteins are produced or that the normal synchronism of protein turnover has been attained. Furthermore, total inhibition of protein synthesis in a selectively vulnerable region does not exclude the possibility that processes requiring proteins with long half-lives continue to operate for a certain period of time. In order to study some of these questions, two series of experiments were carried out: a shortlasting ischemia induced by bilateral carotid occlusion in gerbils (Kirino, 1982), and a prolonged ischemia induced by intrathoracal clamping of the innominate, subclavian and mammary arteries in monkeys (Hossmann and Zimmermann, 1974). In addition, in the monkey studies, histoautoradiography was employed as a supplement to the regional autoradiographic method. In the cerebellar cortex two types of neurons — Purkinje cells and granular cells — are distributed close to each other. In assessing the protein synthesis level in these neurons it was necessary to study them separately because Purkinje cells are highly vulnerable to ischemia while granule cells are resistant neurons. Furthermore, alteration of the neuronal and glial contribution to total amino acid incorporation may occur in the early stages after an ischemic insult.

Material and methods

Cerebral ischemia in gerbils

Adult Mongolian gerbils (50–70 g body weight) and young gerbils (15–17 days old, about 12 g body weight) were loosely immobilized and anesthetized with a mixture of about 70% nitrogen, 30% oxygen, and 1–2% halothane. Femoral veins and arteries were cannulated with polyethylene catheters. Common carotid arteries were exposed bilaterally through a midline cervical incision and Heifetz clips were applied after reducing the anesthesia to 0.5% halothane. After 5 min, blood circulation of the brain was restored by releasing the clips, and halothane was again increased to 1%. Recirculation periods for adult animals were 1 hour (5 animals), 2 hours (4 animals), and 4 hours (4 animals); the recirculation period for young animals was 4 hours (3 animals). Six adult control animals and 2 young control animals were also employed.

Cerebral protein synthesis

For simultaneous measurement of ^{14}C-protein synthesis and tritium amino acid influx (Bodsch and Hossmann, 1983b), 70 μCi ^{14}C-amino acids (carboxyl-labeled phenylalanine, tyrosine, isoleucine, leucine, and methionine) were injected as a bolus intravenously and allowed to incorporate for a period of 45 min. Two minutes before sacrifice of the animal (at 43 min of the labeling scheme) 580 μCi ^{3}H-amino acids (same as above) were infused at a constant rate for a period of 2 min. Upon termination of the infusion, systemic circulation was stopped by intra-arterial injection of saturated potassium chloride solution and the animals were then decapitated. Brains were quickly removed, frozen in methylbutane at $-50°$C and transferred to a cryostat at $-20°$C. Coronal sections of 20 and 200 μm thickness (alternating slices) were cut and the 20 μm sections were dried at 45°C. Five days later these sections were eluted for 12 hours in a solution containing 10% trichloroacetic acid, 70% ethanol and 2% polyvinylpropolidone in order to remove non-incorporated free ^{14}C and ^{3}H amino acids and metabolites from the tissue. Dried sections were placed into X-ray cassettes and exposed to Kodak NMB films for 2 weeks along with ^{14}C-methylmethacrylate standards which previously had been calibrated with standard brain sections containing defined amounts of ^{14}C per gram of brain tissue. The concentration of radioactive tracer in the sections was determined by quantitative autoradiography. Timed plasma samples were collected during the labeling period, counted by liquid scintillation and analyzed for plasma amino acid concentrations by high performance liquid chromatography.

^{3}H- and ^{14}C-labeled free amino acids of brain tissue as well as labeled aminoacyl-tRNA and proteins were measured biochemically in microsamples obtained from the 200-μm sections. The levels of these substances as well as the blood-brain amino acid influx were determined as described previously (Bodsch and Hossmann, 1983a). Separate brain samples were then used to measure methionine adenosyl transferase (MAT) activity (Hiemke and Ghraf, 1981) and ^{35}S-methionine tRNA utilization (in vitro protein incorporation) according to published procedures (Barra et al., 1972).

Protein phosphorylation

Protein phosphorylation was studied in tissue from hippocampal stratum radiatum. The CA1 region was dissected from 200 μm thick coronal sections at $-20°$C, placed in ice-cold 0.32 M sucrose, homogenized and a subcellular fraction termed SP was isolated according to the procedure described by Hoch and Wilson (1984). The SP fraction was suspended in phosphorylation buffer, composed of 50 mM 4-(2-hydroxyethyl)-1-piperazine-ethane sulfonic acid (HEPES) and 10 mM magnesium chloride, pH 7.4, at a protein concentration of 50 μg/ml. Calcium chloride at 50 μM and/or calmodulin (CaM) at 2 μM were present in the assay mixtures as noted. The phosphorylation assay was preincubated (20 μl) for 1 min at 37°C and 5 μl [γ-^{32}P]ATP was added to give a final concentration of 10 μM (10 μCi/assay). The incubation was continued for 30 seconds and the reaction was terminated by the addition of sodium dodecyl sulfate (SDS) and mercaptoethanol to final concentrations of 0.5% and 4%, respectively. Following heating of the incubation solution for 3 min at 95°C, glycerol and bromphenol blue were added to yield final concentrations of 10% and 0.01%, respectively. The phosphorylation assays and separate molecular weight standard proteins were applied in 20-μl aliquots to 12% SDS-polyacrylamide slab gels (Laemmli, 1970) (0.75-mm thickness, 30 cm long) and electrophoresed at 800 V for 5 hours. Gels were fixed and exposed to Kodak NMB film for 14 hours and then stained with Coomassie blue for visualization of molecular weight standards.

Cerebral ischemia in monkeys

Seven adult Rhesus monkeys (*Macaca mulatta*) of both sexes weighing 3.5 to 12.5 kg were used. The animals were tranquilized with 50 to 125 mg ketamine (Ketamnest®), and subsequently anesthetized with 0.4 to 0.8 vol% halothane and 70% nitrous oxide. After immobilization with pancuronium bromide (Pancuronium®) the trachea was intubated and artificial ventilation was maintained throughout the experiment. Both femoral veins were cannulated for intravenous drug administration, and the left femoral artery for continuous recording of arterial blood pressure and intermittent sampling for measurement of blood gases. Body temperature was kept constant at 36.5°C using a feedback controlled heating pad. The head of the animals was fixed in a stereotactic frame, and craniotomy was performed on the right side over the sensory cortex from where the electrocorticogram (ECoG) and somatically evoked potentials (SEP) were recorded. Two animals served as controls. Five animals were thoracotomized and submitted to 1 hour global cerebral ischemia, as described previously (Hossmann and Zimmermann, 1974). Completeness of ischemia was ascertained by intravenous injection of 1 mCi ^{133}Xe per kg just before clamping and recording (with an external scintillation detector) a constant level of radioactivity from the head during the period of ischemia. Immediately after the onset of ischemia, anesthesia was discontinued. Recirculation was initiated by raising arterial blood pressure with dopamine immediately before release of vascular clamps, and by treating the animals with controlled infusions of buffers and osmotically active substances. Recirculation times were 1.5, 3, 6, 12 and 24 hours. At the end of the experiments protein synthesis was estimated. A mixture of five ^{3}H-labeled amino acids (phenylalanine, tyrosine, isoleucine, leucine, methionine, total activity 1 mCi/kg body weight) was infused intravenously for 30 seconds, and the animal was sacrificed by air embolism 45 min later. Immediately before air embolism, the frontal lobe was freeze-clamped in liquid nitrogen for determination of specific activity of free amino acids, aminoacyl-tRNA and proteins. Coronal cryostat sections (10-μm thickness) were also prepared, free amino acids were removed, as described above, and autoradiograms of amino acid incorporation into proteins were obtained by exposing brain sections for 4 weeks to LKB ultrofilm. Finally, the same sections were covered by a photographic dipping film (Rogers, 1979), exposed in the dark for 8 weeks, and then developed and processed for light-microscopic autoradiography.

Results

Short-lasting cerebral ischemia in adult gerbils

Transient forebrain ischemia in the Mongolian gerbil was induced by bilateral occlusion of the common carotid arteries for 5 min. Incorporation of ^{14}C-carboxyl-labeled amino acids into cerebral proteins was measured in vivo in controls and after post-ischemic recirculation times of 1 hour, 2 hours, and 4 hours. As illustrated by the ^{14}C-autoradiograms of amino acid incorporation (Fig. 1), no major changes of protein synthesis were present in any brain region after 1 hour of recirculation. After

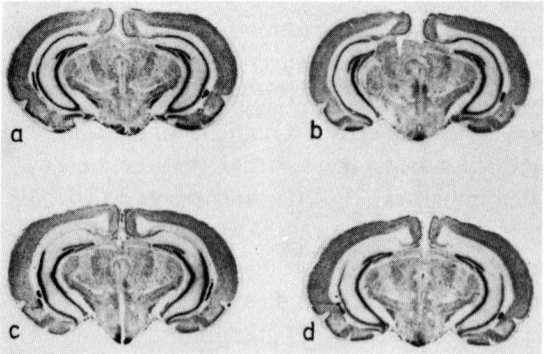

Fig. 1. Autoradiographs of ^{14}C-amino acid incorporation into cerebral proteins of adult gerbil brains. (a) Control, (b–d) after 5 min bilateral occlusion of common carotid arteries and subsequent recirculation for (b) 1 hour, (c) 2 hours, and (d) 4 hours.

TABLE 1

Cerebral protein synthesis in vivo in the adult gerbil hippocampal CA1 region

	Amino acid influx (nmol/g/min)	Brain amino acids (nCi/nmol)	Aminoacyl-tRNA (nCi/nmol)	Proteins (nCi/nmol)
Control ($n = 6$)	9.8 ± 0.9	5.82 ± 0.72	1.27 ± 0.16	20.13 ± 1.24
1 hour[a] ($n = 4$)	9.0 ± 0.8	5.42 ± 0.86	1.36 ± 0.18	19.40 ± 1.06
2 hours[a] ($n = 4$)	9.4 ± 1.0	6.02 ± 0.25	1.42 ± 0.21	1.78 ± 0.23
4 hours[a] ($n = 3$)	10.2 ± 1.3	5.86 ± 0.61	1.28 ± 0.20	0.50 ± 0.07

Values are means ± SD.
[a] Recirculation times following 5 minutes of ischemia.

2 hours however, a remarkable suppression of protein synthesis occurred in the pyramidal cell layer and in the radiatum layer of hippocampal subfield CA1. Compared to the controls a simultaneous increase of amino acid incorporation was visible in the CA2/CA3 pyramidal cell layer adjacent to the CA1 layer which exhibited depressed amino acid incorporation. This dissociation disappeared at 4 hours, where amino acid incorporation remained completely suppressed in the CA1 region while the activity in the CA2/CA3 pyramidal cells returned to normal.

The significance of this finding was further evaluated by measurement of ^{3}H-amino acid influx and of the tracer pools in the brain. As demonstrated in Table 1, neither amino acid influx nor the specific activity of the free amino acid pool nor that of the amino acyl-tRNA pools were significantly affected at any recirculation time. However, after 2 and 4 hours of recirculation the specific activity of proteins from the CA1 region was clearly reduced as compared to controls. Although the blood to brain influx of radioactive tracers was unaffected, reduced ^{14}C-amino acid incorporation at 2 and 4 hours could have been masked by an increased amino acid metabolism which would divert ^{14}C-precursors from the protein incorporation pathway. Determination of the total activity of methionine adenosyltransferase (MAT, the enzyme responsible for metabolism of methionine) argues against this conclusion. MAT activities were unchanged at all recirculation times (Table 2). Instead, the ^{35}S-methionyl-tRNA utilization of tissue from the CA1 region in vitro clearly shows that incorporation into protein was not operative in this region at 2 and 4 hours. While methionyl-tRNA utilization in the cerebral cortex remained between 3.3–4 pmol · min^{-1} · mg^{-1} protein throughout the observation period, a severe decrease by 84% of control levels occurred at 2 hours in the CA1 region.

TABLE 2

Cerebral protein synthesis in vitro in the adult gerbil brain

	Methionine adenosyl transferase activity (nmol/h/mg protein)	^{35}S-Methionyl-tRNA utilization (pmol/min/mg protein)
Control ($n = 6$)		
cortex	3.4 ± 0.4	3.8 ± 0.3
CA1	2.7 ± 0.3	6.4 ± 0.4
2 hours ($n = 4$)[a]		
cortex	3.5 ± 0.5	4.0 ± 0.5
CA1	2.7 ± 0.4	1.0 ± 0.2
4 hours ($n = 3$)[a]		
cortex	3.8 ± 0.6	3.3 ± 0.5
CA1	3.0 ± 0.5	0.2 ± 0.1

Values are means ± SD.
[a] Recirculation times following 5 minutes of ischemia.

Short-lasting cerebral ischemia in young gerbils

Aside from the many biochemical differences between the infant and adult brain there also seems to be a difference in the susceptibility to ischemia induced by carotid ligation in gerbils. Infant gerbils aged 15–17 days do not show the adult vulnerability to depression of cerebral protein synthesis at 4 hours post ischemia (Fig. 2). Even the most vulnerable area of the adult brain, the CA1 sector, was unaffected. Although a number of thalamic nuclei and the cerebral cortex exhibited double the rate of synthesis compared to the same structures in the adult brain, CPSR in the hippocampus were comparable at both stages of development: amino acid incorporation into proteins of the CA1 hippocampus was 20.13 ± 1.24 nCi/nmol in adults (1.27 ± 0.16 nCi/nmol amino acid tRNA) and 23.42 ± 2.02 nCi/nmol in young animals (1.46 ± 0.21 nCi/nmol amino acid tRNA). Values for the cerebral cortex protein incorporation were 16.23 ± 1.02 nCi/nmol in adults (1.38 ± 0.18 nCi/nmol amino acid tRNA) and 37.53 ± 2.18 nCi/nmol in young animals (1.48 ± 0.24 nCi/nmol amino acid tRNA).

Protein phosphorylation in the gerbil hippocampus

Crude synaptic membrane preparations from hippocampal CA1 (stratum radiatum) of control and post-ischemic recirculated adult animals were assayed in the presence of Ca^{2+} and calmodulin (CaM) by the in vitro [γ-^{32}P]ATP phosphorylation assay and subsequent separation of labeled proteins on SDS-polyacrylamide gels. The normal protein phosphorylation pattern obtained from control tissue showed stimulation of phosphorylation upon incubation with Ca^{2+} and a marked CaM-Ca^{2+}-dependent phosphorylation (Fig. 3A). By contrast, neither Ca^{2+} nor CaM plus Ca^{2+} stimulated the phosphorylation of proteins from tissue of stratum radiatum at 2 hours post ischemia. A phosphoprotein pattern considerably different from the two latter was obtained from the hippocampus at 4 hours post ischemia. The major phosphoprotein bands of molecular weight 66 K and 41 K observed in con-

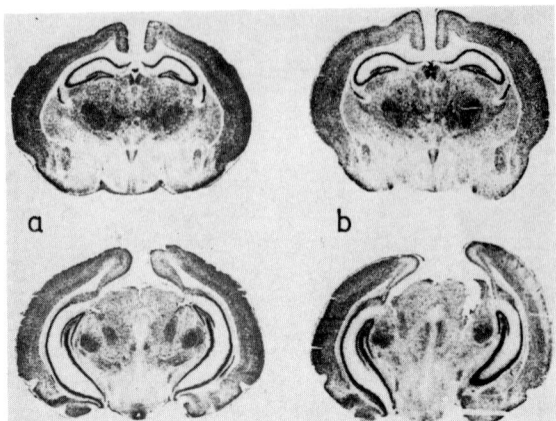

Fig. 2. Autoradiographs of ^{14}C-amino acid incorporation into cerebral proteins of young (15–17 days of age) gerbil brains. (a) Control and (b) 4 hours after recirculation following 5 min transient ischemia.

trol conditions were completely absent. Instead, a band at 21 K, which has been previously shown to present the synaptic vesicle protein (Hoch and Wilson, 1984), was markedly stimulated. However, in the presence of Ca^{2+} as well as CaM, phosphorylation was significantly inhibited. The reproducibility of this finding was further tested on SDS-polyacrylamide gels, which give better resolution of bands in the molecular weight range of 40 to 100 K (Fig. 3B). In the presence of CaM the pattern of phosphoproteins from three different animals at 4 hours post ischemia was comparable. However, differences in the amount of ^{32}P in some bands were obvious and may reflect slightly different degrees of depressed phosphorylation.

Prolonged cerebral ischemia in monkey

The animals were subjected to 1 hour of complete cerebral ischemia, followed by blood recirculation for 1.5 to 24 hours. During ischemia, the electrocorticogram (ECoG) and somatically evoked potentials were completely suppressed. Post-ischemic electrophysiological recovery depended on the duration of recirculation. 1.5 hours after ischemia, the ECoG revealed a return of single spikes followed by a burst-suppression pattern between 3 and 6

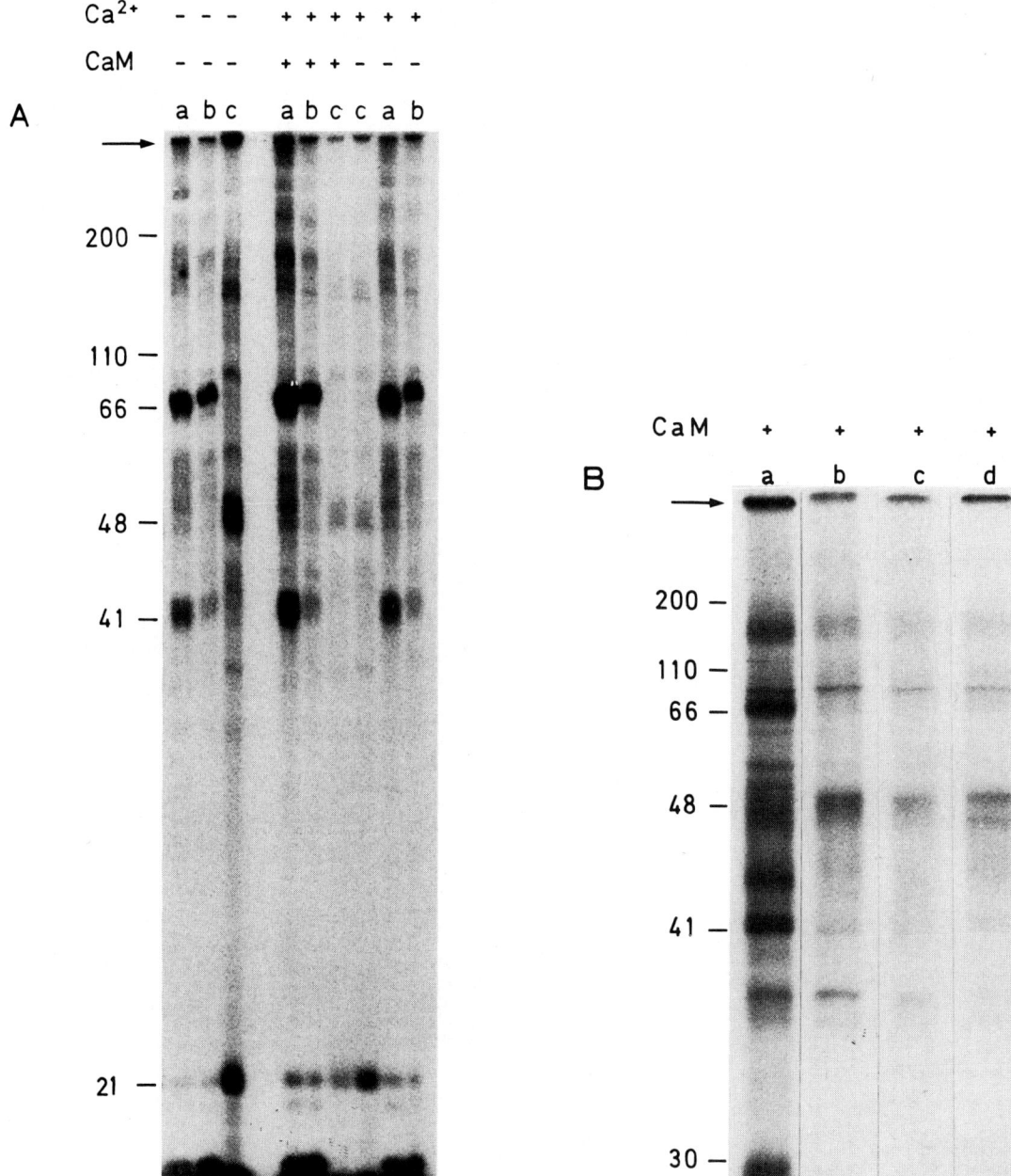

Fig. 3. Protein phosphorylation. (A) 30 cm polyacrylamide gel slab of in vitro γ-^{32}P-ATP incorporation: a, control; b, 2 hours; and c, 4 hours post ischemia. Ca^{2+} and calmodulin (CaM) were present in the incubation mixtures as indicated. (B) 15 cm polyacrylamide gel slab of in vitro γ-^{32}P-ATP incorporation of: a, control, and b–d, from three different animals at 4 hours post ischemia. All incubation media contained CaM.

hours. After longer recirculation times continuous ECoG activity returned with a gradually increasing amplitude and frequency content (Fig. 4). The recovery of somatically evoked potentials was less stereotypical and was observed in only three animals with 1.5, 12 and 24 hours recirculation, respectively.

In the cerebral hemispheres, protein synthesis was distinctly reduced after 1.5 hours recirculation, tracer incorporation being almost homogeneous without differentiation between gray and white matter (Fig. 5b). After recirculation of 6 hours and longer, protein synthesis of gray matter gradually increased until, after 24 hours, an almost normal autoradiogram was obtained (Fig. 5d). Only in thalamic nuclei (with the exception of nucleus reticularis) amino acid incorporation was distinctly lower than in the control animals. Recovery of protein synthesis in cerebellum progressed faster than in cerebral hemispheres. After 1.5 hours of recirculation a distinct differentiation between white and gray matter became visible, and after longer recir-

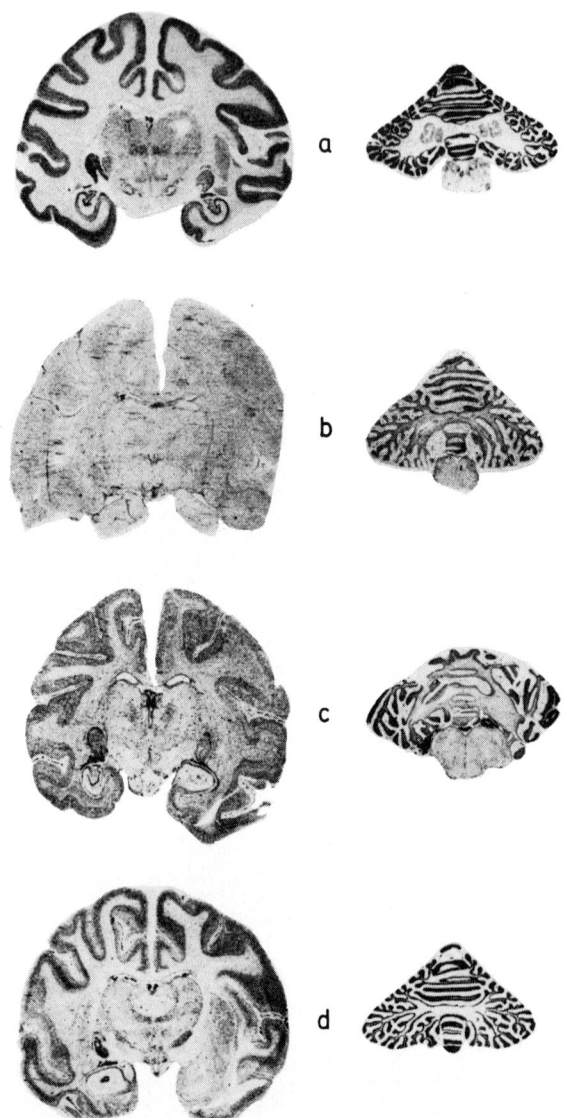

Fig. 5. Autoradiographys of ³H-amino acid incorporation into cerebral proteins of the monkey brain (forebrain and cerebellum): (a) Control, (b–d) after 1 hour of global ischemia and recirculation for (b) 1.5 hours, (c) 6 hours, and (d) 24 hours.

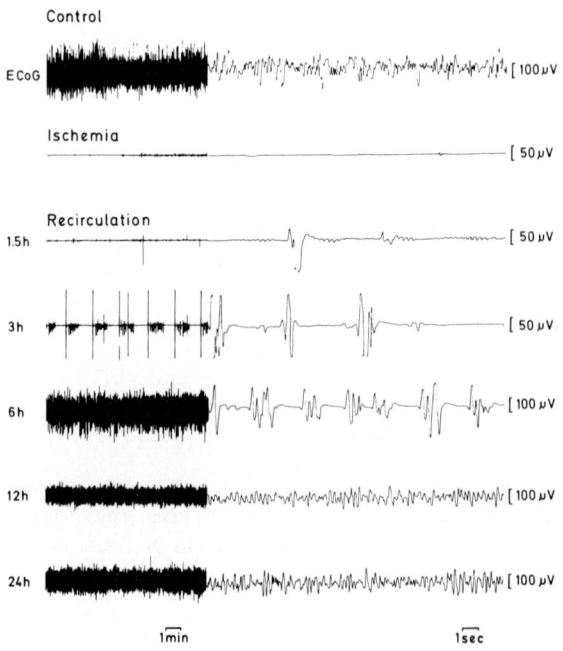

Fig. 4. Suppression and recovery of ECoG after 1 hour of complete ischemia of monkey brain.

culation times autoradiograms were comparable with those of the control animals.

Quantitation of specific activity changes in various amino acid pools is summarized in Table 3. The specific activity integral of plasma amino acids was relatively constant in all animals. Therefore,

TABLE 3

Cerebral protein synthesis in vivo in the monkey brain (freeze-clamped material)

	Specific activity plasma integral (nCi/nmol)	Brain amino acids		Aminoacyl-tRNA (nCi/nmol)	Proteins (nCi/nmol)
		(nmol/g)	(nCi/nmol)		
Control 1	586	422	3.76	0.77	10.26
Control 2	500	408	3.62	0.80	10.08
1.5 hours[a]	516	613	1.73	0.57	1.52
3 hours	492	675	1.37	0.50	2.78
6 hours	581	548	2.26	0.56	4.31
24 hours	492	488	3.02	0.91	9.48

[a] Circulation times after 1 hour of ischemia.

the radioactivity input function to the brain did not change after ischemia. However, while the free amino acid concentration in the brain increased during the first 3 hours post ischemia, the specific activity declined. Interestingly, the decrease of specific activity of the aminoacyl-tRNA pools was less pronounced than that of the free amino acid pools.

At 1.5 hours after ischemia protein-incorporated radioactivity was reduced by 85%. Subsequently, it gradually increased until, after 24 hours, the difference between the controls and the ischemic animal was less than 10% (Table 3).

The spatial distribution of radioactivity incorporated into proteins at the cellular level was de-

TABLE 4

Amino-acid incorporation[a] by monkey brain neurons

	Control	Postischemic recirculation time (hours)				
		1.5	3	6	12	24
Cerebral cortex						
frontal	220.7 ± 83.0	20.1 ± 18.4 (9)	34.1 ± 20.4 (16)	101.3 ± 60.8 (46)	173.4 ± 108.8 (79)	187.2 ± 103.2 (85)
parietal	175.8 ± 71.2	4.0 ± 3.2 (2)	17.7 ± 17.4 (10)	66.8 ± 42.8 (38)	150.0 ± 82.3 (85)	123.2 ± 40.1 (70)
border zone	174.8 ± 67.1	1.1 ± 0.4 (1)	34.1 ± 27.3 (20)	54.2 ± 29.3 (31)	77.5 ± 40.7 (44)	92.9 ± 31.6 (53)
Cerebellar cortex						
Purkinje cells	171.9 ± 49.6	12.4 ± 7.2 (7)	35.5 ± 26.8 (21)	74.5 ± 36.0 (43)	80.9 ± 34.0 (47)	86.7 ± 52.5 (50)
hippocampus						
CA1	77.9 ± 21.1	16.6 ± 12.6 (21)	60.7 ± 28.3 (78)	89.8 ± 27.8 (115)	34.7 ± 12.9 (48)	38.5 ± 11.9 (49)
CA3	131.8 ± 30.0	14.7 ± 8.8 (11)	77.3 ± 24.3 (59)	88.6 ± 23.2 (67)	42.5 ± 12.1 (32)	59.7 ± 16.4 (45)

[a] Expressed as number of silver grains per neuron (means ±SD; percentage of control in parentheses).

termined in various structures of the brain by microscopic autoradiography (Table 4). At 1.5 hours of recirculation, cortical and hippocampal neurons as well as Purkinje cells exhibited depressed abilities to incorporate labeled amino acids (Fig. 6b, f, j). The number of grains per neuron in different parts of the cerebral cortex and in Purkinje cells was only 1–9% of control, while grain counts over CA1 and CA3 pyramidal cells decreased to 21% and 11% of control, respectively. Between 3 and 24 hours post ischemia temporal profiles of cell-labeling of cortical neurons and Purkinje cells were similar insofar as continuous increases were observed in all cases. This results in an increase of 50–53% in the grain counts in the vascular border zones of the cerebral cortex and the cerebellar Purkinje cells, and even higher increases in the counts in the frontal (85%) and parietal (70%) cortices. However, the time course of neuronal labeling of pyramidal cells from CA1 and CA3 was different. Following a rapid recovery to 115% in CA1 and 67% in CA3, at 6 hours secondary suppression occurred between 6 and 12 hours and grain numbers dropped to 49% in CA1 and 45% in CA3 after 24 hours recirculation. The number of grain counts over glial cells was low compared to that of neurons. The control value of 7.0 over oligodendroglia from corpus callosum did not change significantly during the total post-ischemic observation period.

Discussion

Short lasting ischemia in gerbils

A temporary arrest of the circulation affects central nervous system cells by several direct and indirect effects. These changes persist for some time after circulation has been restored and thereby limit recovery of neuronal function. Delayed neuronal death, however, is a phenomenon that develops late during recirculation and seems to be restricted to selectively vulnerable structures, although circulatory arrest affects large areas of the whole brain. Delayed neuronal death has been noted in the hippocampus of different mammalian species (Ito et al., 1975; Kirino, 1982; Pulsinelli et al., 1982) following transient ischemia. It has been demonstrated that neither cerebral blood flow nor glucose utilization limit the metabolic requirements of brain cells throughout the first day of recirculation after a brief ischemia induced by bilateral occlusion of common carotid arteries in the gerbil brain (Suzuki et al., 1983a). Instead, a pronounced hyperactivity in neuronal firing has been detected when spontaneous potentials were recorded from the hippocampal CA1 subfield during this period (Suzuki et al., 1983b). Though several aspects of cerebral metabolism show large variations associated with changes

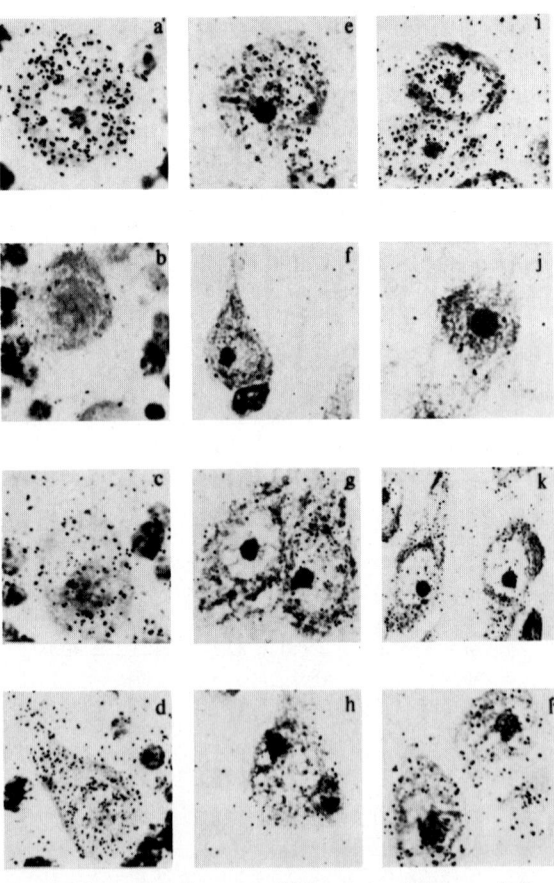

Fig. 6. Histoautoradiograms of ^{3}H-amino acid into cerebellum and hippocampus of monkey before and after 1 hour complete ischemia. (a–d) Purkinje cells; (e–h) pyramidal cells of hippocampus CA1; (i–l) pyramidal cells of hippocampus CA3. a, e, i, control; b, f, j, 1.5 hours recirculation; c, g, k, 6 hours recirculation; d, h, l, 24 hours recirculation. Hematoxylin staining.

in neuronal activity, protein synthesis remains remarkably constant. As pointed out by Ames and Nesbett (1983) this stability makes it a particularly useful measure of the basic metabolic capacity of cerebral tissue. We have recently observed unique biochemical properties of CA1 cells in the gerbil ischemia model with respect to cerebral protein synthesis (Bodsch et al., 1983; Bodsch and Takahashi, 1985). The inability of the selectively vulnerable neurons to maintain their protein synthesis capacity — in the presence of normal RNA synthesis (Bodsch and Takahashi, 1983) — was confined to pyramidal cells in the CA1 subfield long before neuronal death was visible by morphological criteria.

In the hippocampal formation CA1 pyramidal cells send their dendrites into stratum oriens and stratum radiatum. The main afferent, excitatory input to CA1 neurons is mediated by glutamatergic innervation through Schaffer's collaterals from CA3 neurons. Therefore, selective inhibition of protein synthesis in vulnerable CA1 neurons may be accompanied by changes in synaptic transmission at the sites of CA1 innervation in stratum radiatum. We investigated the parallel appearance of selective reductions in protein synthesis and protein phosphorylation. We report here that both protein synthesis of pyramidal CA1 and protein phosphorylation of stratum radiatum CA1 are affected simultaneously between 1 and 2 hours post ischemia in the gerbil model. For up to 1 hour CA1 neurons preserve their protein synthesis capacity, indicating that 5 min of ischemia itself does not cause an immediate reduction in the capacity for cerebral protein synthesis. The sequence of events that emerges from the autoradiographic imaging studies of ^{14}C-amino acid incorporation clearly indicates a simultaneous increase of protein synthesis in CA2/CA3 and a pronounced reduction in CA1 between 1 and 2 hours of recirculation. Four hours after the start of recirculation the protein synthesis activity in CA2/CA3 neurons returned to control level but was completely suppressed in the total CA1 sector. We conclude that intrahippocampal connections contribute to the selective increase in CA3 protein synthesis and decrease in CA1 protein synthesis via the afferent input from CA3 neurons through Schaffer's collaterals.

Alterations in postsynaptic densities have been reported to appear ultrastructurally in synapses of stratum radiatum CA1 in a similar model of transient ischemia in the rat brain (Van Lubitz and Diemer, 1983). Moreover, it was recently demonstrated that the major constituent of the postsynaptic density fraction is the calmodulin-dependent protein kinase (Kennedy et al., 1983) that phosphorylates proteins in synaptic endings, and increasing evidence indicates that changes in synaptic transmission may be mediated, by calmoculin-induced protein phosphorylation (Schulman and Greengard, 1978). Since the active form of calcium for a variety of reactions appears to be the calmodulin-calcium complex, the phosphorylation patterns of proteins from the stratum radiatum were assayed. The state of synaptic proteins was affected during post-ischemic recirculation initially at 2 hours by the loss of the calcium and calcium-calmodulin-dependent regulation of phosphorylation. Further progression (at 4 hours) of neuronal damage in the CA1 sector led to alterations in the phospho-protein pattern and increased phosphorylation sites on substrate proteins. Changes in the protein patterns are likely to be mediated by protease activity. It has been proposed that selectively vulnerable neurons have a tendency to epileptic acitivity and that the resulting calcium influx may trigger a series of molecular events, leading to cellular damage (Siesjö, 1981). Although we did not measure the calcium influx into CA1 neurons, the results of in vitro protein phosphorylation lend support to the thesis that the cellular damage may be the result of intracellular calcium changes because the calcium-calmodulin-dependent phosphorylation was clearly affected. An increase of calcium in damaged hippocampal neurons has, in fact, been demonstrated but it was not clear what the targets of the accumulated calcium, its associated damages and neuronal degenerative processes are about (Simon et al., 1984). We suggest that the most sensitive target for altered intracellular calcium is the calcium-calmodulin-dependent synaptic protein phosphorylation system, which provides the depolarisation-induced trigger for the release of neurotransmitter molecules (DeLorenzo et al., 1979). Excessively high release of glutamate in vulnerable CA1 neurons has been found in post-ischemic conditions (Jørgensen and Diemer, 1982). We, therefore, conclude from our finding that parallel inhibition of protein synthesis and loss of regulation in synaptic calcium-calmodulin-dependent protein phosphorylation change the molecular character of hippocampal CA1 neurons selectively — possibly by affecting synaptic plasticity following abnormal turnover of proteins. This occurs before cellular degeneration processes become visible. Delayed onset of neuronal damage in selective vulnerability thus may be a consequence of failure in replacing damaged molecular structures for normal neuronal activity, which obviously results in neuronal death.

Cerebral protein synthesis during pre- and postnatal development has been reported to proceed at markedly higher rates and to produce qualitatively different sets of proteins (Dunlop et al., 1975), compared to the adult brain. The synthesis of proteins in infant animals is favored over the rate of protein degradation. Our observations support the previous finding (Klatzo, personal communication) that hippocampal CA1 neurons of young animals are less vulnerable to ischemia than those of adults. At present it is not possible to decide if the observed changes are primarily evoked by local biochemical or circulatory factors.

Prolonged ischemia in monkeys

The results of the present investigation on monkey protein synthesis corroborate earlier studies from our laboratory (Kleihues et al., 1975), in which progressive electrophysiological and biochemical recovery were observed after 1 hour of total ischemia of normothermic monkey brain. The improvement in recovery as compared to the earlier series is probably due to better physiological maintenance during the experiment and to the fact that anesthesia was discontinued during reanimation. ECoG activity and protein synthesis are attributes of neuronal viability. While ECoG activity allows the evaluation of electrical function of a certain population of cortical neurons — more precisely of those neurons near to the electrodes — autoradiographic determination of regional cerebral protein synthesis can demonstrate the functional state of all neurons at a given moment. The autoradiographic studies indicate that in the cortex a smal number of neurons seem to die immediately after ischemia while other neurons show only transitory changes. Most of the cortical neurons remained intact at all times, and accordingly, protein synthesis increased gradually to near control levels in the parietal and frontal cortex. Neurons in the vascular border zones of the cerebral cortex, however, exhibited a significant recovery delay (Table 4), with only 53% amino acid incorporation at 24 hours. The reason may be a hemodynamic one as the local blood perfusion pressure of border zone is lower than that in the center of the arterial supplying territories. However, there are also indications of intrinsic differences in cellular vulnerability. In the cerebellum, the Purkinje cells are selectively damaged whereas granule cells remain intact. In CA1 neurons of the hippocampus protein synthesis transiently returned to control levels after 6 hours before a secondary reduction in protein synthesis occurred at 12 hours. This delayed suppression resembled that observed in gerbils after 5 min ischemia but the interval was considerably longer. It should also be noted that recovery of protein synthesis was heterogenous, certain cells showing an increase in protein synthesis being adjacent to others which do not exhibit any recovery of protein synthesis. The variation is also reflected by the high values of standard deviations in Table 4.

The morphologic pattern of selective vulnerability of cerebral ischemia in the gerbil and the rat has been established in detail (Kirino, 1982; Pulsinelli et al., 1982) but not yet for the monkey brain. Studies to clarify these morphologic alterations are under investigation. However, the phenomenon of secondary reduction observed in the monkey hippocampus may prompt some speculations. Although the protein synthesis machinery recovers between

1.5 and 3 hours and a cytoplasmic repair process may develop in these neurons, newly synthesized proteins may not be adequate for keeping the functional state of these neurons intact. Therefore, after a certain period of normal protein synthesis, the cell may form non-functional or non-sense proteins for structural and metabolic repair such that the protein synthesis machinery is reduced again. It may also be that those neurons showing recovery of protein synthesis and which are located next to neurons which do not recover, require a certain amount of trophic support from their neighbours for continued viability. This phenomenon, indeed, has similarities to naturally occurring cell death.

References

Ames, A. and Nesbett, F.B. (1983) Pathophysiology of ischemic cell death. I. Time of onset of irreversible damage; importance of the different components of the ischemic insult. *Stroke*, 14: 219–226.

Barra, H.S., Unates, L.E., Syaredra, M.S. and Caputto, R. (1972) Capacities for binding amino acids by tRNAs from rat brain and their changes during development. *J. Neurochem.*, 19: 2289–2297.

Bodsch, W. (1983) Biochemical prerequisites for measurement of protein synthesis. In: W.D. Heiss and M.E. Phelps (Eds.), Springer, New York-Heidelberg, pp. 229–231.

Bodsch, W. and Hossmann, K.-A. (1983a) A quantitative regional analysis of amino acids involved in rat brain protein synthesis by high performance liquid chromatography. *J. Neurochem.*, 40: 371–382.

Bodsch, W. and Hossmann, K.-A. (1983b) The double-label method of local protein synthesis: autoradiography and protein biochemistry of in vivo labeled proteins. *J. Cereb. Blood Flow Metabol.* 3, Suppl. 1: S468–469.

Bodsch, W. and Takahashi, K. (1983) Selective neuronal vulnerability to cerebral protein- and RNA-synthesis in the hippocampus of the gerbil brain. In: A. Bes, P. Braquet, R. Paoletti and B.K. Siesjö (Eds.), *Cerebral Ischemia*. Elsevier, New York, pp. 197–208.

Bodsch, W., Takahashi, K. (1985) Selective neuronal vulnerability to in vivo protein synthesis and protein phosphorylation. *Proc. Natl. Acad. Sci. USA*, in press.

Bodsch, W., Mies, G. and Hossmann, K.A. (1983) Local rates of protein synthesis and analysis of specific proteins in the gerbil brain following ischemia. *J. Neurochem.*, 41, Suppl. 1: S137.

Chiappinelli, V., Giacobini, E., Pilar, G. and Uchimura, H. (1976) Neuron death and target structure. *J. Physiol.*, 257: 746–766.

Cunningham, T.J. (1983) Naturally occurring neuron death and its regulation of developing neural pathways. *Int. Rev. Cytol.*, 74: 163–186.

DeLorenzo, R.J., Freedman, S.D., Yohe, W.B. and Maurer, S.C. (1979) Stimulation of CA^{2+}-dependent neurotransmitter release and presynaptic nerve terminal protein phosphorylation by calmodulin and a calmodulin-like protein isolated from synaptic vesicles. *Proc. Natl. Acad. Sci. USA*, 76: 1838–1842.

Dienel, G.A., Pulsinelli, W.A. and Duffy, T.E. (1980) Regional protein synthesis in rat brain following acute hemispheric ischemia. *J. Neurochem.*, 35: 1216–1226.

Dunlop, D.S., Van Elden, W. and Lajtha, A. (1975) A method for measuring brain protein synthesis rates in young and adult rats. *J. Neurochem.*, 24: 337–344.

Dwyer, B.E., Donatoni, P. and Wasterlain, C.G. (1982) A quantitative autoradiographic method for the measurement of local rates of brain protein synthesis. *Neurochem. Res.*, 7: 563–576.

Hershkowitz, M., Wilson, J.E. and Glassman, E. (1975) The incorporation of radioactive amino acids into brain subcellular proteins during training. *J. Neurochem.*, 25: 687–694.

Hiemke, C. and Ghraf, R. (1981) Regional distribution of methionine adenosyltransferase in rat brain as measured by a rapid radiochemical method. *J. Neurochem.*, 37: 613–618.

Hoch, D.B. and Wilson, J.E. (1984) Effects of calcium, strontium, and barium ions on phosphorylation of hippocampal proteins in vitro. *J. Neurochem.*, 42: 54–58.

Hossmann, K.-A. and Zimmermann, V. (1974) Resuscitation of the monkey brain after 1 h complete ischemia. I. Physiological and morphological observations. *Brain Res.*, 81: 59–74.

Ito, U., Spatz, M., Walker, J.T. Jr. and Klatzo, I. (1975) Experimental cerebral ischemia in mongolian gerbils. I. Light microscopic observations. *Acta Neuropathol.*, 32: 209–223.

Jørgensen, M.B. and Diemer, N.H. (1982) Selective neuron loss after cerebral ischemia in the rat: possible role of transmitter glutamate. *Acta Neurol. Scand.*, 66: 536–540.

Kennedy, M.B., Bennett, M.K. and Erondu, N.E. (1983) Biochemical and immunochemical evidence that the "major postsynaptic density protein" is a subunit of a calmodulin-dependent protein kinase. *Proc. Natl. Acad. Sci. USA*, 80: 7357–7361.

Kirino, T. (1982) Delayed neuronal death in the gerbil hippocampus following ischemia. *Brain Res.*, 239: 57–69.

Kleihues, P. and Hossmann, K.-A. (1971) Protein synthesis in the cat brain after prolonged cerebral ischemia. *Brain Res.*, 35: 409–418.

Kleihues, P. and Hossmann, K.-A. (1973) Regional incorporation of L-[3-^{3}H]tyrosine into cat brain proteins after 1 hour of complete ischemia. *Acta Neuropathol.*, 25: 313–324.

Kleihues, P., Hossmann, K.-A., Pegg, A.E., Kobayashi, K. and Zimmermann, V. (1975) Resuscitation of the monkey brain after one hour complete ischemia. III. Indications of metabolic recovery. *Brain Res.*, 95: 61–73.

Laemmli, U.K. (1970) Cleavage of structural proteins during the assembly of the head of bacteriophage T4. *Nature*, 227: 680–685.

Merei, F.T. and Gallyas, F. (1964) Quantitative determination of the uptake of ^{35}S-methionine in different regions of the normal rat brain. *J. Neurochem.*, 11: 257–264.

Pulsinelli, W.A., Brierley, J.B. and Plum, F. (1982) Temporal profile of neuronal damage in a model of transient forebrain ischemia. *Ann. Neurol.*, 11: 491–498.

Rennyson, V.M. and Mytilineous, C. (1979) In: O. Deranko (Ed.), *SIF Cells*. DHEW Publ. No. (NIH), pp. 76–94.

Rogers, A.W. (1979) *Techniques of Autoradiography*, 3rd Edn. Elsevier, Amsterdam.

Schulman, H. and Greengard, P. (1978) Stimulation of brain membrane protein phosphorylation by calcium and an endogenous heat-stable protein. *Nature,* 271: 478–479.

Siesjö, B.K. (1981) Cell damage in the brain: a speculative synthesis. *J. Cereb. Blood Flow Metabol.*, 1: 155–185.

Simon, R.P., Griffiths, T., Evans, M.C., Swan, J.H. and Meldrum, B.S. (1984) Calcium overload in selectively vulnerable neurons of the hippocampus during and after ischemia: an electron microscopy study in the rat. *J. Cereb. Blood Flow Metabol.*, 4: 350–361.

Suzuki, R., Yamaguchi, T., Kirino, T., Orzi, F. and Klatzo, I. (1983a) The effects of 5-minute ischemia in mongolian gerbils. I. Blood-brain barrier, cerebral blood flow, and local cerebral glucose utilization changes. *Acta Neuropathol.*, 60: 207–216.

Suzuki, R., Yamaguchi, T., Li, C.L. and Klatzo, I. (1983b) The effects of 5-minute ischemia in Mongolian gerbils. II. Changes of spontaneous neuronal activity in cerebral cortex and CA1 sector of hippocampus. *Acta Neuropathol.*, 60: 217–222.

Van Lubitz, D.K.J.E. and Diemer, N.H. (1983) Cerebral ischemia in the rat: ultrastructural and morphometric analysis of synapses in stratum radiatum of the hippocampal CA-1 region. *Acta Neurophathol.*, 61: 52–60.

Yanagihara, T. (1973) Cerebral anoxia: an improved in vitro model for biochemical study. *Stroke*, 4: 409–411.

Changes in lipid metabolism in traumatized spinal cord

Paul Demediuk[a], Royal D. Saunders[a], Nancy R. Clendenon[a,b], Eugene D. Means[c], Douglas K. Anderson[c] and Lloyd A. Horrocks[a]

Departments of [a]Physiological Chemistry and [b]Neurology, The Ohio State University, Columbus, OH, USA, and [c]The V. A. Medical Center, Cincinnati, OH, USA

Introduction

In 1974, the Insurance Institute for Highway Safety (USA) estimated that the direct and indirect costs of automobile related spinal cord injuries averaged over $150 000 per patient annually (Insurance Institute for Highway Safety, 1976). Using a modest 10% per annum inflation factor, the average annual cost of a spinal cord injury in the United States in 1984 will approach $400 000. Epidemiologic studies have estimated that the annual incidence of spinal cord injuries in the United States averages 40 per million population (Bracken et al., 1981). This represents approximately 10 000 new cases each year at a cost of about 4 billion dollars. In addition to the economic costs, each new case represents a personal tragedy, with the majority of injuries involving active persons between the ages of twenty and thirty-five years (Bracken et al., 1981). At the present time, the biochemical events initiated by blunt traumatic injury to the spinal cord are only beginning to be elucidated. As a result, very little can be done clinically to alleviate the tissue destruction and restore the functional losses which occur after such injuries. In our laboratory we are studying changes in membrane structure and function which occur following spinal cord trauma. We believe these changes are intimately involved in the irreversible, self-propagating cell death that is characteristic of spinal cord trauma.

With brain ischemia, the initiation of the biochemical changes which are proposed to cause tissue damage appears to be due to the lack of blood flow and the resultant drastic reduction in oxygen tension (Siesjö, 1981). In contrast, the initiation of a similar sequence of biochemical changes which occur following blunt spinal cord injuries does not appear to be due to the absence of circulation. Spinal cord blood flow is reduced following impact trauma (Osterholm, 1974; De La Torre, 1982), but a significant level of flow still remains, even at the injury site (Anderson et al., 1982). Therefore, although circulatory reduction may contribute, the primary initiator of tissue destruction may well be the mechanical deformation, either by impact or compression, which the spinal cord undergoes during an accident situation. Following the deformation, the mammalian spinal cord undergoes a progressive series of autodestructive pathological changes, the severity of which depends upon the magnitude of the trauma delivered. A significant loss of motor function occurs in severe cases as a result of hemorrhagic necrosis of central gray matter that begins within minutes of the injury, and the degeneration of long tracts of the white matter is evident within 24 to 36 hours post injury. Although the histopathology of spinal cord trauma has been extensively documented (Osterholm, 1974; De La Torre, 1982), the actual biochemical events which are responsible for initiating and propagating this irreversible autodestructive process have not been identified. A very likely site for posttraumatic molecular damage is the cell membrane, with the permanent loss of function that results from spinal cord injury being associated with marked early alterations of membrane integrity and function. For example, capillary endothelial defects can be observed within 2 minutes after injury (Goodman et al., 1976; 1979; Griffiths, 1978). Such defects are probably caused by metabolites of free arachidonic acid (Kontos et al., 1980). Other early events in traumatized spinal cord include edema and the loss of Na^+, K^+-ATPase and cytochrome oxidase activities (Clendenon et al., 1978; Goodman et al., 1976). The edema is probably related to the loss in ability of cells to pump ions and to make ATP. In spite of these reports, the direct cause(s) of these membrane defects are not known. A possible postinjury mechanism that may damage cell membranes is the free radical induced peroxidation of membrane polyunsaturated fatty acids (PUFA). Free radicals are thought to be generated as the result of "decompartmentalization of endogenous cellular iron", hemorrhage, and hypoxia (Anderson and Means, 1984; Mead, 1976; Seligman et al., 1977; Siesjö, 1981). That lipid peroxidation is involved in the long-term (24 h) destruction of spinal cord tissue following trauma is widely accepted (Demopoulos et al., 1980). However, the role of peroxidation in perturbing cell membranes in the very early stages (from 1 min to 1 h) after injury is not well documented. Perhaps the earliest posttraumatic cellular events involve activation of hydrolytic lipases or proteases. In brain ischemia models, free fatty acid production and phospholipase activation take place within the first few minutes (DeMedio et al., 1980; Bazan et al., 1982; Edgar et al., 1982), whereas activation of proteolytic enzymes within the first hour has not been reported. Thus, it is probably necessary to remove some of the lipid before significant degradation of protein can take place. In addition, lipase products such as free fatty acids (FFA), lysophospholipids, and diglycerides (DG) can significantly perturb the integrity of biomembranes (Allen et al., 1978; Usher et al., 1978; Klausner et al., 1980). Arachidonic acid, which is preferentially released in ischemia, is metabolized to prostaglandins and hydroxy fatty acids; compounds with very potent physiological effects (Gaudet and Levine, 1979; Spagnuolo et al., 1980; Wolfe, 1982). Prostaglandin production has also been observed following experimental spinal cord trauma (Jonsson and Daniell, 1976). The action of some of these lipase products on cell membranes may then render the remaining membrane constituents more susceptible to peroxidative attack, as well as acting to reduce critical membrane enzyme activities and allowing influx of extracellular Ca^{2+} ions (Young et al., 1982; Stokes et al., 1983).

Our recent studies at the Spinal Cord Injury Research Center of The Ohio State University and the Cincinnati Veterans Administration Medical Center have examined the posttrauma production of spinal cord lipolysis products (such as FFA and DG), the metabolism of free arachidonate to biologically active eicosanoids, the degradation of membrane lipids, and the consequences of production of these compounds in the context of membrane function. Dogs and cats were used in these experiments, with both impact trauma and compression trauma being used as models for blunt spinal cord trauma. It is hoped that these experiments will help to identify and clarify the most important aspects of the pathogenesis of membrane perturbations and cellular necrosis that follow spinal cord trauma. Our studies are ultimately aimed at providing a rational basis for the testing of potential therapeutic agents such as phospholipase inhibitors, antioxidants, and inhibitors of eicosanoid biosynthesis.

In particular, we have measured free fatty acid levels, diglyceride levels, membrane ATPase activities, eicosanoid production, cholesterol levels, and phospholipid levels in control and traumatized spinal cord.

Methods

Mongrel cats or dogs were used in all experimental procedures. Cats were used exclusively for compression trauma, whereas dogs were utilized for impact injury. All of the cats were anesthetized with intraperitoneal pentobarbital sodium (30 mg/kg) and muscle paralysis was induced with succinylcholine chloride (1 mg/kg). The vertebral column was exposed in the upper lumbar region and a one segment laminectomy was performed at the level of the second lumbar vertebrae (L-2) (Anderson et al., 1976, 1978). All laminectomies were carefully performed and attention directed toward preventing contact of the dura mater with surgical instruments. During timed periods following laminectomy and/or compression injury, the surgery site was covered with 0.9% NaCl warmed to 37°C. Spinal cord trauma was induced by placing a 170-g weight, extradurally, on the spinal cord for a prescribed length of time (Anderson et al., 1976). The injury apparatus was a stainless steel rod (tip 6 mm in diameter) passed through a guide tube which was positioned directly over and perpendicular to the center of the spinal cord. Spinal cord tissue in the L-1 to L-3 region as frozen in situ with liquid nitrogen (Anderson et al., 1980). Approximately 2 cm of spinal cord at the L-2 site was maximally exposed, removed intact, and stored at −70°C until assayed. Compression trauma animals were placed in one of four different experimental groups. Group 1 consisted of animals in which the vertebral column was exposed and the underlying spinal cord was frozen through the intact bone (i.e., no laminectomy was performed). In group 2, laminectomies were performed and the cats were allowed to recover for either 10, 60, 90, or 120 min before the spinal cords were frozen. Group 3 animals were laminectomized, allowed to recover for 90 min, and then the spinal cord was compressed with a 170 g weight for either 1 min, 3 min, or 5 min. In this group, the spinal cords were frozen immediately upon termination of the compression. In group 4, following laminectomy plus 90 min of recovery, the spinal cords were compressed with 170 g for 5 min, but the spinal cords were not frozen until either 5 min, 15 min, or 30 min after the compression had been terminated.

In experiments involving dogs, each animal was anesthetized with Suritol (thiamylal sodium, 5 mg/kg) and the vertebral column was exposed in the mid-thoracic region. Laminectomies were performed at T-4–T-5. Using the method of Albin et al. (1967), impact trauma was induced by dropping a 20-g weight 20 cm through a tube positioned directly over the exposed spinal cord. During experiments for the determination of ATPase activities, approximately 60 min elapsed between laminectomy and injury, after which the exposed segments were removed at 2, 5, 15, 30, and 60 min. For experiments on lipid components, the excised segments were frozen in liquid N_2 immediately following laminectomy, 90 min post laminectomy, 6 min after injury, and 36 min after injury. Samples were kept at −70°C prior to analysis.

Each dura-free frozen sample of spinal cord was prepared in a −20°C stand-up cold room for subsequent analysis by one of three different methods. Segments used for determination of arachidonic acid metabolites (eicosanoids) were thoroughly cleaned of meninges, scraped free of blood, and then each total sample was extracted for lipids. Segments used for FFA and DG analyses were cleaned as above, and then cored with a flat-ended 14-gauge needle to produce samples that were either predominantly gray matter (central core) or predominantly white matter (outer area). Samples for ATPase analyses were cleaned, dissected into rostral and caudal control areas, and the trauma site, and then separated into gray and white areas as above.

Lipid extraction and analyses were performed as follows. For FFA and DG, total lipids were extracted using a two-phase chloroform/methanol system (Agardh et al., 1981). The total FFA and DG were then separated by thin layer chromatography (TLC) and fatty acid methyl esters (FAME) were prepared (Agardh et al., 1981). The FAME were separated and quantitated by gas-liquid chromatography using 10% Alltech CS-10 as the stationary phase. For eicosanoids, phospholipids, and cholesterol, total lipids were extracted with hexane: 2-propanol and separated on silicic acid columns (Hara and Radin, 1978; Saunders and Horrocks, 1984). Prostaglandins E_2 and $F_{2\alpha}$, thromboxane B_2 (the stable metabolite of thromboxane A_2), and 6-keto prostaglandin $F_{1\alpha}$ (the stable metabolite of prostacyclin) were eluted from the columns with methyl formate and quantitated by radioimmunoassay (Fertel et al., 1981). Phospholipids were separated by TLC (Horrocks and Sun, 1972) and quantitated by the method of Rouser et al. (1969). Cholesterol was determined by the method of Bowman and Wolf (1962).

The method of Hunt and Craig (1973) was followed to measure Na^+-, K^+- and Mg^{2+}-ATPase activities. The rate of ATP hydrolysis was determined by quantitating P_i according to the procedure of Muszbek et al. (1977). Total protein was measured colorimetrically by the method of Lowry et al. (1951). ATPase activities are expressed as nmol P_i released per h per mg protein.

Results

Spinal cord samples that had been frozen through an intact vertebral column were assayed in an attempt to establish "normal" or control values for FFA and DG in the feline spinal cord. Levels of these lipolytic products in spinal cords handled in this fashion were substantially higher (Fig. 1) than those reported for normal brain (Yoshida et al.,

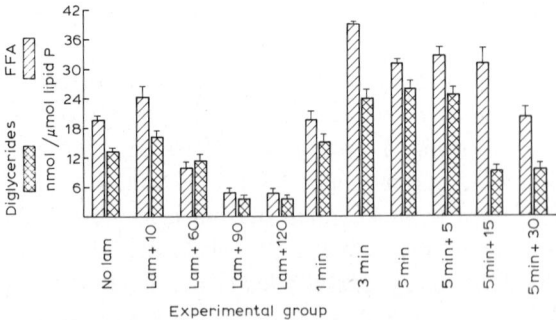

Fig. 1. Total free fatty acids (FFA) and diglycerides from gray matter of cat spinal cord. LAM indicates laminectomy at L-2, with the numbers being the time periods in minutes allowed for recovery before freezing. The injury groups are 1 min of 170 g compression trauma, 3 min of compression, 5 min of compression, and 5 min of compression after which the weight was removed and the cord frozen after an additional 5 min, 15 min, and 30 min. Values are means of four separate determinations ($n = 4$).

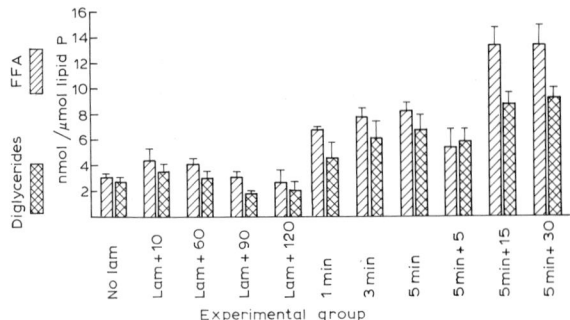

Fig. 2. Total free fatty acids (FFA) and diglycerides from white matter of cat spinal cord. Experiment as described in Fig. 1 ($n = 4$ for all groups).

1982). Laminectomy caused a further elevation in the levels of FFA and DG (Fig. 1). The laminectomy-induced changes in white matter FFA and DG were considerably less pronounced than those seen in gray matter (Fig. 2). Among the individual FFA, free arachidonate was elevated to the greatest degree in both gray and white matter (Figs. 3 and 4).

In both gray and white matter, the postlaminectomy elevations in FFA and DG were transient, falling to levels approximating those seen in brain within 90 min after laminectomy. Consequently, we have used the FFA and DG values from this time period (i.e., laminectomy plus 90 min recovery) as controls, and all cats subjected to compression trauma underwent a 90-min postlaminectomy recovery period before trauma was initiated (the dogs used for eicosanoid analyses had the same recovery period).

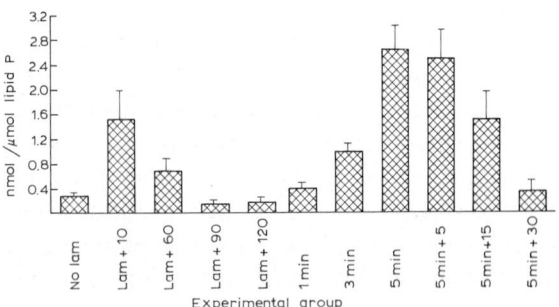

Fig. 3. Free (unesterified) arachidonic acid levels from gray matter of cat spinal cord. Experiment as previously described ($n = 4$).

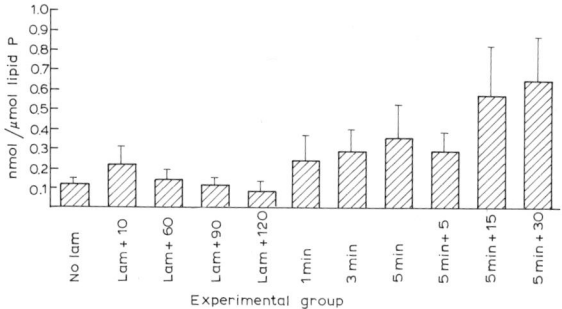

Fig. 4. Free (unesterified) arachidonic acid levels from white matter of cat spinal cord. Experiment as previously described ($n = 4$).

Compression trauma for 1 min caused significant increases in gray matter total FFA and DG levels of 4.2-fold and 4.6-fold, respectively (Fig. 1). increasing the compression time from 3 to 5 min resulted in a further elevation in spinal cord levels of total FFA and DG. All of the individual FFA analyzed were significantly elevated by compression trauma with the largest relative increases occurring in arachidonic acid (Fig. 3). Similarly, all gray matter diglyceride acyl groups were elevated following compression trauma (data not shown). Total FFA and DG were also significantly elevated in white matter by 1, 3, and 5 min of compression trauma, although the magnitude of these increases was less than that seen in gray matter after the same period of compression (Fig. 2).

Recovery from 5 min of compression trauma resulted in a different pattern of FFA and DG in both gray and white matter. By 30 min after the termination of 5 min of compression, the gray matter total FFA had declined approximately 35%, with the largest decreases occurring among the polyunsaturates, particularly arachidonic acid (Fig. 3). By 15 min after termination of compression, the gray matter total DG levels had fallen 65%, remaining at this level for at least 30 min after removing the weight. In contrast, the white matter total FFA and DG were significantly increased at 15 min and 30 min after termination of 5 min of compression (Fig. 2). Free arachidonic acid levels continued to increase at these time periods (Fig. 4). Despite the observed statistically significant increases in free arachidonate levels during 1 min and 5 min of compression injury, no significant increases in the amounts of cat spinal cord eicosanoids were seen at these time periods (Fig. 5). Data are expressed as pmol eicosanoid/μmol sphingomyelin. If the wet weight is used as the denominator, wide variations are seen in the amounts of phosphorus and cholesterol (65.5 to 104.5 and 87.5 to 141.4 μmol/g wet weight respectively) whereas the ratio of cholesterol to phosphorus remains relatively constant (1.33 $\pm$ 0.08, $n = 10$). The fluctuations in the wet weight may be caused by edema occurring in the tissue following injury (Goodman et al., 1976). Therefore, the results are expressed as pmol/μmol sphingomyelin because sphingomyelin is a membrane component with a slow rate of turnover (Hennacy and Horrocks, 1978; DeMedio et al., 1980).

Prostaglandins E_2 and $F_{2\alpha}$ were elevated 24- and 10-fold respectively at 5 min after 5 min of injury. At 30 min, the prostaglandin $F_{2\alpha}$ levels were further increased 24-fold above control levels. Thromboxane levels were increased 10-fold at 5 min after 5 min compression and 14-fold after 30 min. There was no significant increase in 6-keto prostaglandin $F_{1\alpha}$ up to 30 min following injury.

Prostaglandin levels from dog spinal cord that

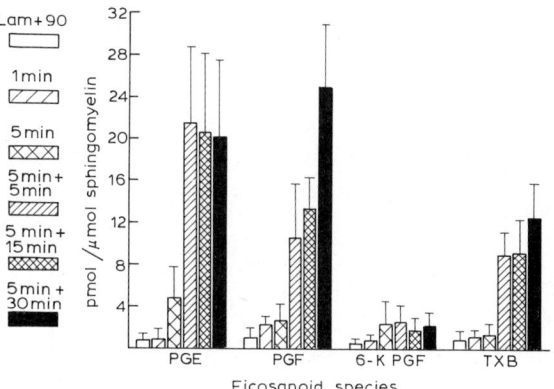

Fig. 5. Prostaglandin, prostacyclin, and thromboxane levels of whole cat spinal cord samples. PGE denotes prostaglandin PGE_2; PGF is prostaglandin $F_{2\alpha}$; 6K-PGF is 6-keto prostaglandin $F_{1\alpha}$, a stable metabolite of prostacyclin; TXB is thromboxane B_2, a stable metabolite of thromboxane A_2. Experiment as described in Fig. 1 ($n = 4$).

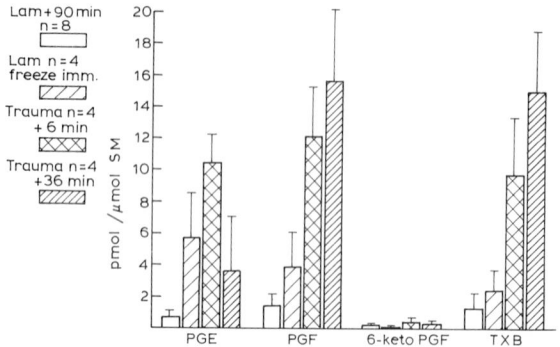

Fig. 6. Prostaglandin, prostacyclin, and thromboxane levels of whole dog spinal cord. LAM indicates laminectomy. Trauma was induced by a 400 g-cm impact at T-4. Abbreviations as in Fig. 5.

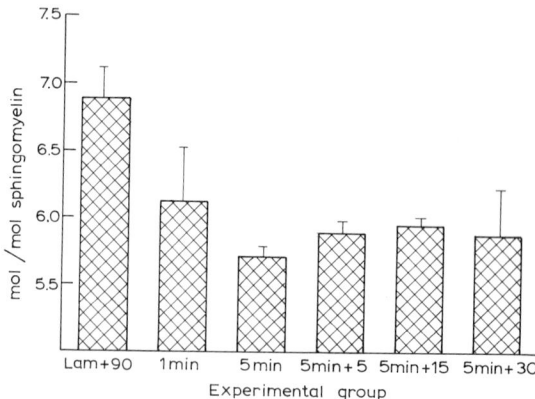

Fig. 8. Cholesterol levels of whole cat spinal cord. Experiment as in Fig. 7 ($n = 4$).

was injured using an impact of 400 g-cm, were very similar to those found in cat spinal cord (Fig. 6). Laminectomy by itself perturbed the spinal cord sufficiently to cause an observable increase in prostaglandins E_2 and $F_{2\alpha}$. At 6 min after impact, prostaglandins E_2 and $F_{2\alpha}$ increased 15- and 8-fold respectively. Prostaglandin $F_{2\alpha}$ further increased to 11-fold above control levels at 36 min following injury, whereas prostaglandin E_2 fell to 5-fold above the control level at this time point. Thromboxane levels were increased 7-fold after 6 min and 11-fold after 36 min following impact. No significant increases were found in the levels of 6-keto prostaglandin $F_{1\alpha}$ up to 36 min following impact injury.

The content of ethanolamine plasmalogens in cat spinal cord was decreased 10% after 1 min of compression and 20% at 30 min after 5 min of compression (Fig. 7). The levels of phosphatidic acid were increased 50% after 5 min of compression trauma and 150% after 30 min (data not shown). There were no significant changes in the content of other phospholipids. The cholesterol content decreased 10% after 1 min of compression trauma but did not change any further at later times (Fig. 8). Because these values were determined for whole spinal cord samples, it was not possible to distinguish whether the major changes were occurring in gray or white matter (or in both). Preliminary re-

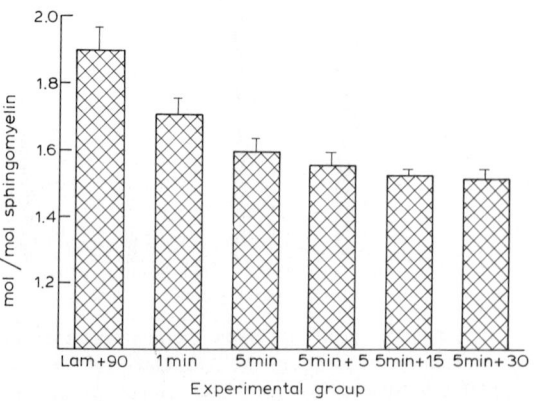

Fig. 7. Ethanolamine plasmalogen levels of whole cat spinal cord. Laminectomy plus a 90-min recovery period acts as control. Injury as in Fig. 1 ($n = 4$).

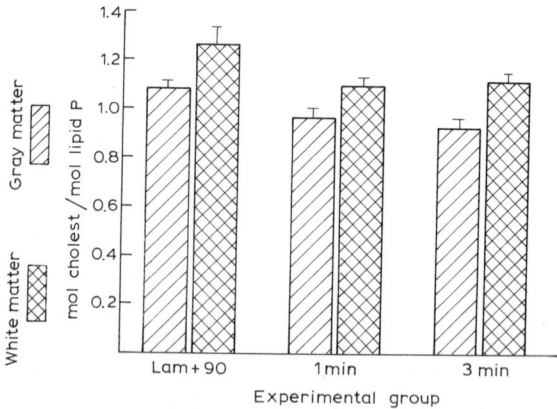

Fig. 9. Cholesterol/phospholipid phosphorus ratio of gray and white matter from cat spinal cord. Laminectomy plus a 90-min recovery period acts as the control for comparison with 1 min and 3 min compression injury ($n = 4$).

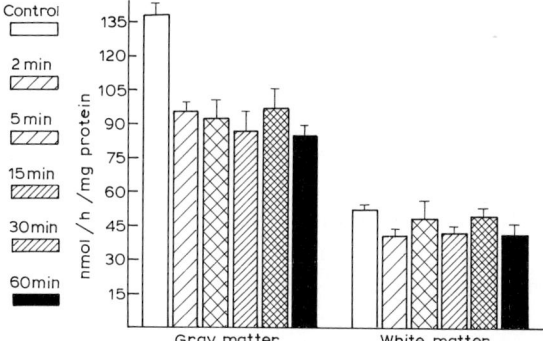

Fig. 10. Na$^+$, K$^+$-ATPase activity of gray and white matter from dog spinal cord. Trauma was initiated by a 400 g-cm impact at T-4. Times indicated are the periods following impact before removal and freezing. Values reported are the average of three determinations each.

sults from cat spinal cord include 12% decreases of cholesterol levels in both gray and white matter after 1 or 3 min of trauma (Fig. 9). Ethanolamine plasmalogen levels were also decreased in both gray and white matter with values for control and 3 min of compression of 1.78 ± 0.04 ($n = 2$) and 1.58 ± 0.02 ($n = 4$) in white matter and of 1.77 ± 0.02 ($n = 2$) to 1.57 ± 0.03 ($n = 4$) in gray matter.

A significant decrease ($p < 0.01$) in Na$^+$, K$^+$-activated ATPase activity was observed in samples of gray matter after 2 min of impact injury of the dog spinal cord (Fig. 10). Specific activities remained at approximately 68% of control for all subsequent time interval studied. By 30 min post injury, Mg^{2+}-dependent ATPase activity was sig-

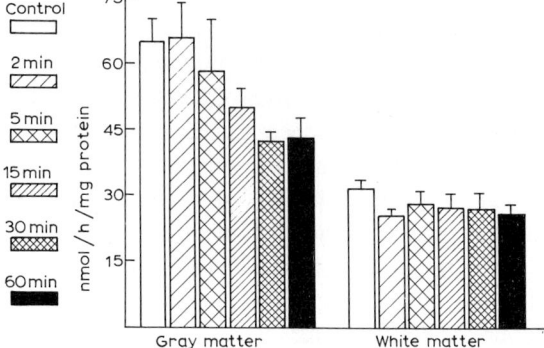

Fig. 11. Mg^{2+}-ATPase activity of gray and white matter from dog spinal cord. Experiment as in Fig. 10.

nificantly inhibited ($p < 0.02$) to 65% of the control value (Fig. 11). No sustained alteration in activity for either ATPase was noted in white matter samples from the trauma site for these time periods. Activities for tissue excised adjacent to the injury site were generally similar to the control values.

Discussion

A pronounced transient elevation of spinal cord FFA, DG, and prostaglandin levels following surgical exposure of the vertebral column and laminectomy was found. This, along with previous demonstrations that laminectomy causes a transient decrease in spinal cord blood flow (Anderson et al., 1978) and Na$^+$, K$^+$-ATPase activity (Anderson and Means, 1983), and increases in tissue levels of ADP and AMP (Anderson et al., 1980), indicates that these surgical procedures perturb biochemical processes in the spinal cord. These are relevant findings because laminectomy is a common neurosurgical procedure for the treatment of clinical disorders, such as tumors within the spinal cord or spinal canal (Gurdjian and Thomas, 1970). The FFA and DG values are, to our knowledge, the first such values to be reported for spinal cord. Prostaglandin levels in cat spinal cord were previously reported (Jonsson and Daniell, 1976). However, the "baseline control" values from this study were determined immediately after laminectomy, and the tissue was not frozen until up to 2 min after removal. Based upon our data, it is obvious that freezing with liquid N$_2$ in situ and a stabilization period after surgery are necessary to obtain baseline levels.

The concentrations of total FFA in spinal cord gray matter after surgical exposure of the vertebral column (480 nmol/g wet weight) were similar to those seen in brain subjected to bicuculline-induced seizures (440 nmol/g), but were approximately 50% lower than the levels reported for brain during other pathological conditions such as ischemia and hypoglycemia (800 nmol/g) (Siesjö, 1981; Siesjö et al., 1982; Horrocks et al., 1984). The levels of total DG in gray matter measured at 10 min post laminectomy (320 nmol/g) were also elevated compared with "control" values for brain (100–170 nmol/g), but were lower than the levels measured in brain tissue at 30 min post mortem (450 nmol/g) (Sun, 1970; Keough et al., 1972; Banschbach and Geison, 1974). Levels of FFA and DG in white matter were lower than those in gray matter, as they are in monkey and rat brain (Bazan, 1971a; Bazan et al., 1971). Between 10 and 90 min after laminectomy there was a dramatic reduction in both FFA (480 and 95 nmol/g wet weight) and DG (320 and 65 nmol/g wet weight concentrations). The spinal cord FFA values after recovery are higher than the lowest reported values of Yoshida et al. (1982) (64 nmol/g wet weight) for rat brain, but are less than the typical range of FFA concentrations in brain tissue typically found in the literature (i.e. 140–170 nmol/g), including the most recent results from Yoshida et al. (1984). The increases in spinal cord FFA and DG following surgical exposure of the vertebral column and/or laminectomy suggest that membrane lipases are activated, probably as the result of mechanical manipulation of the spinal cord during the surgical procedures. However, these laminectomy-induced elevations in FFA and DG were transient, recovering to "normal" control levels within 90 min after laminectomy with no apparent permanent damage to the tissue.

Compression of the feline spinal cord with 170 g for 5 min (which results in extensive tissue necrosis and sensorimotor loss) caused an 8-fold elevation in gray matter FFA and DG (i.e. to 800 nmol/g and 520 nmol/g, respectively). These increases were similar to those seen in post-mortem rodent brain tissue and during complete cerebral ischemia (FFA: 800–1200 nmol/g; DG: 450 nmol/g) (Keough et al., 1972; Banschbach and Geison, 1974; Bazan, 1971b; Bazan et al., 1971). All individual FFA were significantly increased by trauma, including arachidonate. The levels of arachidonic acid in traumatized spinal cord were similar to those seen in brain tissue subjected to insults causing cellular damage (i.e., prolonged ischemia or hypoglycemia), but were substantially greater than the FFA changes in brain tissue that occur subsequent to insults that do not cause any apparent permanent damage (i.e., bicuculline-induced seizures and electroconvulsive shock) (Yoshida et al., 1982; Agardh et al., 1981; Rodriguez de Turco et al., 1983; Siesjö et al., 1982). The magnitude of the posttraumatic increase was approximately the same for all DG acyl groups. This resembles the pattern of change in ischemic brain, but was different from that seen following induced convulsions. In white matter, FFA and DG also increased as a result of compression trauma, but the magnitude of these changes was considerably less than that seen in gray matter.

At 5 and 15 min after termination of 5 min of compression, total FFA in spinal cord gray matter were still elevated. However, by 30 min, total FFA had begun to decrease falling almost 40% from the previous time periods. The declines were more rapid for the long-chain PUFA, particularly arachidonate. The magnitude and time course of this recovery in spinal cord FFA are similar to that seen in gerbil brain following 30 min of ischemia, and in rat brain following bicuculline-induced seizures (Yoshida et al., 1982; Siesjö et al., 1982; Rehncrona et al., 1982; Yoshida et al., 1980).

Total DG levels in spinal cord remained elevated for 5 min after termination of compression. However, by 15 min, total DG had decreased 65%. This pattern of change in spinal cord DG was similar to that reported for rat brain following bicuculline-induced seizures (Rodriguez de Turco et al., 1983).

The time course of post-compression alterations in white matter FFA and DG were out of phase with those in gray matter. At 15 and 30 min after compression was terminated, total FFA and DG were significantly elevated in white matter whereas in gray matter these lipolysis products were declining (vide supra). This biochemical data is consistent with histological findings demonstrating that posttraumatic damage to spinal cord is seen first in gray matter, then spreads radially outward to white matter (Osterholm, 1974; De La Torre, 1982).

The endogenous levels of unesterified arachidonic acid, prostaglandins, and thromboxanes in the central nervous system are extremely low but rise markedly in response to insult (Wolfe, 1978). Products of arachidonic acid metabolism have been implicated in the response of the central nervous system to injury. Most of these studies have been done using models of brain injury and include drug-induced convulsions and electroshock (Bazan, 1971b), ischemia (Gaudet and Levine, 1979; Shohami et al., 1983), cold injury (Pappius and Wolfe, 1983) and concussive injury (Ellis et al., 1981). The only previous report on prostaglandins in spinal cord injury was for prostaglandins E_2 and $F_{2\alpha}$ (Jonsson and Daniell, 1976). Prostaglandin $F_{2\alpha}$ levels increased 11-fold as compared to animals pretreated with indomethacin. In that study however, the earliest time point was 60 min after trauma by dropping a weight on the cord, and the spinal cord was not allowed to stabilize following laminectomy.

The changes seen in ethanolamine plasmalogen levels in cat and dog spinal cord following trauma were previously observed in isolated myelin at 10, 30, and 60 min following spinal cord injury in primates (Horrocks et al., 1973). These plasmalogen decreases are also similar to those which occur as a result of brain ischemia in the rat (Dorman et al., 1983). The decreased cholesterol levels that we have found are in agreement with the results of Demopoulos et al. (1980), who proposed that such a decrease may result from lipid peroxidation initiated by trauma to the spinal cord. No comparable reports are available for brain trauma. An increase in phosphatidic acid has not been observed previously after central nervous system trauma.

There are a number of potential sources for the FFA and DG that accumulate in spinal cord following blunt trauma. Analogous increases which occur in cerebral tissue as a result of brain injury have been proposed to arise primarily from the hydrolysis of membrane glycerophospholipids as the result of the activation of various lipases and the reversal of certain biosynthetic enzymes (Siesjö, 1981; Yoshida et al., 1982; Agardh et al., 1981; Dorman et al., 1983). One potential source could be phospholipases of the A type which may be activated by Ca^{2+}, by direct covalent modification, or by the covalent modification of an inhibitor such as lipomodulin. This could result in the hydrolysis of choline and ethanolamine glycerophospholipids with subsequent release of FFA (Aveldaño and Bazan, 1975; Bazan, 1976; Marion and Wolfe, 1979; Van den Bosch, 1980; Edgar et al., 1982). A second probable source of FFA is the degradation of ethanolamine plasmalogens by plasmalogenase, followed by removal of the acyl group from the 2-position of the resultant lysophospholipid by a lysophospholipase (Horrocks and Fu, 1978). The observed decrease in ethanolamine plasmalogen with spinal cord trauma supports this mechanism as a source of FFA. A third possibility, whereby both DG and FFA could arise, is the sequential action of phospholipase C, diglyceride lipase, and monoglyceride lipase acting upon inositol and choline glycerophospholipids. Phospholipase C activity has been found to increase in cat brain after experimental concussive injury (Wei et al., 1982). DG can also be formed from glycerophospholipids by reversal of the synthetic enzyme 1,2-diacylglycerol:CDPcholine cholinephosphotransferase, which catalyzes the reaction of CMP with phosphatidylcholine to produce CDPcholine and DG (Goracci et al., 1981, 1983). Finally, in traumatized spinal cord tissue with reduced blood flow and tissue energy reserves, the reacylation of liberated fatty acids may be impeded (Sun et al., 1979) and thus contribute to the injury-induced rise of FFA (Bazan et al., 1971a). Based upon our data, it is not possible at the present time to pinpoint the source of FFA and DG production. A combination of lipase activities is probably responsible.

The decreases seen in spinal cord FFA and DG following the termination of compression may also be due to several mechanisms (Yoshida et al., 1982) including equilibration with the FFA in blood and cerebrospinal fluid, oxidation of the fatty acids as an energy source, reacylation into glycerophospholipids, and enzymic and non-enzymatic peroxidation of arachidonate (Kimes et al., 1983; Agardh et al., 1981; Sun, 1977; Gaudet and Levine, 1979; Horrocks et al., 1981). The enzymic peroxidation of free arachidonic acid can produce prostaglandins, thromboxanes, and leukotrienes. Increases in prostaglandins and thromboxanes have been observed, making it probable that the liberated arachidonate is acting as a source for these eicosanoids. However, the amounts of eicosanoids produced do not account for the magnitude of the observed decline in free arachidonate. The decrease in DG could occur due to their sequential hydrolysis by diglyceride lipase and monoglyceride lipase and/or by direct phosphorylation by diglyceride kinase to produce phosphatidic acid (Lapetina and Cuatrecasas, 1979). The latter mechanism may also account for at least part of the observed rise in phosphatidic acid. Phosphatidic acid is an intermediate in the synthesis of other phospholipids. Its synthesis may reflect an attempt by the injured cord to replace degraded phospholipids.

The potential consequences of the observed membrane lipid changes are quite diverse. The decreases in Na^+, K^+-ATPase activity that we have reported with spinal cord injury provide one prime example of such consequences in the context of membrane damage. This enzyme is membrane bound and phospholipid dependent, with its activity requiring an intact membrane structure (Fourcans and Jain, 1974; Goldman and Albers, 1973; Wheeler et al., 1975). Membrane damage would be expected to alter the structural configuration of the Na^+, K^+-ATPase, with resultant reduction in enzymatic activity.

Elevations in FFA and DG following spinal trauma may damage cells and affect physiological processes by altering membrane sturcture and fluidity. At low concentrations, FFA and DG readily intercalate into membranes producing significant changes in the packing and acyl group motion of the constituent lipid molecules. Typical control values of both FFA and DG are approximately 0.4 mol % of the pool of total phospholipids. In our model of spinal cord trauma these values increase to approximately 4 mol % each, a level at which fatty acids have been shown to perturb both model and biological membranes as determined by fluorescence polarization, differential scanning calorimetry, and enzymic assays (Usher et al., 1978; Klausner et al., 1980; Karnovsky et al., 1982; Hill et al., 1983). Also, DG which can undergo rapid transmembrane flip-flop (unlike phospholipids), may affect membrane curvature (Sheetz and Singer, 1974; Allan et al., 1978).

Physiologically, a number of membrane-related effects of FFA and DG have been observed. In erythrocytes, low levels of FFA stabilize cells against osmotic fragility, whereas higher concentrations facilitate osmotic hemolysis in hypotonic medium (Raz and Livne, 1973). Free fatty acids have also been shown to inhibit calcium uptake by sarcoplasmic reticulum vesicles from rabbit skeletal muscle (Katz et al., 1982). In addition, FFA inhibit the Na^+-dependent synaptosomal uptake of proline, aspartate, glutamate, and gamma-aminobutyric acid, and reduce synaptosomal Na^+, K^+-ATPase activity (Raz and Livne, 1973; Rhoads et al., 1982). Intracerebral injections of arachidonic acid in rats selectively destroy the outer leaflet of capillary plasma membranes in white matter (Wakai et al., 1982). Diglycerides stimulate transepithelial sodium transport in frog skin epithelium (Yorio et al., 1980) and the Ca^{2+}-activated, phospholipid-dependent protein kinase C from rat brain (Mori et al., 1982). Diglycerides also markedly increase phospholipase-catalyzed hydrolysis of phospholipid bilayers (Dawson et al., 1983).

Due to the variety of actions attributed to arachidonic acid metabolites, the eicosanoids may be involved in the irreversible loss of spinal cord function. In addition to their roles in cellular inflammation, eicosanoids have effects on central nervous system vascular homeostasis (White and Hagan, 1982). Thromboxane A_2 is a potent vasoconstrictor and promotor of platelet aggregation whereas prostacyclin is a vasodilator and antiaggregant. The increase in thromboxane synthesis relative to that of prostacyclin may be involved in the decrease in blood flow (Means et al., 1978) and platelet aggregation (Demopoulos et al., 1980) observed following spinal cord injury. Because prostacyclin synthetase is localized in endothelial cell microsomes, the failure of prostacyclin to be synthesized may be explained by the vascular endothelial cell injury observed after trauma (Goodman et al., 1976; Nelson et al., 1977). Prostaglandin $F_{2\alpha}$ is also a vasoconstrictor but the effects of prostaglandin E_2 are controversial (White and Hagan, 1982).

Proper membrane structure is essential for impulse conduction in the central nervous system. The myelin sheath, derived from the plasma membrane of oligodendroglia, surrounds the long tracts of the spinal cord and expedites nerve conduction. Therefore, alterations in membrane structure will have detrimental effects on central nervous system function. The degradation of ethanolamine plasmalogens may be related to the dissociation of myelin observed following spinal cord injury in primates (Horrocks et al., 1973; Toews et al., 1980). The decrease in cholesterol may also have effects on membrane structure. Cholesterol is known to have a condensing effect on the acyl chain region of fluid lipid bilayers, producing a more ordered rigid structure. This effect is important in the passive diffusion of water and small molecules through the bilayer. A decrease in cholesterol increases the passive permeability of lipid bilayers to water and other small molecules and ion such as K^+, Na^+, Ca^{2+}, glucose, glycerol, and indoles (Blok et al., 1977; Houslay and Stanley, 1982).

With regard to the temporal sequence of biochemical events which result in irreversible cell death after spinal cord trauma, very little is clearly understood. Two important questions in this context are: (1) at what time point has the cell gone beyond the point of rescue? and (2) what is the combination of factors which together produce this irreversibility? One prevalent theory regarding the pathophysiology of spinal cord trauma is that ischemia plays a central role in the autodestruction of spinal cord tissue. It has been suggested that a reduction in the delivery of oxygen to the injured cord leads to the disruption of tightly coupled electron transport with subsequent production of oxygen free radicals within cell and organelle membranes. The free radicals are then thought to lead to peroxidative attack on polyunsaturated fatty acids within those membranes. Although this hypothesis certainly has merit in regard to long-term (> 2 h) pathogenesis, recent evidence suggests that the earliest events (between 1 min and 1 h) leading to cell death are not circulatory in nature but are membrane lipid related. We postulate that mechanical deformation of the spinal cord initiates (in some as yet unknown manner) activation of membrane lipases, particularly the plasmalogenase, within the first minute. The hydrolysis products then act to perturb membrane structure resulting in increases in membrane permeability and decreases in ion pumping capability. Membrane perturbations may also be intimately involved with the observed decreases in extracellular Ca^{2+} activity by allowing the influx of this ion (Young et al., 1982; Stokes et al., 1983). Some accumulation of hydrolytic products (FFA, DG, eicosanoids) is reversible as was seen after laminectomy. Perhaps if the levels of membrane lipid hydrolysis products can be kept below a certain point through the use of therapeutic agents, within an hour or less of injury, the overall damage and loss of function can be greatly reduced. Membrane lipid changes may be causative agents in producing the reduced blood flow. Closely paralleling the release of FFA is the conversion of arachidonate to eicosanoids. These potent bioactive molecules are probably important factors in reduction of spinal cord blood flow, which in the cat falls to 20% of control values in gray matter at 30 min after 5 min of compression (Means et al., 1978). Associated with the reduction in blood flow there is also a dramatic reduction in the tissue content of high-energy phosphate compounds (Anderson et al., 1980, 1982; Locke et al., 1971; Walker et al., 1979). This drop in energy charge is mirrored by an elevation of lactate levels within the injured tissue (Anderson et al., 1980, 1982; Braughler and Hall, 1983). Such changes in metabolism reflect the lowered blood flow and tissue oxygen delivery and contribute to the pathological deterioration of the injured tissue. At the cellular level, peroxidative mechanisms are most probably causing further membrane damage, thereby completely compromising the ability of the cells to regulate the ionic gradients across the membrane. This will result in loss of cellular water, dissolution of transmembrane chemical and electrical potentials, and ultimately in cell death. With the loss of oligodendroglia, there is consequent demyelination and permanent loss of sensory and motor function. This sequence of events spreads radially outward, beginning in the central gray matter and (depending upon the degree of trauma delivered) encompassing varying degrees of the surrounding white matter.

In the context of this forum on ischemic brain damage, a comparison and contrast of ischemic insult to the brain and blunt spinal cord trauma is appropriate. As previously stated, available evidence indicates that the initiating factors leading to irreversible tissue damage with these two types of injury are quite different. The pathophysiological reactions of spinal trauma appear to begin immediately after mechanical deformation and before there is any significant decrease in blood flow. This is in contrast to brain ischemia where damage begins with lowered tissue oxygen and glucose levels which result from circulatory deficits. Both brain ischemia (Bazan, 1976; Bazan et al., 1976; DeMedio et al., 1980; Yoshida et al., 1980, 1982, 1984) and spinal trauma are characterized by release of free fatty acids (particularly arachidonate) and diglycerides and loss of ethanolamine plasmalogens. The decrease in plasmalogen levels is greater in spinal cord than in brain. In addition, there is a loss of choline glycerophospholipids in brain ischemia that is not seen with spinal injury (DeMedio et al., 1980). We have also observed decreases in cholesterol content that are unique to spinal cord trauma. In brain and spinal cord, released arachidonic acid acts as a substrate for cyclooxygenase with resultant biosynthesis of prostaglandins and thromboxane A_2 (Gaudet and Levine, 1979; Jonsson and Daniell, 1976). For both types of injury, membrane damage is indicated by declines in the activities of ion-pumping enzymes such as the Na^+, K^+-ATPase (Clendenon et al., 1978; Schwartz et al., 1976). Further indication of membrane perturbation comes from the influx of extracellular Ca^{2+} that occurs in brain and spinal cord (Stokes et al., 1983; Young et al., 1982; Siesjö, 1984; Wieloch and Siesjö, 1982). However, this influx is much more dramatic in spinal cord, where the extracellular Ca^{2+} concentration falls to about 1 μM, a level that is almost undetectable (Stokes et al., 1983). Although spinal cord trauma does result in a lowered blood flow and lowered tissue oxygen levels (Anderson et al., 1982), the magnitude of these changes is not as great as in ischemia, which is defined by severe hypoperfusion and hypoxia. Because there is less blood flow and oxygen availability associated with these injuries, the energy charge of both ischemic brain tissue and traumatized spinal cord tissue is reduced (Anderson et al., 1982; Walker et al., 1979; Siesjö, 1984). Due to the greater severity of hypoxia in ischemic brain, this effect is more pronounced in brain ischemia than in spinal cord injury. Lactate accumulation occurs in approximately the same degree in brain and spinal cord (Braughler and Hall, 1983; Siesjö, 1984). Thus, although there are similarities between ischemic brain damage and spinal cord trauma, there are also significant differences in the pathophysiological reactions of brain and spinal cord. It is important that the differences be considered when designing potential clinical therapies for these insults to the central nervous system.

In conclusion, at the present time a great deal of active experimental interest is being focused on elucidating the molecular mechanisms whereby a mechanical injury to the spinal cord causes irreversible tissue destruction and physical disability in so many active young persons worldwide. An important adjunct to this research, in order to develop rational clinical therapies, is the identification of the time point at which these mechanisms become irreversible. It is hoped that the research presented here will provide ideas for further investigations which may result in methods to greatly reduce the severity of such tragic and costly injuries.

Acknowledgements

The authors wish to thank Mr. Thomas Waters and Mr. Ronald Yates for their performance of the delicate surgical procedures required for these studies. The work conducted at The Ohio State University was supported in partly by research Grants NS-08291 and NS-10165 and Training Grant NS-07091 from the National Instituess of Health.

References

Agardh, C.-D., Chapman, A.A., Nilsson, B. and Siesjö, B. (1981) Endogenous substrates utilized by rat brain in severe insulin-induced hypoglycemia, *J. Neurochem.*, 36: 490–500.

Albin, M.S., White, R.J., Yashon, D. and Harris, L.S. (1969) Effects of localized cooling on spinal cord trauma. *J. Trauma*, 9: 1000–1008.

Allan, D., Thomas, P. and Michell, R.H. (1978) Rapid transbilayer diffusion of 1,2-diacylglycerol and its relevance to control of membrane curvature. *Nature*, 276: 289–290.

Anderson, D.K. and Means, E.D. (1983) The effect of laminectomy on spinal cord blood flow, energy metabolism, and ATPase activity. *Acta Intl. Symposium Spinal Cord Biochemistry*, 1: 23–31.

Anderson, D.K. and Means, E.D. (1984) Lipid peroxidation in spinal cord. $FeCl_2$ induction and protection with antioxidants. *Neurochem. Pathol.*, 1: 249–264

Anderson, D.K., Prockop, L.D., Means, E.D. and Hartley, L.E. (1976) Cerebrospinal fluid lactate and electrolyte levels following experimental spinal cord injury. *J. Neurosurg.*, 44: 715–722.

Anderson, D.K., Nicolosi, G.R., Means, E.D. and Hartley, L.E. (1978) Effects of laminectomy on spinal cord blood flow. *J. Neurosurg.*, 48: 232–238.

Anderson, D.K., Means, E.D. and Waters, T.R. (1980) Spinal cord energy metabolism in normal and post laminectomy cats. *J. Neurosurg.*, 52: 387–391.

Anderson, D.K., Means, E.D., Waters, T.R. and Green, E.S. (1982) Microvascular perfusion and metabolism in injured spinal cord after methylprednisolone treatment. *J. Neurosurg.*, 56: 106–113.

Aveldaño, M.I. and Bazan, N.G. (1975) Differential lipid deacylation during brain ischemia in a homeotherm and a poikilotherm. Composition and content of free fatty acids and triacylglycerols. *Brain Res.*, 100: 99–110.

Banschbach, M.W. and Geison, R.L. (1974) Post-mortem increase in rat cerebral hemisphere diglyceride pool size. *J. Neurochem.*, 23: 875–877.

Bazan, N.G. (1971a) Free fatty acid production in cerebral white and gray matter of the squirrel monkey. *Lipids*, 6: 211–212.

Bazan, N.G. (1971b) Changes in free fatty acids of brain by drug-induced convulsions, electroshock, and anaesthesia. *J. Neurochem.*, 18: 1379–1386.

Bazan, N.G. (1976) Free arachidonic acid and other lipids in the nervous system during early ischemia and after electroshock. *Adv. Exp. Med. Biol.*, 72: 317–335.

Bazan, N.G., Bazan, H.E.P., Kennedy, W.G. and Joel, C.D. (1971) Regional distribution and rate of production of free fatty acids in rat brain. *J. Neurochem.*, 18: 1387–1394.

Bazan, N.G., Aveldaño de Caldironi, M.I. and Rodriguez de Turco, E.B. (1982) Rapid release of free arachidonic acid in the central nervous system due to stimulation. *Prog. Lipid Res.*, 20: 523–529.

Blok, M.C., Van Deenen, L.L.M. and De Gier, J. (1977) The effect of cholesterol incorporation on the temperature dependence of water permeation through liposomal membranes prepared from phosphatidylcholines. *Biochim. Biophys. Acta*, 464: 509–518.

Bowman, R.E. and Wolf, R.C. (1962) A rapid ultramicro method for total serum cholesterol. *Clin. Chem.*, 8: 302–309.

Bracken, M.B., Freeman, D.H. and Hellenbrand, K. (1981) Incidence of acute traumatic hospitalized spinal cord injury in the United States, 1970–1977. *Am. J. Epidemiol.*, 113: 615–622.

Braughler, J.M. and Hall, E.D. (1983) Lactate and pyruvate metabolism in injured cat spinal cord before and after a single large intravenous dose of methylprednisolone. *J. Neurosurg.*, 59: 256–261.

Clendenon, N.R., Allen, N., Gordon, W.A. and Bingham, W.G. (1978) Inhibition of Na^+, K^+-activated ATPase activity following experimental spinal cord trauma. *J. Neurosurg.*, 49: 563–568.

Dawson, R.M.C., Hemington, N.L. and Irvine, R.F. (1983) Diacylglycerol potentiates phospholipase attack upon phospholipid bilayers: possible connection with cell stimulation. *Biochem. Biophys. Res. Comm.*, 117: 196–201.

De La Torre, J.C. (1982) Spinal cord injury. Review of basic and applied research. *Spine*, 6: 315–335.

DeMedio, G.E., Goracci, G., Horrocks, L.A. et al., (1980) The effect of transient ischemia on fatty acid and lipid metabolism in the gerbil brain. *Ital. J. Biochem.*, 29: 412–432.

Demopoulos, H.B., Flamm, E.S., Pietronigro, D.D. and Seligman, M.L. (1980) The free radical pathology and the microcirculation in the major central nervous system disorders. *Acta Physiol. Scand.*, Suppl. 492: 91–118.

Dorman, R.V., Dabrowiecki, Z. and Horrocks, L.A. (1983) Effects of CDPcholine and CDPethanolamine on the alterations in rat brain lipid metabolism induced by global ischemia. *J. Neurochem.*, 40: 276–279.

Edgar, A.D., Strosznajder, J. and Horrocks, L.A. (1982) Activation of ethanolamine phospholipase A_2 in brain during ischemia. *J. Neurochem.*, 39: 1111–1116.

Ellis, E.F., Wright, J.F., Wei, E.P. and Kontos, H.A. (1981) Cyclooxygenase products of arachidonic acid metabolism in cat cerebral cortex after experimental concussive brain injury. *J. Neurochem.*, 37: 892–896.

Fertel, R., Yetiv, J.Z., Coleman, M.A., Schwarz, R.D., Greenwald, J.E. and Bianchine, J.R. (1981) Formation of antibodies to prostaglandins in the yolk of chicken eggs. *Biochem, Biophys. Res. Comm.*, 102: 1028–1033.

Fourcans, B. and Jain, M.K. (1974) Role of phospholipids in transport and enzymatic reactions. *Adv. Lipid Res.*, 12: 146–166.

Gaudet, R.J. and Levine, L. (1979) Transient cerebral ischemia and brain prostaglandins. *Biochim. Biophys. Res. Comm.*, 86: 893–901.

Goldman, S.S. and Albers, R.W. (1973) Sodium-potassium activated adenosine triphosphatase. IX. The role of phospholipids. *J. Biol. Chem.*, 248: 876–874.

Goodman, J.H., Bingham, W.G. and Hunt, W.E. (1976) Ultrastructural blood-brain barrier alterations and edema formation in acute spinal cord trauma. *J. Neurosurg.*, 44: 418–424.

Goodman, J.H., Bingham, W.G. and Hunt, W.E. (1979) Platelet aggregation in experimental spinal cord injury – ultrasturctural observations. *Arch. Neurol.*, 36: 197–201.

Goracci, G., Francescangeli, E., Horrocks, L.A. and Porcellati, G. (1981) The reverse reaction of choline phosphotransferase in rat brain microsomes: a new pathway for degradation of phosphatidylcholine. *Biochim. Biophys. Acta,* 664: 373–379.

Goracci, G., Francescangeli, E., Horrocks, L.A. and Porcellati, G. (1983) The effect of CMP on the release of free fatty acids of rat brain in vitro. *Neurochem. Res.,* 8: 971–981.

Griffiths, I.R. (1978) Ultrastructural changes in spinal cord microvasculature after impact injury. *Adv. Neurol.,* 20: 415–422.

Gurdjian, E.S. and Thomas, L.M. (1970) *Operative Neurosurgery.* Williams and Wilkins, New York, pp. 371.

Hara, A. and Radin, N.S. (1978) Lipid extraction of tissues with a low-toxicity solvent. *Anal. Biochem.,* 90: 420–426.

Hennacy, D.M. and Horrocks, L.A. (1978) Recent developments in the turnover of proteins and lipids in myelin and other plasma membranes in the central nervous system. *Bull. Molec. Biol. Med.,* 3: 207–221.

Hill, D.J., Dawidowicz, E.A., Andrews, M.L. and Karnovksy, M.J. (1983) Modulation of microsomal glucose-6-phosphatase translocase activity by free fatty acids: implications for lipid domain structure in microsomal membranes. *J. Cell Physiol.,* 115: 1–8.

Horrocks, L.A. and Sun, G.Y. (1972) Ethanolamine plasmalogens. In: N. Marks and R. Rodnight (Eds.), *Research Methods in Neurochemistry, Vol. 1.* Plenum, New York, pp. 223–231.

Horrocks, L.A. and Fu, S.C. (1978) Pathway for hydrolysis of plasmalogens in brain. In: S. Gatt, L. Freysz, and P. Mandell (Eds.), *Advances in Experimental Biology and Medicine, Vol. 101: Enzymes of Lipid Metabolism.* Plenum, New York, pp. 397–406.

Horrocks, L.A., Toews, A., Yashon, D. and Locke, G.E. (1973) Changes in myelin following trauma of the spinal cord in monkeys. *Neurobiology,* 3: 256–263.

Horrocks, L.A., VanRollins, M. and Yates, A.J. (1981) Lipid changes in the aging brain. In: A.N. Davison and R.H.S. Thompson (Eds.), *The Molecular Basis of Neuropathology.* Edward Arnold, London, pp. 601–630.

Horrocks, L.A., Dorman, R.V. and Porcellati, G. (1984) Fatty acids and phospholipids in brain during ischemia. In: A. Bes, P. Braquet, R. Paoletti and B.K. Siesjö (Eds.), *Cerebral Ischemia, ICS 654.* Excerpta Medica, Amsterdam-New York-Oxford, 211–222.

Houslay, M.D. and Stanley, K.K. (1982) *Dynamics of Biological Membranes. Influence on Synthesis, Structure, and Function.* Wiley, New York, pp. 71–81.

Hunt, W.A. and Craig, C.R. (1973) Alterations in cation levels and Na^+, K^+-ATPase activity in rat cerebral cortex during the development of cobalt-induced epilepsy. *J. Neurochem.,* 20: 559–567.

Insurance Institute for Highway Safety (1976) *The Cost of Spinal Cord Injuries.* Status report II, No. 20, Washington, DC.

Jonsson, H.T. and Daniell, H.B. (1976) Altered levels of PGF in cat spinal cord tissue following traumatic injury. *Prostaglandins,* 11: 51–61.

Karnovsky, M.J., Kleinfeld, A.M., Hoover, R.L. and Klausner, R.D. (1982) The concept of lipid domains in membranes. *J. Cell Biol.,* 94: 1–6.

Katz, A.M., Nash-Adler, P., Watras, J., Messine, F.C., Takenaka, H. and Louis, C.F. (1982) Farry acid effects on calcium influx and efflux in sarcoplasmic reticulum vesicles from rabbit skeletal muscle. *Biochim. Biophys. Acta,* 687: 17–26.

Keough, K.M.W., MacDonald, G. and Thompson, W. (1972) A possible relation between phosphoinositides and the diglyceride pool in rat brain.*Biochim. Biophys. Acta,* 270: 337–347.

Kimes, A.S., Sweeney, D., London, E.D. and Rapoport, S.I. (1983) Palmitate incorporation into different brain regions in the awake rat. *Brain Res.,* 274: 291–301.

Klausner, R.D., Kleinfeld, A.M., Hoover, R.L. and Karnovsky, M.J. (1980) Lipid domains in membranes., Evidence derived from structural perturbations induced by free fatty acids and lifetime heterogeneity analysis. *J. Biol. Chem.,* 255: 1286–1295.

Kontos, H.A., Wei, E.P., Povlishock, J.T., Dietrich, W.D., Magiera, C.J. and Ellis, E.F. (1980) Cerebral arteriolar damage by arachidonic acid and prostaglandin G_2. *Science,* 209: 1242–1245.

Lapetina, E.G. and Cuatrecasas, P. (1979) Stimulation of phosphatidic acid production precedes the formation of arachidonate and parallels the release of serotonin. *Biochim. Biophys. Acta,* 573: 394–402.

Locke, G.E., Yashon, D. and Feldman, R.A. (1971) Ischemia in primate spinal cord injury. *J. Neurosurg.,* 36: 614–617.

Lowry, O.H., Rosebrough, N.J., Farr, A.L. and Randall, R.J. (1951) Protein measurement with the Folin phenol reagent. *J. Biol. Chem.,* 193: 265–275.

Marion, J. and Wolfe, L.S. (1979) Origin of the arachidonic acid released post-mortem in rat forebrain. *Biochim. Biophys. Acta,* 574: 25–32.

Mead, J.F. (1976) Free radical mechanisms of lipid damage and consequences for cellular membranes. In: W. A. Pryor (Ed.), *Free Radicals in Biology, Vol. 1.* Academic Press, New York, pp. 51–68.

Means, E.D., Anderson, D.K., Nicolosi, G. and Gaudsmith, J. (1978) Microvascular perfusion experimental spinal cord injury. *Surg. Neurol.,* 9: 353–360.

Mori, T., Takai, Y., Yu, B., Takahashi, J., Nishizuka, Y. and Fujikara, T. (1982) Specificity of the fatty acyl moieties of diacylglycerol for the activation of calcium-activated phospholipid-dependent protein kinase. *J. Biochem.*, 91: 427–431.

Muszbek, L., Szabo, T. and Fesus, L. (1977) A highly sensitive method for the measurement of ATPase activity. *Anal. Biochem.*, 77: 286–288.

Nelson, E., Gertz, S.D., Rennels, M.L., Ducker, T.B. and Blaumanis, O.R. (1977) The role of vascular damage in the pathogenesis of central hemorrhagic necrosis. *Arch. Neurol.*, 34: 332–333.

Osterholm, J.L. (1974) The pathophysiological response to spinal cord injury. The current status of related research. *J. Neurosurg.*, 40: 5–33.

Pappius, H.M. and Wolfe, L.S. (1983) Functional disturbances in brain following injury: search for underlying mechanisms. *Neurochem. Res.*, 8: 63–72.

Raz, A. and Livne, A. (1973) Differential effects of lipids on the osmotic fragility of erythrocytes. *Biochim. Biophys. Acta*, 311: 222–229.

Rehncrona, S., Westerberg, E., Akesson, B. and Siesjö, B.K. (1982) Brain cortical fatty acids and phospholipids during and following complete and severe incomplete ischemia. *J. Neurochem.*, 38: 84–93.

Rhoads, D.E., Kaplan, M.A., Petersen, N.A. and Raghupathy, E. (1982) Effects of free fatty acids on synaptosomal amino acid uptake systems. *J. Neurochem.*, 38: 1255–1260.

Rodriguez de Turco, E.B., Morelli de Liberti, S. and Bazan, N.G. (1983) Stimulation of free fatty acid and diacylglycerol accumulation in cerebrum and cerebellum during bicucullinc-induced status epilepticus. Effect of pretreatment with α-methyl-*p*-tyrosine and *p*-chlorophenylalanine. *J. Neurochem.*, 40: 252–259.

Rouser, G., Siakotus, V. and Fleischer, S. (1969) Quantitative analysis of phospholipids by thin layer chromatography and phosphorus analysis of spats. *Lipids*, 1: 85–86.

Saunders, R.D. and Horrocks, L.A. (1984) Simultaneous extraction and preparation for HPLC of prostaglandins and phospholipids. *Anal. Biochem.*, in press.

Schwartz, J.P., Mrsulja, B.B., Mrsulja, B.J., Passonneau, J.V. and Klatzo, I. (1976) Alteration of cyclic nucleotide-related enzymes and ATPase during unilateral ischemia and recirculation in gerbil cerebral cortex. *J. Neurochem.*, 27: 101–107.

Seligman, M.L., Flamm, E.S., Goldstein, B.D., Poser, R.G., Demopoulos, H.B. and Ransohoff, J. (1977) Spectrofluorescent detection of malonaldehyde as a measure of lipid free radical damage in response to ethanol potentiation of spinal cord trauma. *Lipids*, 12: 945–950.

Sheetz, M.P. and Singer, S.J. (1974) Biological membranes as bilayer couples. A molecular mechanism of drug-erythrocyte interactions. *Proc. Natl. Acad. Sci. USA*, 71: 4457–4461.

Shohami, E., Rosentahl, J. and Lavy, S. (1983) The effect of incomplete cerebral ischemia on prostaglandin levels in rat brain. *Stroke*, 13: 494–499.

Siesjö, B.K. (1981) Cell damage in the brain: a speculative synthesis. *J. Cereb. Blood Flow Metabol.*, 1: 155–185.

Siesjö, B.K. (1984) Cerebral circulation and metabolism. *J. Neurosurg.*, 60: 883–908.

Siesjö, B.K., Ingvar, M. and Westerberg, E. (1982) The influence of bicuculline-induced seizures on free fatty acid concentrations in cerebral cortex, hippocampus, and cerebellum. *J. Neurochem.*, 39: 796–802.

Spagnulo, C., Sautebin, L., Galli, G., Ralagni, G., Galli, C., Mazzari, S. and Finesso, M. (1980) PGF_2^z, thromboxane B_2 and HETE levels in gerbil brain cortex after ligation of common carotid arteries and decapitation. *Prostaglandins*, 18: 53–61.

Stokes, B.T., Fox, P. and Hollinden, G. (1983) Extracellular calcium activity in the injured spinal cord. *Exp. Neurol.*, 80: 561–572.

Sun, G.Y. (1970) Compositio of acyl groups in the neutral glycerides from mouse brain. *J. Neurochem.*, 17: 445–446.

Sun, G.Y. (1977) Metabolism of arachidonate and stearate injected simultaneously into the mouse brain. *Lipids*, 12: 661–665.

Sun, G.Y., Su, K.L., Der, O.M. and Tang, W. (1979) Enzymic regulation of arachidonate metabolism in brain membrane phospholipids. *Lipids*, 14: 229–235.

Toews, A.D., King, J.S., Yashon, D. and Horrocks, L.A. (1980) Myelin and microsomes from Rhesus monkey spinal cord: isolation and effects of trauma. *Neurol. Res.*, 1: 271–279.

Usher, J.R., Epand, R.M. and Papahadjopoulos, D. (1978) The effect of free fatty acids on the thermotropic phase transition of dimyristroyl glycerophosphocholine. *Chem Phys. Lipids*, 22: 245–253.

Van den Bosch, H. (1980) Intracellular phospholipases A. *Biochim. Biophys. Acta*, 604: 191–246.

Wakai, S., Aritake, K., Asano, T. and Takakura, K. (1982) Selective destruction of the outer leaflet of the capillary endothelial membrane after intra-cerebral injection of arachidonic acid. *Acta Neuropathol.*, 58: 303–306.

Walker, J.G., Yates, R.R. and Yashon, D. (1970) Regional canine spinal cord energy state after experimental trauma. *J. Neurochem.*, 33: 397–401.

Wei, E.P., Lamb, R.G. and Kontos, H.A. (1982) Increased phospholipase C activity after experimental brain injury. *J. Neurosurg.*, 56: 695–698.

Wheeler, K.P., Walker, J.A. and Barker, D.M. (1975) Lipid requirement of the membrane sodium-plus-potassium ion-dependent adenosine triphosphatase system. *Biochem. J.*, 146: 713–722.

White, R.P. and Hagan, A.A. (1982) Cerebrovascular actions of prostaglandins. *Pharmacol. Ther.*, 18: 313–331.

Wieloch, T. and Siesjö, B. (1982) Ischemic brain injury: the importance of calcium, lipolytic activities, and free fatty acids. *Pathol. Biol.*, 30: 269–277.

Wolfe, L.S. (1978) Some facts and thoughts on the biosynthesis of prostaglandins and thromboxanes in brain. In: F. Coceani and P. M. Olley (Eds.), *Advances in Prostaglandin and Thromboxane Research, Vol. 4*. Raven Press, New York, pp. 215–220.

Wolfe, L.S. (1982) Eicosanoids: prostaglandins, thromboxanes, leukotrienes, and other derivatives of carbon-20 unsaturated fatty acids. *J. Neurochem.*, 38: 1–14.

Yorio, T., Torres, S. and Tarapoom, N., (1980) Alterations in membrane permeability by diacylglycerol and phosphatidylcholine containing arachidonic acid. *Lipids,* 18: 96–99.

Yoshida, S., Inoh, S., Asano, T., Sano, K., Kubota, M., Shimazaki, H. and Ueta, N. (1980) Effect of transient ischemia on free fatty acids and phospholipids in the gerbil brain. Lipid peroxidation as a possible cause of post ischemic injury. *J. Neurosurg.*, 53: 323–331.

Yoshida, S., Abe, K., Busto, R., Watson, B.O., Kogure, K. and Ginsberg, M.D. (1982) Influence of transient ischemia on lipid-soluble antioxidants, free fatty acids, and energy metabolites in rat brain. *Brain Res.,* 245–307–316.

Yoshida, S., Harik, S., Busto, R., Santiso, M., Martinez, E. and Ginsberg, M.D. (1984) Free fatty acids and energy metabolites in ischemic cerebral cortex with noradrenaline depletion. *J. Neurochem.,* 42: 711–717.

Young, W., Yen, V. and Blight, A. (1982) Extracellular calcium ion activity in experimental spinal cord contusion. *Brain Res.,* 253: 105–113.

Cellular and molecular effects of polyunsaturated fatty acids in brain ischemia and injury

Pak Hoo Chan, Robert A. Fishman, Susan Longar, Sylvia Chen and Albert Yu

Brain Edema Clinical Research Center, Department of Neurology, University of California School of Medicine, San Francisco, CA 94143, USA

Introduction

It is generally recognized that the level of free polyenoic fatty acids (PUFAs) is very low in brain in situ. These PUFAs are usually localized at C-2 position of glycerol backbond in membrane phospholipids. It has been demonstrated that free PUFAs, especially arachidonic acid and docosahexaenoic acid are rapidly released following ischemia, electroconvulsive seizures and various pathological insults (Bazan, 1970, 1971; Bazan et al., 1971; Marion and Wolfe, 1979; Gardiner et al., 1981; Rehncrona et al., 1982; Tang and Sun, 1982; Yoshida et al., 1982; Chan et al., 1983a; Yoshida et al., 1983). The release of and accumulation of PUFAs arachidonic acid in particular is due the activation of phospholipase A_2 (Edgar et al., 1982; Au et al., 1985). It has been suggested that phosphatidylinositol-specific phospholipase C is also involved in the formation of diacylglycerols, the metabolic precursors of arachidonic acid (Sun et al., 1984). Other inositol phospholipids including phosphatidylinositol-4-phosphate and phosphatidyl-4,5-biphosphate may also be involved in the production of diacylglycerols (Nishizuka, 1984).

The role of polyunsaturated fatty acids in brain edema and injury

Free PUFAs, and arachidonic acid in particular, have both physiological and pathological effects on cellular systems. It has been demonstrated that free arachidonic acid readily intercalates into the membrane and produces significant changes in the packing of the lipid molecules (Usher et al., 1978; Klausner et al., 1980a, b). PUFA-induced membrane fluidity has been associated with the stimulation of chloride transport in corneal epithelium (Schaeffer and Zadunaisky, 1979) and it enhanced activities of both membrane-associated adenylate cyclase and guanylate cyclase (Wallach and Pastan, 1976; Anderson and Jaworski, 1977; Asakawa, 1978). Furthermore, free arachidonic acid has been postulated as a potential second messenger since it causes Ca^{2+} metabolization (Cheah, 1981) and activates Ca^{2+}-dependent protein kinase C (Mc Phail et al., 1984). These physiological functions of arachidonic acid are summarized in Fig. 1. Although the physiological effects of unsaturated fatty acids on various cellular systems are well documented, little is known about the pathological effects of high level PUFAs on CNS metabolism and function.

Using single cortical slices of the rat brain as a bioassay system in vitro, we have demonstrated that PUFAs, including linoleic acid (18:2), linolenic acid (18:3) and arachidonic acid (20:4) are potent inducers of cellular (cytotoxic) edema (Chan and Fishman, 1978; Chan et al., 1980). In these experiments, the edematous brain slices were characterized by increased sodium and decreased potassium contents. The [^{3}H]inulin space, an extracellular space marker, was also decreased significantly. Cel-

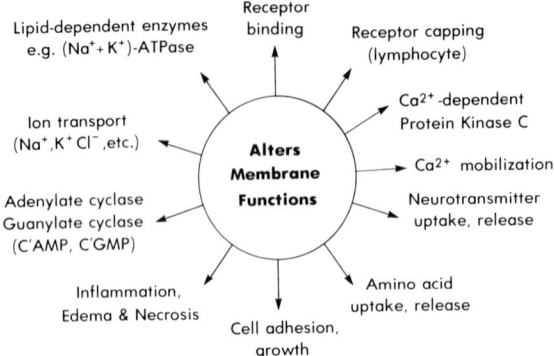

Fig. 1. Physiological and pathological functions of arachidonic acid in cellular systems.

lular metabolism was also affected: lactic acid levels were increased and high energy nucleotides were reduced. Both saturated fatty acids and monounsaturated fatty acids were not effective (Table 1).

From our in vitro studies we have concluded that high levels of PUFAs from damaged cell membrane are associated with the development of cellular brain edema. We have further studied the local effects of arachidonic acid on vasogenic edema in rats in vivo. Animals were infused with 0.05 mmol of saturated, monounsaturated or polyunsaturated fatty acids into thalamus, and the edema and cation levels were studied at 24 hours following the injection. Among the fatty acids, arachidonic acid was the most potent fatty acid in inducing cerebral edema concomitant with the increase in sodium and decrease in potassium contents (Table 2). A lesser degree of change in hemispheric water, sodium and potassium contents was seen after injection of linolenic acid (18:3). Oleic acid (18:1), palmitic acid (16:0) and nonanoic acid (9:0) were ineffective in inducing brain edema. Furthermore, arachidonic acid and linolenic acid caused 3-fold and 2-fold increases, respectively in [^{125}-I]albumin space at 24 hours in the injected hemisphere when compared with Krebs-Ringer (Table 2). Oleic acid, palmitic acid and nonanoic acid were not effective in altering blood-brain barrier permeability (Chan et al., 1983b).

Gross examination revealed that the hemispheres injected with PUFA were swollen, with evidence of compression of the ipsilateral ventricle. The edema dissected along the ipsilateral corpus callosum, expanding it two to three times its normal width. Microscopic examination of hemispheres injected with PUFA revealed a consistently abnormal area

TABLE 1

The role of polyunsaturated fatty acids in the development of cellular edema in brain slices

Fatty acid	Swelling (%)	Inulin space (%)	Lactic acid (mmol/kg dry wt)	Na$^+$ (mEq/kg dry wt)	K$^+$ (mEq/kg dry wt)
Control	11.3	46.11	236	599	393
Palmitic acid (16:0)	9.4	46.12	258	838^b	387
Oleic acid (18:1)	11.0	41.07^b	278^a	694^a	419
Linoleic acid (18:2)	32.5^b	33.47^b	519^b	1340^b	92^b
Linolenic acid (18:3)	26.0^b	42.88^b	391^b	949^b	188^b
Arachidonic acid (20:4)	35.2^b	32.6^b	527^b	1239^b	140^b
Docosahexaenoic acid	33.5^b	41.47^b	543^b	1215^b	77^b

Data obtained from Chan and Fishman, 1978.
^{a} $p < 0.02$, ^{b} $p < 0.001$, Student's t test.

TABLE 2

The role of polyunsaturated fatty acids in the development of vasogenic brain edema

Fatty acid	Water content (%)	[^{125}I]BSA space (%)	Na$^+$ (mEq/kg dry wt)	K$^+$ (mEq/kg dry wt)
Krebs-Ringer (Control)	79.5 ± 0.2	2.04 ± 0.1	241 ± 1	556 ± 2
Nonanoate (9:0)	79.1 ± 0.07	21.7 ± 0.02	248 ± 1	554 ± 1
Palmitate (16:0)	79.3 ± 0.07	2.30 ± 0.13	255 ± 1[a]	546 ± 1[a]
Oleate (18:1)	79.1 ± 0.08	2.40 ± 0.01[a]	265 ± 1[a]	536 ± 2[a]
Linolenate (18:3)	79.8 ± 0.04	4.25 ± 0.02[a]	278 ± 1[a]	320 ± 1[a]
Arachidonate (20:4)	80.6 ± 0.2[a]	6.68 ± 0.29[a]	284 ± 1[a]	258 ± 2[a]

Data obtained from Chan et al., 1983b.
All values are expressed as means ± SE of the mean.
[a] $p < 0.01$, compared to control group, Student's t test.

of neuropil 3 to 4 mm in diameter and centered at the tip of the needle (Fig. 2). The neuropil in this region stained poorly and contained cystic spaces. Ventriculocisternal perfusion with arachidonic acid produced a characteristic acute lesion consisting of ependymal disruption, subependymal edema, and local blood-brain barrier disruption as evidenced by Evans blue leakage from periventricular capillaries. Ventriculocisternal perfusion with Krebs-Ringer, or nonanoic acid did not cause any apparent periventricular injury (Martin et al., 1982). These morphological data indicate that PUFAs are potent inducers of membrane damage and may cause development of vasogenic edema.

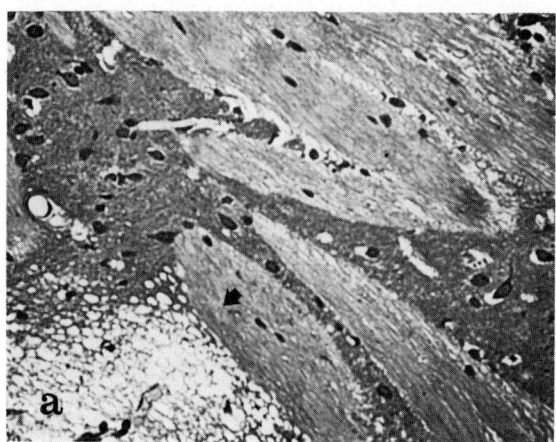 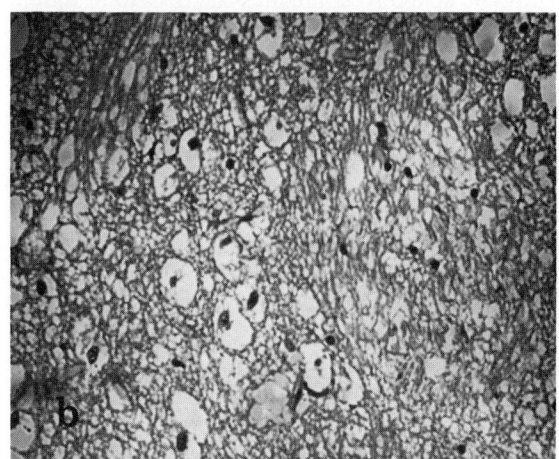

Fig. 2. Effects of arachidonic acid on microscopic morphology of corpus striatum at 24 hours. (a) Control animals injected with Krebs-Ringer buffer, arrow indicates area damaged by needle insertion; (b) animals injected with arachidonic acid (both × 160). (Data from Chan et al., 1983b.)

Molecular mechanisms of arachidonic acid induced brain edema

The molecular mechanisms of PUFA-induced cellular edema were studied further in our in vitro cortical slices system. The amphiphilic nature of the PUFA lead us to raise the question whether the development of brain edema is due to the alteration of membrane integrity by arachidonic acid. Our approach to this problem was to study neurotransmitter uptake and $(Na^+ + K^+)$-ATPase activity which are known to be associated with membrane functions. We have demonstrated that the addition of arachidonic acid (0.5 mM) caused a significant reduction of high affinity uptake of neurotransmitters GABA (γ-aminobutyric acid) and glutamate in brain slices and in synaptosomes (Chan et al., 1983c). However, the uptake of α-aminoisobutyric acid (AIBA), the non-metabolized amino acid, was not inhibited by arachidonic acid. The ID_{50} values for glutamic acid and GABA were 3.3×10^{-5} M and 4.1×10^{-5} M respectively, in synaptosomal preparations. This inhibitory effect of GABA uptake was partly counteracted by the membrane-stabilizing antioxidant, α-tocopherol (0.1 mM). These data suggest that 20:4-induced membrane perturbations play an important role in affecting GABA uptake. It has been shown by others that free arachidonic acid also stimulates the release of amino acids from synaptosomes (Rhoads et al., 1983a, 1983b). In order to address the question regarding the specificity of cellular vulnerability in various types of brain cells, we have recently developed primary cell cultures of both astrocytes and neurons from rats (Yu et al., 1985). Our preliminary studies have shown that arachidonic acid (0.01 mM) caused a significant reduction in GABA uptake in GABAergic neuronal cultures. The uptake of GABA in primary astrocytes was not affected. Furthermore, arachidonic acid also stimulates the release of prelabelled [^{3}H]GABA from primary neurons (Yu et al., 1985). These pilot experiments suggest that primary cell cultures are useful tools to study the functional vulnerability of various cell types in the central nervous system affected by arachidonic acid and other cellular factors.

Besides the uptake and release of neurotransmitter amino acids, we have also studied the effect of PUFAs on membrane-bound enzyme $(Na^+ + K^+)$-ATPase. Sodium arachidonate (20:4) and docosahexaenoate (22:6) were more effective in the reduction of $(Na^+ + K^+)$-ATPase in synaptosomes (Chan et al., 1983c). The inhibition of $(Na^+ + K^+)$-ATPase activity by arachidonic acid is temperature dependent. The transition temperature of 20°C and 25°C was obtained from the Arrhenius plot for control and 20:4-treated enzyme, respectively. These data indicate that the lipid fluidity of the membrane was affected by 20:4. The mechanism of the change is not clear since the incorporation of PUFA into membranes would increase membrane fluidity. These opposing findings suggest that the PUFA metabolites, especially oxygen radicals may be involved in causing the alteration of membrane integrity and fluidity.

Arachidonic acid as a precursor of oxygen radicals

Arachidonic acid, once released from membrane phospholipids, is readily metabolized to prostaglandins, thromboxanes via cyclooxygenase or to hydroxy, hydroperoxy fatty acids and leukotrienes (Gaudet and Levine, 1979; Ellis et al., 1983; Moskowitz et al., 1984). Prostaglandins and leukotrienes are involved in numerous physiological and pathological functions such as inflammation, membrane permeability, chemotaxis, microcirculating response, receptor binding, platelet aggregation and hormonal effects (Fig. 3) (Kuehl and Egan, 1980; Samuelsson, 1983). Furthermore, it has been proposed that a highly reactive oxygen radical species is formed during the conversion from PGG_2 to PGH_2 or from 5-hydroperoxyeicosatetroneic acid (5HPETE) to leukotriene A_4 (LTA_4) (Samuelsson et al., 1979; Kuehl and Egan, 1980). These active oxygen radical species further participate in radical propagation and membrane protein and lipid peroxidation, which are associated with degrading of membrane integrity (Mead, 1976; Freeman and Crapo, 1982). However, there was no direct

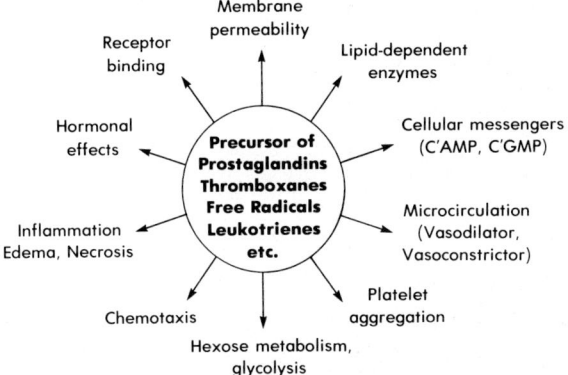

Fig. 3. Physiological and pathological functions of arachidonic acid metabolites in cellular systems.

TABLE 3

Superoxide radicals and lipid peroxidation in arachidonic acid incubated brain slices

Fatty acid	$O_2 \cdot -$ (nmol NBF/mg protein)	Malondialdehyde (nmol/mg protein)
Krebs Ringer (Control)	9.7 ± 0.6	5.3 ± 0.5
Palmitic acid (16:0)	10.1 ± 0.5	N.D.
Oleic acid (18:1)	9.0 ± 1.2	6.6 ± 0.9
Linoleic acid (18:2)	13.1 ± 1.3[a]	11.2 ± 0.6[a]
Linolenic acid (18:3)	14.4 ± 0.9[a]	N.D.
Arachidonic acid (20:4)	12.9 ± 0.7[a]	13.5 ± 0.7[a]
Docosahexaenoic acid (22:6)	N.D.	12.8 ± 1.7[a]

Data obtained from Chan and Fishman, 1980.
Mean ± SE. [a] $p < 0.001$, Students t test. N.D. not determined.

experimental evidence regarding the existence of oxygen-free radicals associated with arachidonic acid metabolism in the central nervous system (CNS). Our experimental approach to this problem was to investigate the possible formation of oxygen radicals and lipid peroxidation in arachidonic acid incubated CNS tissues. We have demonstrated that linoleic acid, linolenic acid, arachidonic acid and docosahexaenoic acid caused both significant increases in superoxide ($O_2 \cdot -$) formation and lipid peroxidation as measured by thiobarbituric acid reactive malondialdehyde (Table 3) (Chan and Fishman, 1980). Palmitic acid and oleic acid were not effective.

The role of oxygen radicals in membrane phospholipid degradation and brain edema

Lipid peroxidation has been shown to occur in cellular membranes of cerebral tissues in vitro (Kovachich and Mishra, 1980; Dirks and Faiman, 1982) and in vivo (Kogure et al., 1982; Watson et al., 1984). It has been hypothesized to be associated with membrane damage and increased endothelial permeability following ischemia and injury (Demopoulos et al., 1978, 1979, 1982; Willmore and Rubin, 1982; Yoshida et al., 1982). Little is known regarding the direct effect of oxygen radicals on cellular injury in CNS. Using an enzymatic free radical generating system including xanthine oxidase, hypoxanthine and ferric ions, we have studied the effects of oxygen radicals in cellular edema, lipid peroxidation, membrane phospholipid degradation and free fatty acid levels in rat brain slices. We have demonstrated that oxygen radicals produced by this enzymatic system stimulated both tissue swelling and malondialdehyde formation in incubated brain slices (Chan et al., 1982). Furthermore, membrane phospholipids were degraded concomitantly with the increases with PUFA in free fatty acid pool, as identified and measured by high performance liquid chromatography (HPLC) and capillary gas chromatography. The increased level of PUFA could be partially blocked by phospholipase A_2 inhibitors chloroquine and mepecrine, indicating that phospholipase A_2 was involved in free radical-mediated fatty acid release processes (Au et al., 1985). These in vitro data suggest a cyclic route for both arachidonic acid and oxygen radicals in cerebral tissue which may play a role in the delayed development

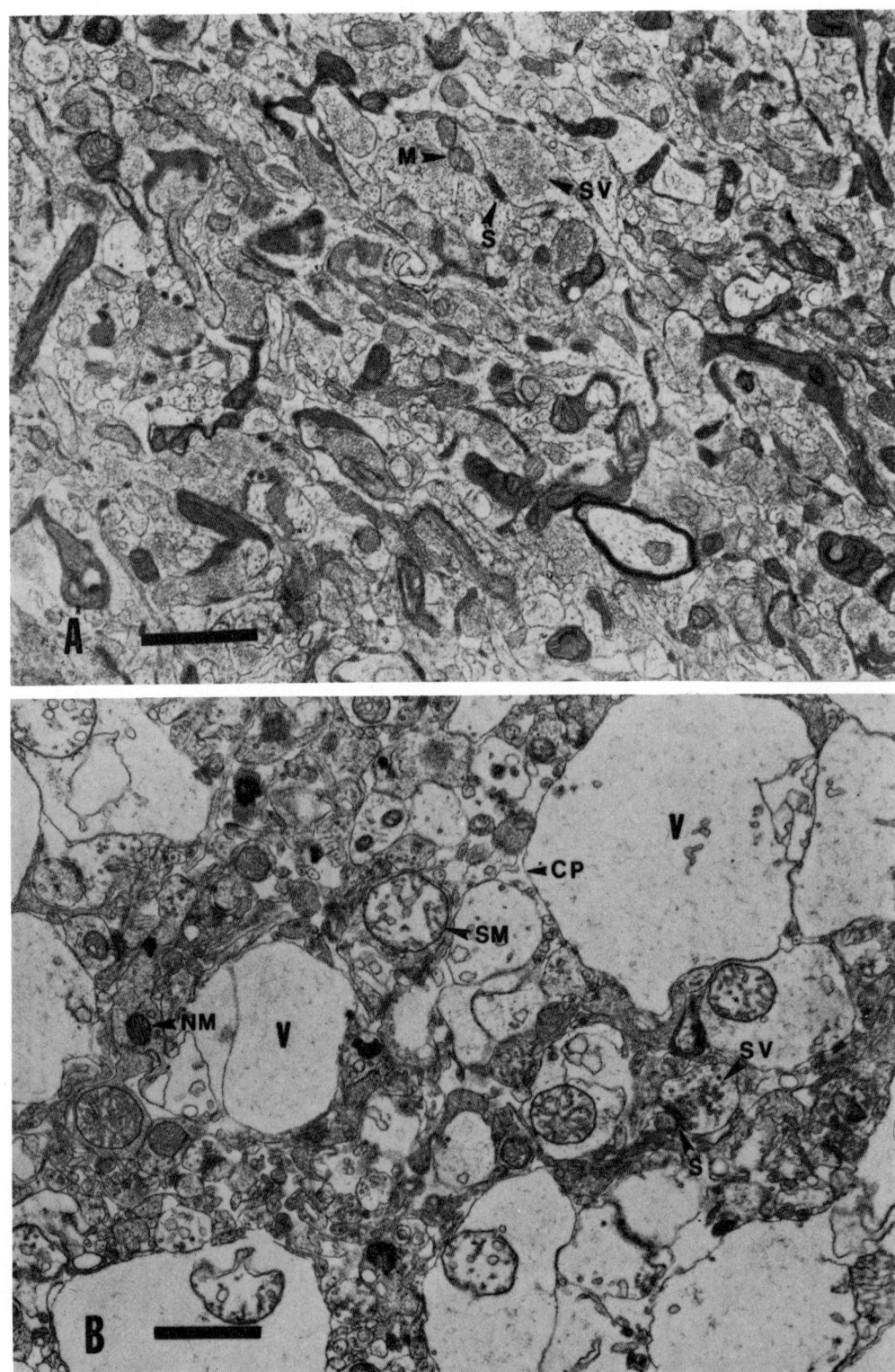

Fig. 4. Effects of oxygen radicals on ultrastructure of cortical slices. (A) Slice incubated in cortical medium for 60 min; M, normal mitochondria; S, synapse; SV, synaptic vesicles; scale bar, 5 μm. (B) Slice incubated in xanthine oxidase-Fe^{3+} system; CP, swollen cellular processes; NM, normal mitochondria; SM, swollen mitochondria; S, synapse; SV, synaptic vesicles; V, vacuole; scale bar, 5 μm. (Data from Chan et al., 1984a.)

of brain edema following in vivo injury. The ultrastructure of the molecular layer of slices exposed to the free radical generating system for 30 and 60 min was dominated by many obviously swollen cellular processes. These were generally empty, save for a few remnants of what appeared to be membranes and abnormal mitochondria. Most mitochondria were grossly swollen, with loss of normal electron density and fragmentation of cristae (Fig. 4).

The in vivo cerebral effects of oxygen radicals were further studied. Xanthine oxidase system was infused into caudate putamen followed by rapid in situ freezing (Pontén et al., 1973). Brain water and sodium content increased significantly concomitantly with decreased potassium content at 24 hours and 48 hours after the infusion. The degree of brain edema and injury depends on the dose of xanthine oxidase. Morpholgical studies further demonstrated that oxygen radicals damage both endothelial cells of blood-brain barrier as well as neurons and glia. The time course of cellular injury and edema was similar to that of the edema induced by cold injury (Chan et al., 1983) or by intracerebral infusion of arachidonic acid (Chan et al., 1983; Chan and Fishman, 1984). Staining of edematous region with fluorescent Evans blue was noted at 2 hours but little or no extravasation of Evans blue was observed at 24 hours or later, indicating that endothelial cell damage, perhaps mediated by free radicals, is an early event (Chan et al., 1984). Biochemical analysis of oxygen-injured caudate putamen further indicated the high level of free fatty acids, especially arachidonic acid and docosahexaenoic acid (Chan and Fishman, 1985a). These data thus support our in vitro studies that oxygen radicals stimulate the release of unsaturated fatty acids from membrane phospholipids. We have hypothesized that the arachidonic acid oxygen radical cycle may play an important role in cellular damage and the development of edema and necrosis following brain ischemia and injury (Chan and Fishman, 1985a) (Fig. 5).

Our studies have suggested that PUFAs, es-

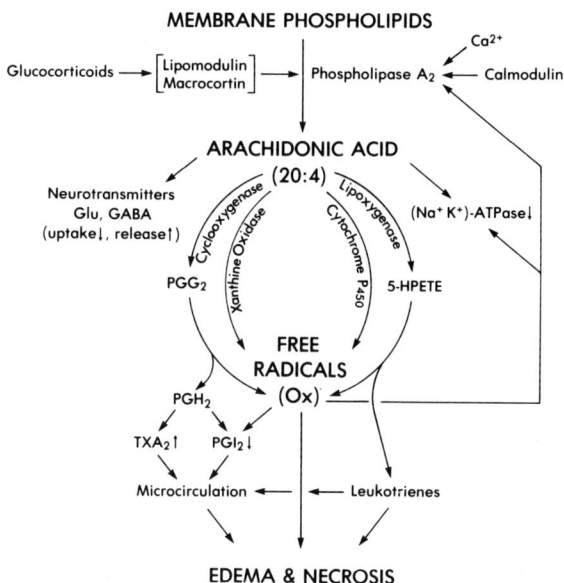

Fig. 5. Biochemistry of brain ischemia and injury.

pecially arachidonic acid, play a key role in membrane damage and the development of edema following ischemia and injury. The availability of residual oxygen during incomplete ischemia as well as the abundant oxygen during reperfusion will convert arachidonic acid to oxygen radicals (oxygen radicals could also be formed from disrupted mitochondria electron transport chain) which may then activate the membrane phospholipase A_2 (Chan and Fishman, 1985b). The latter step will generate more PUFAs (Fig. 5). However, this general hypothesis does not address the question of selective cellular vulnerability (e.g. neurons vs. glia, GABAergic neurons vs. glutamatergic neurons etc.) following ischemia and reperfusion. The use of various primary neuronal and glial cell cultures may be useful to address these questions.

Acknowledgements

This study was supported by USPHS Grant NS-14543. The assistance of Sheryl Colwell in the preparation of the manuscript is gratefully acknowledged.

References

Anderson, W.B. and Jaworski, C.J. (1977) Modulation of adenylate cyclase activity of fibroblasts by free fatty acids and phospholipids. *Arch. Biochem. Biophys.*, 180: 374–383.

Asakawa, T., Takenoshita, M., Uchida, S. and Tanaka, S. (1978) Activation of guanylate cyclase in synaptic plasma membranes of cerebral cortex by free fatty acids. *J. Neurochem.*, 30: 161–166.

Au, A.M., Chan, P.H. and Fishman, R.A. (1985) Stimulation of phospholipase A_2 activity by oxygen-derived free radicals in isolated brain capillaries. *J. Cell. Biochem.*, 27: 449–453.

Bazan, N.G. (1970) Effects of ischemia and electroconvulsive shock on free fatty acid pool in the brain. *Biochim. Biophys. Acta*, 218: 1–10.

Bazan, N.G. (1971) Changes in free fatty acids of the brain by drug-induced convulsions, electroshock and anesthesia. *J. Neurochem.*, 18: 1379–1385.

Bazan, N.G., Bazan, H.E.P., Kennedy, W.G. and Joel, C.D. (1971) Regional distribution and rate of production of free fatty acids in rat brain. *J. Neurochem.*, 18: 1387–1393.

Chan, P.H. and Fishman, R.A. (1978) Brain edema: induction in cortical slices by polyunsaturated fatty acids. *Science*, 201: 358–360.

Chan, P.H. and Fishman, R.A. (1980) Transient formation of superoxide radicals in polyunsaturated fatty acid-induced brain swelling. *J. Neurochem.*, 35: 1004–1007.

Chan, P.H. and Fishman, R.A. (1982) Alterations of membrane integrity and cellular constituents by arachidonic acid in neuroblastoma and glioma cells. *Brain Res.*, 248: 151–157.

Chan, P.H. and Fishman, R.A. (1984) The role of arachidonic acid in vasogenic brain edema. *Fed. Proc.*, 43: 210–213.

Chan, P.H. and Fishman, R.A. (1985a) Free fatty acids, oxygen free radicals and membrane alterations in brain ischemia and injury. In: F. Plum and W. Pulsinelli (Eds.), *Cerebrovascular Diseases* (14th Research Princeton Conference). Raven Press, New York, pp. 161–169.

Chan, P.H. and Fishman, R.A. (1985b) In: A. Lajtha (Ed.), *Handbook of Neurochemistry*, Vol. 10. Plenum Publ. Corp., New York, pp. 153–174.

Chan, P.H., Fishman, R.A., Lee, J. and Quan, S. (1980) Arachidonic acid-induced swelling in incubated rat brain cortical slices: effect of bovine serum albumin. *Neurochem. Res.*, 5: 629–640.

Chan, P.H., Yurko, M. and Fishman, R.A. (1982) Phospholipid degradation and cellular edema induced by free radicals in brain cortical slices. *J. Neurochem.*, 38: 525–531.

Chan, P.H., Longar, S. and Fishman, R.A. (1983a) Phospholipid degradation and edema development in cold-injured rat brain. *Brain Res.*, 277: 329–337.

Chan, P.H., Fishman, R.A., Caronna, J., Schmidley, J.W., Prioleau, G. and Lee, J. (1983b) Induction of brain edema following intracerebral injection of arachidonic acid. *Ann. Neurol.*, 13: 625–632.

Chan, P.H., Kerlan, R. and Fishman, R.A. (1983c) Reductions of γ-aminobutyric acid and glutamate uptake and $(Na^+ + K^+)$-ATPase activity in brain slices and synaptosomes by arachidonic acid. *J. Neurochem.*, 40: 309–316.

Chan, P.H., Fishman, R.A., Schmidley, J.W. and Chen, S.F. (1984a) Release of polyunsaturated fatty acids from phospholipids and alteration of brain membrane integrity by oxygen-derived free radicals. *J. Neurosci. Res.*, 12: 595–605.

Chan, P.H., Schmidley, J.W., Fishman, R.A. and Longar, S.M. (1984b) Brain injury, edema and vascular permeability changes induced by oxygen-derived free radicals. *Neurology*, 34: 315–320.

Cheah, A.M. (1981) Effect of long chain unsaturated fatty acids on the calcium transport of sarcoplasmic reticulum. *Biochim. Biophys. Acta*, 648: 113–119.

Demopoulous, H.B., Yoder, M., Gutman, E.G., Seligman, M.L., Flamm, E.S. and Ransohoff, J. (1978) The fine structure of endothelial surfaces in the microcirculation of experimentally injured feline spinal cords. *Scan. Electr. Microsc.*, 2: 667–682.

Demopoulous, H.B., Flamm, E.S., Seligman, M.L., Mitamura, J.A. and Ransohoff, J. (1979) Membrane perturbations in central nervous system injury: theoretical basis for free radicals damage and a review of the experimental data. In: A.J. Popp, R.S. Bourke, L.R. Nelson and H.K. Kimelberg (Eds.), *Neural Trauma*. New York, Raven Press, pp. 63–78.

Demopoulos, H.B., Flamm, E.S., Seligman, M.L. and Pietronigro, D.D. (1982) Oxygen free radicals in central nervous system ischemia and trauma. In: A.P. Autor (Ed.), *Pathology of Oxygen*. Academic Press, London, pp. 127–155.

Dirks, R.C. and Faiman, M.D. (1982) Free radical formation and lipid peroxidation in rat and mouse cerebral cortex slices exposed to high oxygen pressure. *Brain Res.*, 248: 355–360.

Edgar, A.D., Strosznajder, J. and Horrocks, L.A. (1982) Activation of ethanolamine phospholipase A_2 in brain during ischemia. *J. Neurochem.*, 39: 1111–1116.

Ellis, E.F., Wright, K.F., Wei, E.P. and Kontos, H.A. (1983). Cyclooxygenase products of arachidonic acid metabolism in cat cerebral cortex after experimental concussive brain injury. *J. Neurochem.*, 37: 892–696.

Freeman, B.A. and Crapo, J.D. (1982) Biology of disease. Free radicals and tissue injury. *Lab. Invest.*, 47: 412–426.

Gardiner, M., Nilsson, B., Rehncrona, S. and Siesjö, B.K. (1981) Free fatty acids in the rat brain in moderate and severe hypoxia. *J. Neurochem.*, 36: 1500–1505.

Gaudet, R.J. and Levine, L. (1979) Transient cerebral ischemia and brain prostaglandins. *Biochem. Biophys. Res. Commun.*, 86: 893–901.

Klausner, R.D., Bhalla, D.K., Dragsten, P., Hoover, R.L. and Karnovsky, M.J. (1980a) Model for capping derived from inhibition of surface receptor capping by free fatty acides. *Proc. Natl. Acad. Sci. USA*, 77: 437–441.

Klausner, R.D., Kleinfeld, A.M., Hoover, R.L. and Karnovsky, M.J. (1980b) Lipid domains in membranes. Evidence derived from structural perturbations induced by free fatty acids and lifetime heterogeneity analysis. *J. Biol. Chem.*, 255: 1286–1296.

Kogure, K., Watson, B.D., Busto, R. and Abe, K. (1982) Potentiation of lipid peroxides by ischemia in rat brain. *Neurochem. Res.*, 7: 437–454.

Kovachich, G.B. and Mishra, O.P. (1980) Lipid peroxidation in rat brain cortical slices as measured by the thiobarbituric acid test. *J. Neurochem.*, 35: 1449–1452.

Kuehl, F.A. and Egan, R.N. (1980) Prostaglandins, arachidonic acid, and inflammation. *Science*, 210: 978–984.

Marion, J. and Wolfe, L.S. (1979) Origin of the arachidonic acid released post-mortem in rat forebrain. *Biochim. Biophys. Acta*, 574: 25–32.

Martin, N.A., Schmidley, J.W., Wissig, S.L., Fishman, R.A. and Chan, P.H. (1982) Cerebral injury and blood brain barrier disruption induced by arachidonic acid: histopathology. *Ann. Neurol.*, 12: 110.

Mc Phail, L.C., Clayton, C.C. and Snyderman, R. (1984) A potential second messenger role for unsaturated fatty acids: activation of Ca^{2+}-dependent protein kinase. *Science*, 224: 622–625.

Mead, J.F. (1976) Free radicals mechanisms of lipid damage and consequences for cellular membranes. In; W.A. Pryor (Ed.), *Free Radicals in Biology*. Academic Press, New York, pp. 51–68.

Moskowitz, M.A., Kiwak, K.J., Herkimin, K. and Levine, L. (1984) Synthesis of compounds with properties of leukotrienes C_4 and D_4 in gerbil brains after ischemia and reperfusion. *Science*, 224: 886–889.

Nishizuka, Y. (1984) Turnover of inositol phospholipids and signal transduction. *Science*, 225: 1365–1370.

Pontèn, V., Ratcheson, R.A., Salford, L.G. and Siesjö, B.K. (1973) Optimal freezing conditions for cerebral metabolites in rats. *J. Neurochem.*, 21: 1127–1138.

Rehncrona, S., Westerberg, E., Åkesson, B. and Siesjö, B.K. (1982) Brain cortical fatty acids and phospholipids during and following complete and severe incomplete ischemia. *J. Neurochem.*, 38: 84–93.

Rhoads, D.E., Ockner, R.K., Peterson, N.A. and Raghupathy, E. (1983a) Modulation of membrane transport by free fatty acids: inhibition of synaptosomal sodium-dependent amino acid uptake. *Biochemistry*, 22: 1965–1970.

Rhoads, D.E., Osburn, L.D., Peterson, N.A. and Raghupathy, E. (1983b) Release of neurotransmitter amino acids from synaptosomes: enhancement of calcium-independent efflux by oleic and arachidonic acids. *J. Neurochem.*, 41: 531–537.

Samuelsson, B. (1983) Leukotrienes: mediators of immediate hypersensitivity reactions and inflammation. *Science*, 220: 568–575.

Samuelsson, B., Hammarstrom, S. and Borgeat, P. (1979) Pathway of arachidonic acid metabolism. *Adv. Inflam. Res.*, 1: 405–411.

Schaeffer, B.E. and Zadunaisky, J.A. (1979) Stimulation of chloride transport by fatty acids in corneal epithelium and relation to changes in membrane fluidity. *Biochim. Biophys. Acta*, 556: 131–143.

Sun, G.Y., Tang, W., Huang, S.F.-L. and Foudin, L. (1984) Is phosphatidylinositol involved in the release of free fatty acids in cerebral ischemia? In: J.E. Bleasdale, J. Eichberg and G. Hauser (Eds.), *Inositol and Phosphoinositides: Metabolism and Biological Regulation*. Humana Press, Clifton, New Jersey, in press.

Tang, W. and Sun, G.Y. (1982) Factors affecting the free fatty acids in rat brain cortex. *Neurochem. Int.*, 4: 269–273.

Usher, J.R., Epand, R.M. and Papahadjopoulos, D. (1978) The effect of free fatty acids on the thermotropic phase transition of dimyristoyl glycerophosphocholine. *Chem. Phys. Lipids*, 22: 245–253.

Wallach, D. and Pastan, I. (1976) Stimulation of guanylate cyclase of fibroblasts and free fatty acids. *J. Biol. Chem.*, 251: 5802–5809.

Watson, B.D., Busto, R., Goldberg, W.J., Santiso, M., Yoshida, S. and Ginsberg, M.D. (1984) Lipid peroxidation in vivo induced by reversible global ischemia in rat brain. *J. Neurochem.*, 42: 268–275.

Willmore, L.J. and Rubin, J.J. (1982) Formation of malonaldehyde and focal brain edema induced by subpial of $FeCl_2$ into rat isocortex. *Brain Res.*, 246: 113–119.

Yoshida, S., Abe, K., Busto, R., Watson, B D., Kogure, K. and Ginsberg, M.D. (1982) Influence of transient ischemia on lipid-soluble antioxidants, free fatty acids and energy metabolites in rat brain. *Brain Res.*, 245: 307–316.

Yoshida, S., Inoh, S., Asano, T., Sano, K., Shimasaki, H. and Ueta, N. (1983) Brain free fatty acids, edema, and mortality in gerbils subjected to transient, bilateral ischemia, and effect of barbiturate anesthesia. *J. Neurochem.*, 40: 1278–1286.

Yu, A.C.H., Chan, P.H. and Fishman, R.A. (1985) Arachidonic acid effect on amino acid uptake in cultured brain cells. *Trans. Am. Soc. Neurochem.*, 16: 197.

Free radical damage of the brain following ischemia

Kyuya Kogure[a], Hiroyuki Arai[a], Koji Abe[a] and Minoru Nakano[b]

[a]Department of Neurology, Institute of Brain Diseases, Tohoku University School of Medicine, 1-1 Seiryo-machi, Sendai 980, [b]College of Medical Care and Technology, Gunma University, 3-39-15 Showa-machi, Maebashi 371, Japan

Part I. Introduction — a background review

The human body mainly consists of lipids, proteins, and carbohydrates, but the brain largely consists of lipids, which account for 50% of the dry weight of this organ. Because the alkyl chain of lipids does not have polarity and because lipids are relatively inactive in vivo, they are one of the principal structural materials of living cells. For example, it is generally known that plasma membrane and membranes of intracellular micro-organelles are made of layers of lipid molecules (Van Deenen, 1966; Singer and Nicholson, 1972; Coleman, 1973). However, because a double bond of unsaturated fatty acid has high reactivity, it is liable to combine with hydrogen or other atoms and to split at the double bond due to oxidant action, for example, lipids become peroxide after combining with oxygen. If oxygen combines with $-CH_2-$ of saturated fatty acid in biomembrane, polarity of the area increases, and this part becomes more hydrophilic and chemically reactive, so that the membrane either functions abnormally or is destroyed.

On the other hand, oxygen molecules have high physical affinity for lipids, since oxygen has no polarity in the ground state. Therefore, it is thought that oxygen is brought to the vascular wall and tissue mainly solubilized in fatty membranes of erythrocyte and endothelium, and lipoproteins in plasma after the oxygen has dissociated from hemoglobin, and that membranes abundant in lipids are utilized as the route of oxygen transport from vascular walls to tissues and cells. As a result, partial pressure of oxygen in the hydrophobic part of the membrane (an alkyl chain of fatty acid) is higher than that in the rest of the cell, and this pressure (oxygen concentration) around mitochondria, which reduces oxygen to water by means of cellular respiration, is lower. In such circumstances, there may be the possibility of oxygen being nonspecifically captured by the biological membrane, especially by a part of the double bond, and of lipid peroxidation. In fact, it is well known that "nonspecific oxidation-induced injury of biological compound by oxygen", namely, hyaline degeneration of collagen fibers of the lung and the retina or hemolysis, occurs when a premature baby or animal which is artificially subjected to vitamin E deficiency is exposed to a high concentration of oxygen (Balentine, 1977). A small percentage of oxygen, which is in the ground state and comes into the body by systemic respiration, is activated or captured by free radical organic substances, and, as a result, can induce peroxidative reaction of lipids and proteins.[a]

---

[a] Oxygen peroxidizes the substrate in vivo by means of a reaction catalyzed by oxygenase. The dissociation energy of the oxygen molecule ($O=O$) is 118 kcal/mole and rather small (dissociation energy of $C=C$, $C=O$ and $N=N$ is 146, 178 and 225 kcal/mole, respectively). Organic compounds constituting the living body easily react with oxygen and disintegrate into oxygenate (CO_2 and water) and inorganic salt, given conditions of relatively low activation energy (for example, heating). These observations would indicate that oxygen is chemically ac- →

The process of destruction of biological membrane caused by free radical reaction or peroxidation is theoretically summarized in Fig. 1, and an autoxidation process in which alkyl radicals capture oxygen and proliferate, is explained as follows (Pryor, 1976) (see also Fig. 2):

(1) Initiation
$RH-H\cdot \rightarrow R\cdot$

(2) Propagation
$R\cdot + O_2 \rightarrow ROO\cdot$

$ROO\cdot + RH \longrightarrow ROOH + R\cdot$

(3) Termination
$R\cdot + R\cdot \rightarrow RR$
$R\cdot + ROO\cdot \rightarrow ROOR$
$ROO\cdot + ROO\cdot \rightarrow ROOR + O_2$

However, we have not yet been able to prove whether or not alkyl radicals ($R\cdot$) or alkoxy radicals ($ROO\cdot$) are produced in vivo in conditions of low oxygen concentration, because we could not observe production of conjugated diene, an index of peroxidation of lipids, when homogenates of fresh rat brains were incubated under anaerobic and anoxic conditions (Kogure et al., 1982). On the other hand — although there have been a number of reports regarding the formation of peroxidized lipids by active oxygen — what reaction is related to what entity has not yet been clarified, and this issue is still a topic of lively discussion among investigators.

→
tive. On the contrary, in fact, spontaneous reaction of the oxygen molecule in the ground state with an organic compound is not initiated in vivo without a catalyst. However, oxygen can be activated by metallic ion, e.g. iron, copper, etc., which generally exist in vivo (metal-O_2 complex, for example, $Fe^{2+}O_2 \rightleftarrows Fe^{3+}O_2$). And, after an organic compound becomes a free radical after hydrogenation catalyzed by metal, and especially after it produces a free radical with a carbon atom as the center, the compound can easily capture oxygen. Therefore, peroxidation of organic compounds can be expected to occur at any time and anywhere in a bio active subject with oxygen respiration. As a result, all living beings which utilize oxygen, necessarily need an adjusted defence line against oxygen toxicity.

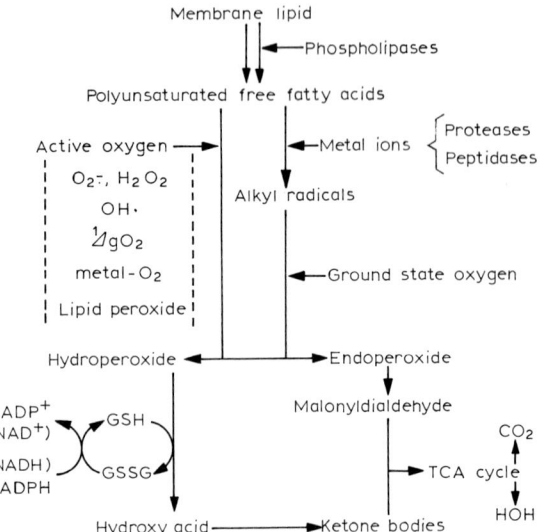

Fig. 1. Peroxidation of free fatty acids by hydroperoxide formation.

When an occlusive cerebrovascular accident occurs, the brain suffers from injury due to several mechanisms. Because the serum level of malondialdehyde is higher and that of vitamin E is lower in

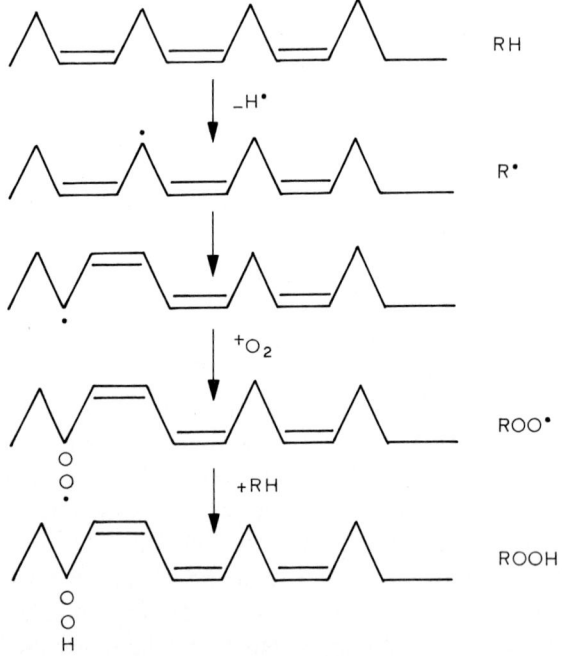

Fig. 2. Peroxidation of polyunsaturated fatty acid.

a patient with cerebrovascular injury as compared with levels in normal subjects, and because increases of conjugated diene, malondialdehyde and GSSG/GSH or decreases of vitamin C and E are observed in cerebral tissues of experimental animals, peroxidation of lipids is thought to be at least partially related to ischemic injury of the brain (Kogure et al., 1982; Demopoulos et al., 1977; Flamm et al., 1978).[b]

Demopoulos et al. (1977) have explained the mechanism of production of peroxidized lipids as follows: rapid oxygen deficiency induces electron stagnation in the mitochondrial electron transport system, and alkyl radicals (R·) are produced when coenzyme Q, which is reduced by one (unpaired) electron has left the chain of the electron transport system and removes hydrogen atoms from the unsaturated fatty acid of lipids composing the mitochondrial inner membrane. Therefore, the increasing level of R· results in the capture of the oxygen remaining in tissues, and autocatalytically facilitates peroxidation of lipids (Demopoulos et al., 1977; Flamm et al., 1978). These authors have suggested that enough oxygen molecules exist in ischemic tissues to cause a chain reaction in the stage of propagation. However, as previously described, the oxygen concentration around mitochondria, especially during ischemia, might be significantly lower than the mean concentration of oxygen in a tissue, and our experiment could not support their hypothesis. Provided that initiation of the reaction is independent of the production of alkyl radicals, peroxidized lipids should be generated by active oxygen species; however, this hypothesis can not be proved until the mechanism of activation of oxygen in ischemic tissues is defined. In order to clarify this issue, we have experimented using the rat cerebral ischemic model, Pulsinelli and Brierley.

Intra- and post-ischemic events

Rapid embolization of some of the cerebral vessels reduces blood flow in this area and results in ischemic lesions. However, since blood flow in the ischemic area is simultaneously restored by the collateral channel of the rami communicantes between the surrounding patent arteries and the peripheral site of the occluded ones, it is usually observed that such lesions gradually become smaller and that the degree of ischemia lessens. Fig. 3 represents examples of changes in rat cerebral blood flow just after the occurrence of embolization according to the embolic stroke model (Kogure et al., 1974). It is clear that metabolic abnormalities and processes resulting in tissue injury are remedied by the resumption of blood flow at a given time, at least, in areas surrounding the ischemic lesion.

If changes occurring at the point of ischemic lesion are considered, after being classified into intra-ischemic and post-ischemic changes, the approximate process of biological changes of a cell or a tissue existing at this point after occlusion can be generally observed using a model in which global brain ischemia is easily induced and blood flow is resumed optionally. In the present study, the model of Pulsinelli et al. (unpublished data) was adopted with the above factors in mind. However, there was a clear difference between the degree of recircula-

---

[b] Although the existence of peroxidized lipids in a sample is proved, it is unclear whether such lipids contribute to the destruction of the tissue or to the prevention of the destruction of the tissue. For example, in the rat embolic stroke model (Kogure et al., 1974) conjugated dienes significantly increase in the lesion about 4 hours after embolization (Kogure et al., 1982). This result is explained by the fact that some of oxygen brought by collateral channels is activated in ischemically injured tissue, and that this active oxygen peroxidizes free fatty acid which is thus removed from the biological membrane previously damaged by ischemia (Yoshida et al., 1980). However, it has not been clarified whether capture of active oxygen by free fatty acid prevents biological membrane injured by ischemia from being peroxidized, i.e., prevents enlargement of the injury by peroxidation, or whether peroxidized lipids themselves produced by this reaction contribute to secondary enlargement of membrane injury after the lipids initiate chain reactions of autoxidation which abstract hydrogen atoms from lipids constituting the membrane (cf. Fig. 3). Considering hydroperoxide and endoperoxide to be active oxygen species as shown in Fig. 2, we would like to discuss this question in this review.

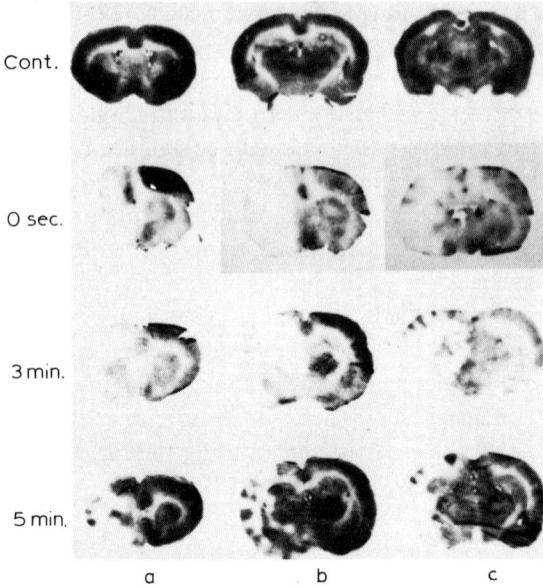

Fig. 3. Sequential cerebral blood flow changes in the rat brain following microsphere embolization.

tion in the brain and the degree of chronotropic change dependent on the duration of ischemia (Fig. 4), and this complicated the interpretation of the obtained biochemical data. Taking changes in cerebral blood flow and in biochemical indices in a preparatory experiment into consideration, we set the duration of ischemia at 5 min, 30 min and 2 hours, and observed changes 10 min and 1 hour after recirculation. These data were compared with those of the control groups. Initiation of energy metabolism in cerebral cells involves a reaction in which electrons are removed from glucose molecules by several processes. Namely, electrons are removed from substrates both in the protoplasmic glycolysis system and in the mitochondrial TCA cycle, and then flow into the electron transport-enzyme coenzyme system, which is located within the lipid layer of the mitochondrial inner membrane having a mosaic structure (Coleman, 1973), resulting in the reduction of oxygen to water in the terminal (cytochrome aa_3). Energy of this electron flow is utilized in the reaction which couples ADP and inorganic phosphorus in several steps and converts them to ATP. Four electrons are necessary for

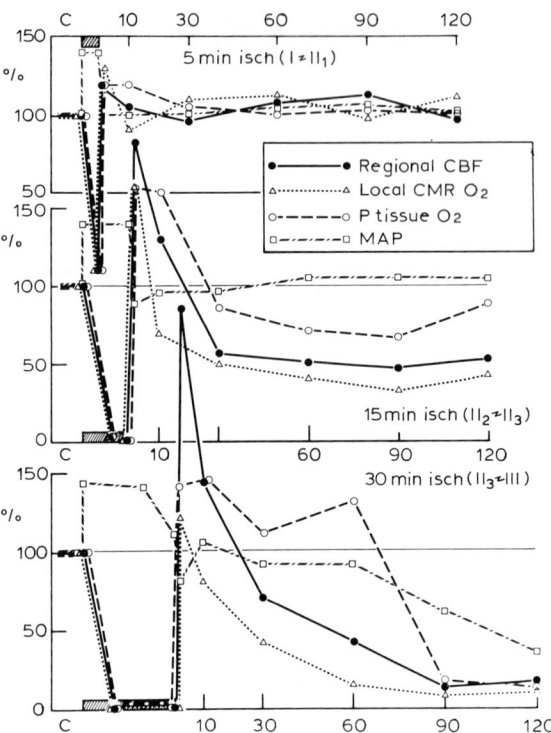

Fig. 4. Post-ischemic changes in cerebral blood flow, CMR O_2, $PO_{2(cortex)}$ and blood pressure in the modified Pulsenelli-Brierley preparation.

an oxygen molecule to be reduced to water by cytochrome aa_3. Intermediates produced by one-electron reduction (O_2^-) or two-electron reduction (H_2O_2 and $OH \cdot$) are chemically unstable and are regarded as being highly active oxygen species. Since ischemia decreases the supply of oxygen, electrons do not flow and are accumulated in the electron transport system. This increasing ratio of $[e^-]/[O_2]$ during ischemia is not thought to enhance production of active oxygen species. Therefore, we have speculated that active oxygen species are generated in the post-ischemic stage when oxygen is resupplied to the ischemic lesion by collateral circulation. In this case, three possible mechanisms of incomplete reduction (activation) of oxygen molecules are considered, namely (a) ischemia-induced metabolic injury prevents removal of electrons from substrates, so that only a small number of electrons are combined with oxygen (a decrease in ratio of $[e^-]/[O_2]$. (b) Although electrons flow into the electron transport system after removal from the substrate, the leakage of electrons from ischemically injured electron transport system (mitochondrial inner membrane) reduces oxygen heterotopically and incompletely, or (c) an obnormal change in cytochrome aa_3 during ischemia prevents electrons from normal transport to oxygen molecules, i.e. oxygen is not reduced or removed from oxygenase and remains a reduction intermediate.

In the first mechanism, the electron transport system is suspected of being empty, i.e., overoxidized. In the second and third mechanisms, redox state in the electron transport system are thought to be normal or rather reduced in the face of re-oxygenation. Therefore, we determined the redox state of the electron transport system in post-ischemia by means of NADH tissue fluorescent photography (Welsh et al., 1977a, 1977b).

NADH tissue fluorescent photography

Data of NADH tissue fluorescent photography are shown in Fig. 5(a, b, and c). Because fluorescent photographs taken at the end of 5 min of ischemia and at the end of 10 min of recirculation were normal, the redox state of the $NADH/NAD^+$ system in mitochondria in those cases was suspected of being normal. Since decapitation resulted in an instantaneous increase in fluorescent intensity in these brains which were frozen with liquid nitrogen 0 seconds after decapitation, electron flow in their electron transport system was assumed to be sufficient as compared with that in the control. On the contrary, NADH fluorescent intensity obtained 10 min after recirculation following ischemia for 30 min was weaker and increased more slowly after decapitation as compared with results for the control. These results suggested that the amount of electrons which the substrate in the brain could release into the electron transport system significantly decreased following ischemia for 30 min (example shown in Fig. 6, ①, and that the electron transport system was overoxidized. In case of recirculation for 10 min following ischemia for 2 hours (Fig. 5c), NADH tissue fluorescent photography still had

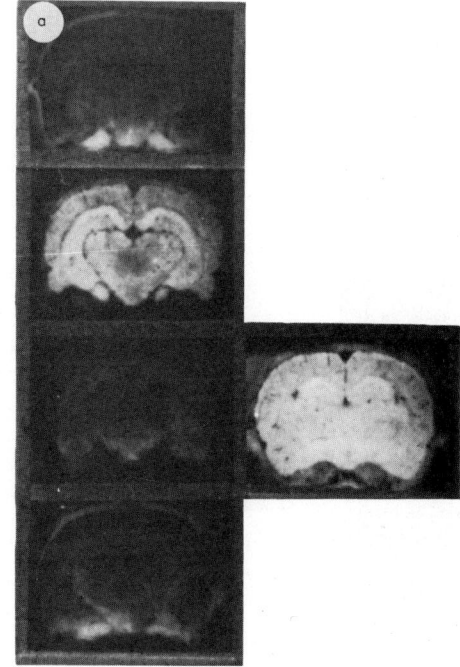
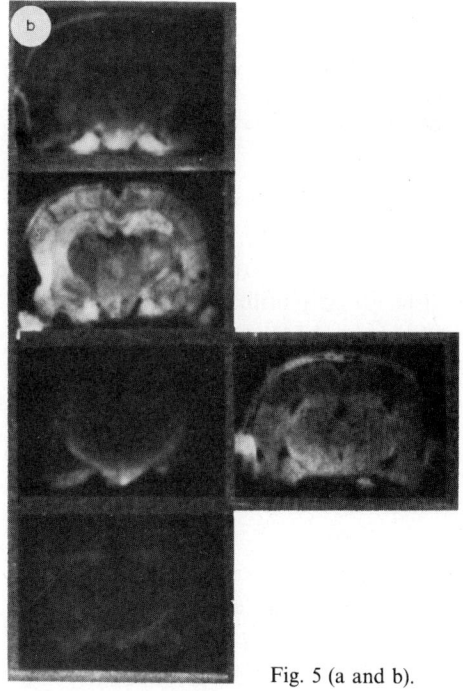

Fig. 5 (a and b).

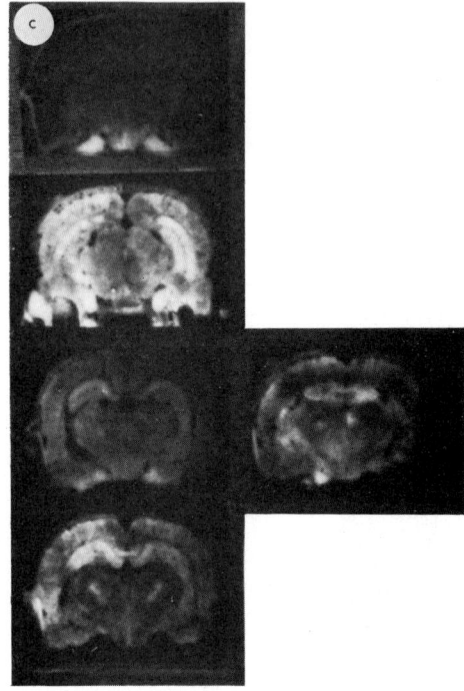

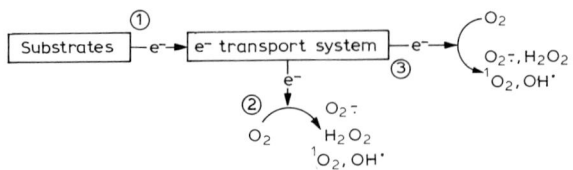

Fig. 6. Three hypothetical steps in the electron transport system which may cause superabundant active oxygen formation during post-ischemic tissue perfusion: ① inhibition of dehydrogenases by ischemic products, ② leakage of electrons from the respiratory chain, ③ ischemic injury in cytochrome oxidase.

Fig. 5 (a, b and c). Representatives of the series of NADH tissue fluorescent pictures from the control brain (top of the left column), taken at the end of 5 min (a), 30 min (b) and 120 min (c) of ischemia (2nd on the left column), 10 min (3rd row) and 60 min (bottom of the left column of each set) after recirculation, and at zero time after decapitation at the end of 10 min of recirculation (attached to the right side of the 10-min recirculation pictures). This photographic method should not be used for quantitative assessment of the change.

great intensity and showed no change after decapitation. It is clearly indicated that almost none of the oxygen transported by recirculation after ischemia (cf. Fig. 4) was utilized: in fact, cerebral oxygen consumption (CMR O_2) was zero. It is assumed that the electron transport system which could carry electrons following ischemia for 30 min, as shown by the fact that the resupply of oxygen resulted in a decrease in ratio of $2e^-$ production/$2e^-$ clearance and in overoxidation of the electron carriers, was destroyed and could not carry electrons after ischemia for 2 hours, and apparent increase in $2e^-$ production/$2e^-$ clearance. If electron leakage from the electron transport system and heterotopic reduction of oxygen due to this leakage were to take place as shown in Fig. 6, ②, this phenomenon would be observed in this stage. Since few electrons are removed from substrates and there is hardly any flow of electrons into cytochrome aa_3 in this stage, there may be a little incompletely reduced oxygen as shown in Fig. 6, ③.

Inhibition of glycolysis by ischemia and its significance

Why is oxidation of substrates not smoothly resumed after recirculation following ischemia? In order to answer this question, we investigated changes in intermediates of cerebral energy metabolism mainly in the electron transport system during and after ischemia. Fig. 7 indicates variation of glucose-6-phosphate (G-6-P) in the first step of glycolysis and of pyruvate, the terminal product of glycolysis. Concentration of G-6-P decreases by half during the 5 min duration of ischemia, but only slightly during the following 25 min. Oxygen deficiency in cellular respiration facilitates glycolysis according to the Pasteur effect (Krebs, 1972; Duffy et al., 1972). However, the data shown in Fig. 7 suggest that activity of facilitated glycolysis decreases for some reason 5 min after ischemia. (Concentration of pyruvate significantly decreases, while G-6-P concentration is constant. It is thought that pyruvate decreases because removal of electrons from intermediates of glycolysis is inhibited and conversion to pyruvate does not occur.) When oxygen deficiency terminates cellular respiration, the cell oxidizes cytoplasmic NADH to NAD^+ by means of the reduction of pyruvate to lactate.

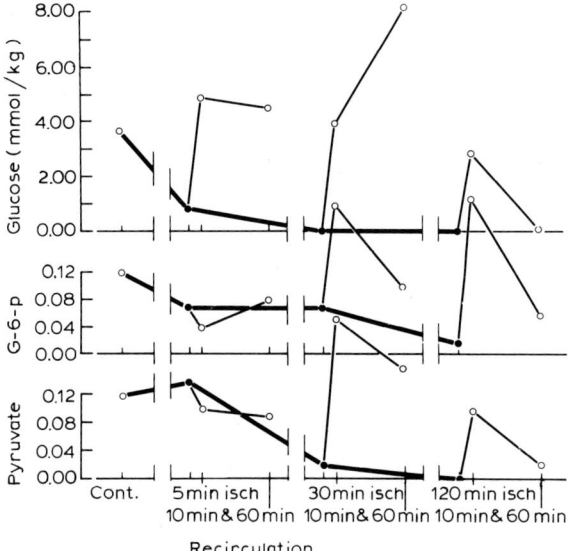

Fig. 7. Changes in glucose, glucose-6-phosphate and pyruvate content in the rat brain at the end of 5 min, 30 min, and 120 min of ischemia, and 10 and 60 min after recirculation in the modified Pulsinelli-Brierley preparation.

Therefore, it has been thought that glycolysis can be continued as long as substrates are available for conversion into pyruvate. In fact, Fig. 8 shows that the concentration of lactate rises to a level 7 times that of the normal level 5 min after ischemia. However, it is unlikely that oxidation of NADH (i.e.,

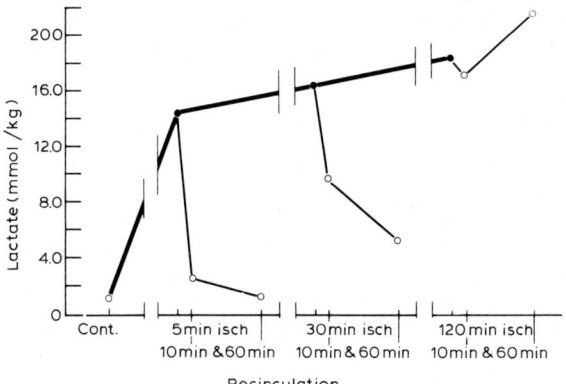

Fig. 8. Changes in lactic acid concentration in the rat brain at the end of 5 min, 30 min, and 120 min of ischemia, and 10 and 60 min after recirculation in the modified Pulsinelli-Brierley preparation. Lingering lactic acid following 120 min of ischemia could be a sign of mitochondrial dysfunction.

reduction of pyruvate) occurred to that degree by lactate dehydrogenase (1, 1, 1, 27) during ischemia from 5 min to 30 min after onset, when the rate of increase of lactate was only 10%. Pyruvate is not only reduced to lactate but is also transaminated to alanine, and converted into malate after carboxylation by NADH-malate dehydrogenase (1, 1, 1, 40), or directly converted into oxaloacetate after carboxylation by pyruvate carboxylase (6, 4, 1, 1), a reaction which occurs in mitochondria in need of ATP and acetyl-CoA and inhibited by accumulation of ADP. Additionally, phosphoenolpyruvate is converted into oxaloacetate by phosphoenolpyruvate carboxylase (4, 1, 1, 32). When these reactions are stimulated during ischemia, even if temporarily (Fig. 9), the amount of pyruvate available for the oxidation of cytoplasmic NADH seems to

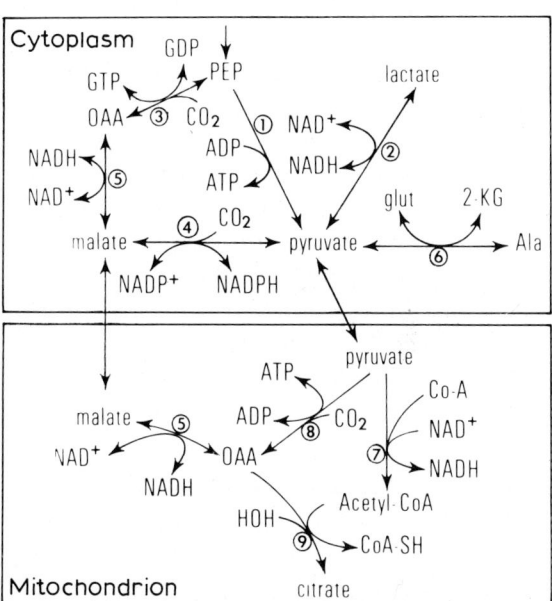

Fig. 9. Reactions of pyruvic acid. PEP, phospho-enolpyruvate; OAA, oxaloacetic acid; Ala, alanine; ①, pyruvate kinase (2, 7, 1, 40); ②, L-lactate dehydrogenase (1, 1, 1, 27); ③, phosphoenolpyruvate carboxylase (4, 1, 1, 32); ④, malate dehydrogenase (1, 1, 1, 40); ⑤, malate dehydrogenase (1, 1, 1, 37); ⑥, alanine aminotransferase (2, 6, 1, 2); ⑦, pyruvate dehydrogenase (1, 2, 4, 1); ⑧, pyruvate carboxylase (6, 4, 1, 1); ⑨, citrate synthetase (4, 1, 3, 7). Aspartate aminotransferase (2, 6, 1, 1) which catalyzes OAA ↔ aspartic acid, also plays an important role in reactions of pyruvic acid.

be insufficient. These reactions would result in a decrease in cytoplasmic NAD^+, and finally inhibit glycolysis as oxidation (electron abstraction) by glyceraldehyde-3-phosphate dehydrogenase (1, 2, 1, 12) becomes a new rate-limiting step. These hypotheses are well supported by the following observation: CO_2 and NH_3 accumulate in ischemic tissues and concentrations of alanine and malate significantly increase in such tissues (Duffy et al., 1972; Norberg et al., 1975; Folbergrová et al., 1974). Since these changes seem to be completed in a comparatively early stage in about the first 10 min in Pulsinelli's model (unpublished data), we have regarded this stage as being the first phase in the second biochemical disease stage of ischemia.

There are not thought to be any other disorders of the electron transport system in this phase. After oxygen is resupplied by recirculation, cytoplasmic NADH is oxidized to NAD^+ by the H_2-transport shuttle system and by the mitochondrial electron transport system. Because this reaction smoothly resumes oxidation of substrates and enables the electron transport system to supply oxygen with sufficient electrons (normal ratio of $[e^-]/[O_2]$), oxygen is scarcely activated by incomplete reduction. Partial pressure of oxygen in the tissue and in the sinus venosus is rapidly normalized.

Metabolic dissociation of cytoplasma and mitochondria

Fig. 10 shows changes in the concentration of α-ketoglutarate (2-KG) and oxaloacetate (OAA), compounds which make up the H_2-transport system, during ischemia. It indicates that 2-KG and OAA decrease by half during the first 5 min of ischemia and almost disappear during the next 25 min. Therefore, recirculation in this stage cannot result in cellular oxidation of cytoplasmic NADH. And, since there is an insufficient flow of electrons in the mitochondrial electron transport system, the ratio of $[e^-]/[O_2]$ in cytochrome aa_3 decreases, and oxygen is liable to be activated by this incomplete reduction[c]. Incidentally, the TCA cycle can not be operated under the conditions described above, because mitochondrial oxidation of pyruvate has a stoichiometric relation to the oxidation of cytoplasmic NADH by the H_2-transport system and mitochondrial electron transport system (Williamson et al., 1971). Recirculation occurring in the second phase of the second disease stage of ische-

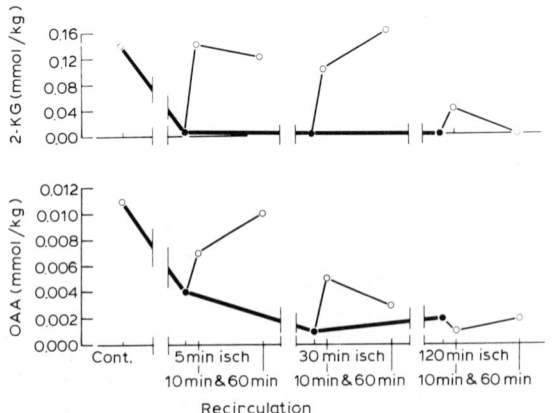

Fig. 10. Changes in α-ketoglutarate and oxaloacetic acid concentrations in the rat brain at the end of 5 min, 30 min, and 120 min of ischemia, and 10 and 60 min after restoration of blood flow in the modified Pulsinelli-Brierley preparation.

---

[c] Several biological defensive mechanisms against toxicity caused by active oxygen have developed during evolution. For example, superoxide dismutase defends against O_2, and glutathione peroxide acts against H_2O_2 and hydroperoxide. α-Tocopherol (vitamine E), β-carotene and hydroquinone counteract O_2. (In case of HO, its scavenger is an entity which does not injure biological functions or structures after oxidation of several kinds of carbohydrates, fatty acids, amino acids and proteins. Cf. Footnote [b]). Additionally, there is a mechanism controlling the quantity of oxygen (oxygen concentration): oxygen is transported to oxygen-reducing protein, namely, mitochondria and enzymes (not mentioned in this report) located in the endoplasmic reticulum, etc., thus preventing oxygen from increasing to more than the K_m value of these enzymes. This is one of the most important defensive mechanisms. This consideration indicates the importance of cells in the consumption of oxygen, as well as the importance of their role as gates in the oxygen pathway. Destruction of cells largely indicates a partial lack of the defence line described above. There is a possibility of secondary expansion of an injury by oxygen in such cells.

mia is characterized by a significant decrease in NADH fluorescent intensity (Fig. 5b) and in cerebral oxygen consumption, and by red bright venous blood (Waltz, 1969; Sundt et al., 1969).

Taking into account the relation of the disease stages to the solid structure of the lesion, it is thought that the disease stage does not reach this point in areas where recirculation by collateral circulation is resumed at an early point. Formation of active oxygen in the second phase of the second disease stage and a resulting dangerous state of peroxidation of lipids may occur in areas where resumption of collateral circulation is delayed or in areas with incomplete ischemia where recirculation is insufficient for tissue demand. Especially, in the latter case, ischemia is thought to be gradually completed over a period of several hours or several days.

Mitochondrial injury and formation of active oxygen

When the mitochondrial electron transport system is injured by ischemia, accumulated electrons in this system cannot flow into cytochrome aa_3 in spite of the resupply of oxygen by recirculation: oxygen is not reduced in this system (Fig. 6, ③). The degree of NADH tissue fluorescent intensity after recirculation is as great as that during ischemia, as shown in Fig. 5c. In this stage, lactate concentration does not decrease after recirculation; this seems to prove the existence of mitochondrial injury (Siesjö, 1978). If lipids are peroxidized by undirected radicals from the electron transport system — one electron reduction according to the mechanism suggested by Demopoulos et al. (1977) — it is likely that such peroxidation does not occur during ischemia, but rather after recirculation in the third phase of the second disease stage of ischemia. And in this case, there is the possibility that the oxygen reaction resulting in the abstraction of electrons precedes the reaction which results in the removal of electrons from lipids. Oxygen molecules resupplied through the hydrophobic lipid layer react with metal[d] and produce active oxygen (metal-O_2 complex) in protein in which hydroxylation is initiated by lysosomal enzymes

$$\text{metal}^{n+}*O_2 \rightleftarrows \text{metal}^{(n+1)} + O_2^-$$

It seems natural that cells would be irreversibly injured in this stage. However, since there are hundreds of mitochondria in a cell and their disorders vary, we regard the necrosis phase as being the one after the second disease stage of ischemia when cells themselves break up. We suspect that, practically, such severely injured tissue is perfused or that some vessels carry blood to remote areas through such tissue. Therefore, such lesions probably injure neighbouring tissues because the active oxygen and/or its pathological products passing through the vessel wall induces abnormality of the coagulant system in the circulating blood.

Our investigation has indicated that (a) when an ischemic focus develops in the brain, part of this lesion is exposed to post-ischemic perfusion by collateral circulation; and that (b) when restoration of recirculation is delayed, secondary extension of the ischemic lesion may be brought about by peroxidation of the tissue after activation of resupplied oxygen. However, what we have presented here, including my opinion and conjecture, shows the only possibility to be that cerebral ischemic lesions activate oxygen. Neither production of active oxygen species, nor the process of lipid peroxidation by active oxygen has been experimentally proved. What we really want to know has not yet been clarified.

Part II. Lipid-protein interaction in peroxidation of the brain tissue

Most of the free radicals generated are very transient and readily disappear in the biological system, which makes their in vivo detection especially difficult. If excited species are generated in the process of free radical reactions, some of them will emit light during their return to the ground state. At least two excited species have been reported to be produced during lipid peroxidation in which lipid peroxy rad-

---

[d] $*O_2$ is thought to be active oxygen (Pryor, 1976), to which the d electron of metal is pushed by half and whose electron arrangement is similar to $^1\Delta_g O_2$. On the other hand, O_2^- is not thought to oxidize lipids.

icals (ROO·) are involved. These are excited carbonyl and singlet molecular oxygen (Sugioka and Nakano, 1976). Free radical damage to the central nervous system is thought to occur after multiple embolization in the injured hemisphere (Kogure et al., 1982). Thus, it may be possible to investigate the free radical reactions, such as lipid peroxidation, which occur in the brain of living animals, using a photon counting system.

The present work was undertaken to detect and measure the chemiluminescence emitted from the brain surface subjected to embolic cerebral stroke. To investigate and examine the source of excited species in such a brain, chemiluminescence and its detailed spectrometry were undertaken during the oxygenation of a brain homogenate. In addition, lipid peroxidation and protein denaturation were also investigated in the homogenate. The possibility of the generation of free radicals during lipid peroxidation was also presented.

Materials and methods

(1) Chemiluminescence measurement using an in vivo system

Male Wistar rats weighing 250–300 g, which had been maintained on a commercial diet, were used in this study. Animals were immobilized by an intraperitoneal injection of pancuronium bromide (0.8 mg/kg) under light ether anesthesia. The rats were then tracheotomized and connected to a rodent respirator for artificial ventilation. Rectal temperature was controlled 37°C by means of a heat mat. The right internal carotid artery was selectively cannulated with PE-50 polyethylene tube with no interference to the common carotid flow (Kogure et al., 1974). The right parietal and temporal bones were carefully removed with a dental drill so that the dura underlying was untouched. Thereafter, the right femoral artery was cannulated for blood sampling. After heparinization through the femoral cannula, $P_{a(O_2)}$ $P_{a(CO_2)}$ and pH were maintained at 105 ± 10, 40 ± 4 and 7.4 ± 0.005 mmHg, respectively. Then, the head of the animal was accomodated in the chemiluminescence analyzer (OX-71, Tohoku Electronic Company, Japan) in a prone position (Inaba et al., 1982). A bundle of fibre optics as a light guide was positioned just above the exposed brain surface so that the photons emitted from the brain could reach the photomultiplier without diffusion. When a steady control state was achieved, photons from the brain were counted continuously throughout the experiment. Latex microspheres, 40 μm in diameter, suspended in the rats' own serum, were then injected slowly into the brain through the carotid tube. The chemiluminescence was measured during 4 hours after embolization in the dark.

(2) Preparation of brain homogenate

In order to exclude the uncertain effects of blood in the intracranial vessels, a small amount of ice-cold 0.15 M KCl was perfused through the outflow tract of left ventricle. After decapitation brain was rapidly removed within 2 min. The cerebellum and the caudal portion from midbrain were not used in the present study. After weighing the brain, a 10% brain homogenate (w/v) was prepared in 0.1 M Tris-HCl buffer at pH 7.4, using a motor-driven glass pestle homogenizer. Two or three ml of 10% homogenate were used for luminescence measurements.

(3) Treatment of brain homogenate with organic solvents

Lipid was extracted according to the method of Folch (Folch et al., 1957). Thirty ml of chloroform-methanol (2:1, v/v) was added to 1 ml of 10% brain homogenate. After shaking vigorously, the mixture was centrifuged at 3000 rpm for 20 min to obtain the lipid-rich fraction (chloroform layer). The methanol-water layer (the supernatant) was then washed with 0.9% NaCl and the resulting upper layer was washed with chloroform. Both chloroform layers were combined (lipid fraction) and stored at −20°C under N_2 before use. An acetone powder of the brain homogenate was prepared at low temperature by the method of Morton (Morton, 1955) and stored in a vacuum desiccator at −20°C. Just before chemiluminescence measurements were made, organic solvent in the lipid fraction was evaporated in vacuo and the resulting lipid film in 0.1 M Tris-HCl buffer (pH 7.4) was treated with a sonic oscillator to prepare liposomes (Sugioka and Nakano, 1976) and the acetone powder was suspended in 0.1 M Tris-HCl buffer (pH 7.4) and dispersed with the aid of a sonic oscillator.

(4) Measurement of chemiluminescence intensity and its spectrum using brain homogenate and extracts

Brain homogenate, liposomes or acetone powder in Tris-HCl buffer were placed at the front of the photomultiplier and the resulting luminescence was measured by flushing 100% oxygen continuously in the dark, using the same chemiluminescence analyzer as mentioned above. Chemiluminescence intensity in the visible region was expressed as counts per 10 seconds. The integrated light intensity was observed by tracing the light intensity change (as a function of time) on homogeneous paper and weighing. The luminescence spectrum was taken as previously described (Nakano et al., 1975; Inaba et al., 1979).

(5) SDS-polyacrylamide gel electrophoresis for brain proteins

10% brain homogenate (2 ml) was mixed with pure ethanol (10 ml) and kept at $-20°C$ for 12 hours. After centrifuging at 3000 rpm for 15 min, the resulting pellet was washed twice with ethanol-water (4:1, v/v). An aliquot of the ethanol suspension was evaporated to dryness in a vacuum desiccator. Dried protein was then dissolved in 0.0625 M Tris-HCl buffer (pH 6.8) containing 9 M urea, sodium dodecyl sulfate (SDS, 0.1%), α-mercaptoethanol (0.5%) and bromophenol blue (0.01%). The sample was electrophoresed on a slab gel electrophoretic apparatus according to the method of Laemmli (Laemmli, 1970). The protein bands on the gel were stained by brilliant blue 250. The protein was determined according to the method of Lowry (Lowry et al., 1951).

(6) Electron spin resonance (ESR) spectrometry

ESR spectra were taken at room temperature with a Varian E-109 spectrometer at 100 kHz field modulation. ESR settings were a magnetic field of 3371 G, a microwave power of 12 mW, a microwave frequency of 9.438 GHz and a modulation amplitude of 1.25 G.

(7) Other assays

Thiobarbituric acid reactive substance (TBARS), -SH group content and ascorbate (oxidized and reduced form) content were measured according to the methods of Ohkawa et al. (1979), Grassetti and Murray (1967) and Roe et al. (1948), respectively. Fatty acid composition was determined by a modification of the method described by May and McCay (May and McCay, 1968; Sugioka et al., 1981).

Results

(1) Chemiluminescence from brain surface

As shown in Fig. 11, a detectable light emmission appeared from the surface of rat brain promptly after the embolization and lasted at least 4 hours.

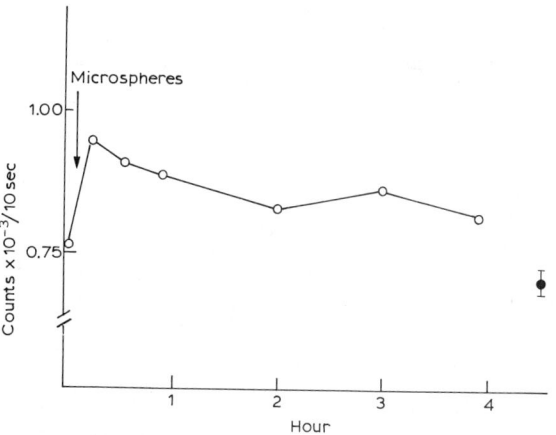

Fig. 11. Chemiluminescence from the surface of rat brain subjected to cerebral infarction (○–○). An arrow indicates the time at which the microspheres were injected through the right internal carotid artery. Closed circle, near the right edge of the figure, indicates background count. Each open circle is the mean value of 10 continuous countings.

This indicates that excited species are generated during the early ischemic stage when the ischemic tissue is faced to an abundant collateral circulation. Unfortunately, extensively low level luminescence from the brain made it difficult to analyze the chemiluminescence spectrum by our filter-type spectrometer.

(2) Chemiluminescence from oxygenated brain homogenate

When brain homogenate was exposed to molecular oxygen by flushing 100% O_2 continuously, the system emitted light which reached a maximum after 1 hour (Fig. 12, curve 1). To investigate the properties of these excited species, the effects of the following substances on the luminescence were tested (data not shown). Flushing with 100% N_2 instead of O_2 completely ceased light emission, indicating the requirement of O_2 for the generation of excited species. When 1×10^{-5} M 2,5-dimethylfuran, a colorless l-scavenger (Noguchi et al., 1977), was added to the emitting system at the time at which maximal light emission was obtained, it did not quench the luminescence, suggesting there was no involvement of singlet oxygen in the emission. When 0.1 mM di-*tert*-butylhydroquinone, a widely used radical scavenger, was added to the system prior to the incubation, it completely terminated the luminescence from the homogenate, suggesting the involvement of a radical mediated reaction for the production of the excited species. 1 mM EDTA or 10^{-6} M desferrioxamine also completely inhibited the luminescence from the brain homogenate, suggesting the requirement of transition metals, particularly iron, for the emission. A triplet sensitizer, 9,10-dibromoanthracene sulfonate or eosin Y at the concentration of 10^{-6}–10^{-5} M added to the homogenate prior to the initiation of the reaction, did not enhance the light emission in the visible region during the autoxidation of brain homogenate, suggesting there was no generation of excited carbonyl during the reaction (Sugioka and Nakano, 1976).

(3) Requirements for cofactors and the protein moiety for chemiluminescence

NADPH-dependent cytochrome P-450 reductase is known to catalyze the reduction of an iron-chelate (Svingen et al., 1976; Sugioka and Nakano, 1982). The resulting Fe^{2+}-chelate would be converted to an active iron-oxygen complex which stimulates lipid peroxidation (Sugioka et al., 1983). Brain parenchymal cells should contain NADPH, NADPH-dependent cytochrome P-450 reductase and suitable iron-chelates. These components, however, should be markedly diluted by homogenization. If one of the components such as Fe^{2+}-chelate or NADPH was supplemented to the homogenate, it should act to stimulate chemiluminescence involved in lipid peroxidation. As expected, chemiluminescence from oxygenated brain homogenate was significantly enhanced by the addition of NADPH, prior (Fig. 12, curve 1 and 2) or during (Fig. 12, curve 1 and 3) the reaction. The addition

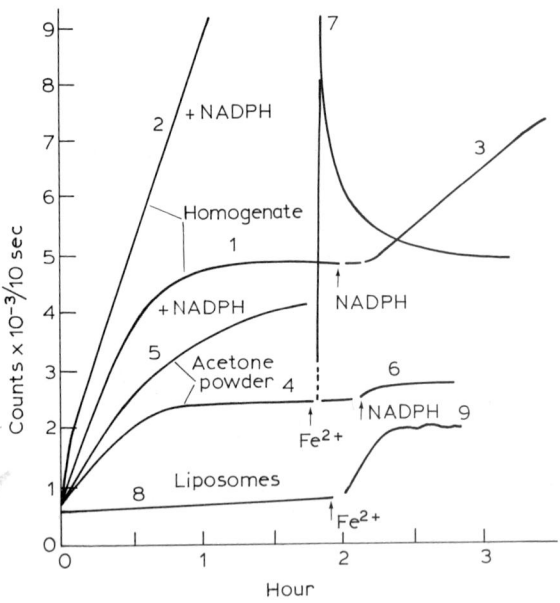

Fig. 12. Chemiluminescence from oxygenated brain homogenate, acetone powder suspension and liposomes. Brain homogenate, acetone powder or liposomes in 0.1 M Tris-HCl buffer at pH 7.4 was used. The 2 mM NADPH were added to the system before flushing O_2 or during the incubation at the time indicated (arrow). Fe^{2+} was added to the system at the time indicated (arrow). Chemiluminescence was measured as described in "Materials and methods".

of iron salt also enhanced chemiluminescence (data not shown). To investigate which fraction, lipid or protein-rich fraction (acetone powder), is essential for the luminescence in the oxygenated brain homogenate, both fractions were exposed to 100% O_2. Acetone powder suspended in Tris-HCl buffer (pH 7.4) in which undenatured protein including NADPH-dependent cytochrome P-450 reductase and cofactors (NADPH, iron and phospholipid, etc.) are present to a greater extent and lesser extent, respectively, emitted light corresponding to approximately 1/2 of that of the homogenate in terms of total light intensity (integrated light intensity) (Fig. 12, curves 1 and 4). The luminescence, however, was slightly enhanced by NADPH (Fig. 12, curves 4, 5 and 6) and significantly elevated by Fe^{2+} (Fig. 12, curves 4 and 7). Thus, the luminescence from the acetone powder suspension would be mainly involved in autoxidation, probably initiated by trace metal iron, but not by an enzymatically induced reaction. Little or no luminescence, however, occurred in the oxygenated liposome suspension (Fig. 12, curve 8). Detectable luminescence only appeared after the addition of Fe^{2+} (Fig. 12, curves 8 and 9). These results suggest that a protein and lipid interaction is required for the luminescence from oxygenated brain homogenate.

It is well known that the ascorbate at an adequate concentration stimulates lipid peroxidation, probably by reducing transition metal irons to produce metal-O_2 complex (Gutteridge et al., 1979). As shown in Fig. 13, ascorbate at 1×10^{-3} M strikingly enhanced chemiluminescence and TBARS value in the oxygenated brain homogenate, but at 1×10^{-2} M completely inhibited them. The latter effect may be due to the inhibition of lipid peroxidation by the known radical scavenging activity of ascorbate at high concentrations.

(4) Light emission spectrum from oxygenated brain homogenate

In an attempt to elucidate the excited species which emits visible light during oxygenation of brain homogenate, the spectrum was recorded using the spectrometer with a filter analyzer. As

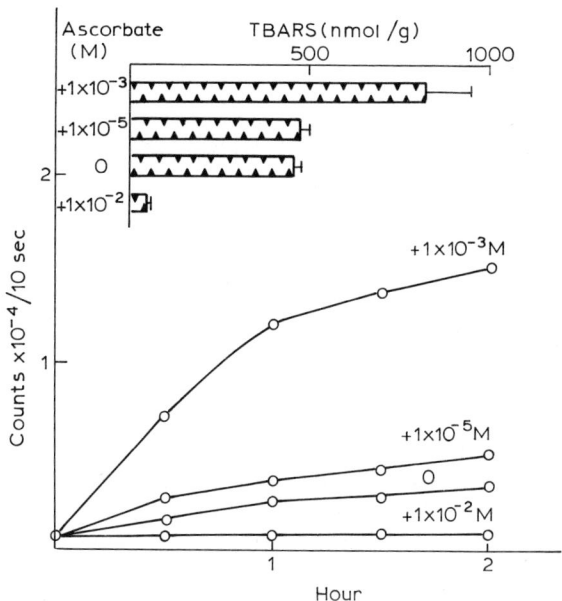

Fig. 13. Effect of ascorbate on chemiluminescence and TBARS formation in the oxygenated brain homogenate. Ascorbate, at the concentration indicated, was added to the brain homogenate before flushing with O_2. TBARS values, obtained at 2 hours incubation, are expressed as mean ± SD ($n = 4$).

shown in Fig. 14, the luminescence spectrum during oxygenation of brain homogenate (Emax: near 520, 550 and 580 nm) was distinguishable from that of singlet oxygen molecules (pairs of metastable $1\Delta g$ in binary emission) as obtained in NaOCl-H_2O_2 system (Emax: 520, 578 and 633 nm) and in microsomal lipid peroxidation (Nakano et al., 1975; Sugioka and Nakano, 1976). However, the spectrum resembled that observed in a tryptophan-prostaglandin hydroperoxidase-hematin-prostaglandin synthetase (Yoshimoto et al., 1980), indole-acetic acid-H_2O_2-myeloperoxidase system at physiological pH (Kobayashi et al., 1980) or in photochemical reactions of indole compounds (Fig. 14) (Vladimirov et al., 1970).

(5) Relationship between chemiluminescence and lipid peroxidation

In order to know the relationship between chemiluminescence and lipid peroxidation, the brain homogenate was placed at the front of a photo-

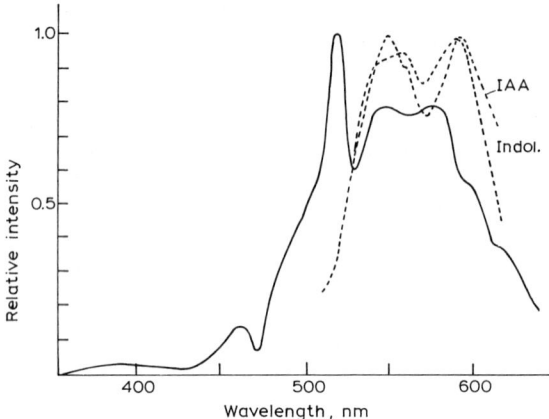

Fig. 14. Chemiluminescence spectrum in the visible region from brain homogenate. Measurement of the chemiluminescence spectrum was started at the time at which maximal light intensity was obtained and continued for 15–20 min. (———), the present experiment; (– – –), phosphorescence from IAA (indole acetic acid) and INDOL (indoles) obtained by Vladimirov et al. (1970).

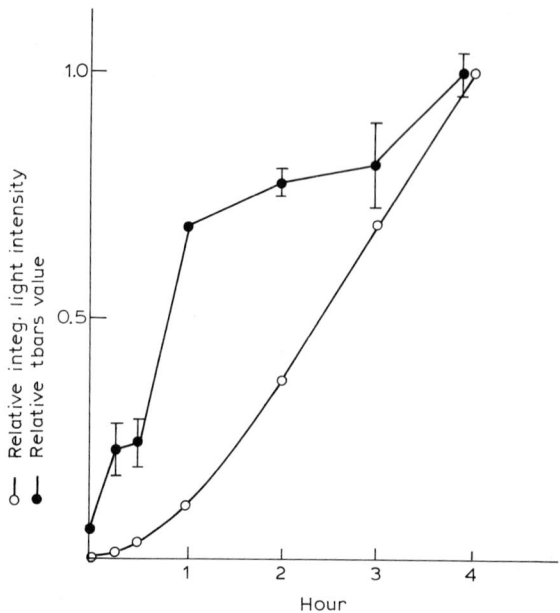

Fig. 15. Comparison of TBARS with integrated light intensity. Chemiluminescence from the brain homogenate was measured flushing with O_2, and another homogenate was incubated under the same conditions and an aliquot (0.2 ml) was taken from the incubation mixture for the determination of TBARS.

multiplier, followed by flushing with 100% O_2 to take chemiluminescence measurement. An aliquot was taken at the time cited for the estimation of TBARS. As shown in Fig. 15, there are some differences between TBARS and integrated light intensity. First, integrated light intensity increased linearly after a short period, while TBARS accumulated rapidly without a lag period. Second, only about 10% of total photons detected were observed within the first 1 hour, whereas about 70% of total TBARS were already formed after 1 hour. Thus, the formation of TBARS appears to proceed that of excited species.

TBARS is a measure of both early and late stages of lipid peroxidation. However, most of the TBA-activity can be ascribed to the breakdown of lipid peroxides to malondialdehydes during the acid-heating stage of the test. Since fatty acids with 2 or more double bonds contribute to most of TBARS, it is important to know the change of fatty acid composition of the brain homogenate during oxygenation. However, arachidonic acid which has four double bonds in a molecule was not significantly changed after oxygenation of brain homogenate (Fig. 16). It, therefore, seems likely that lip-

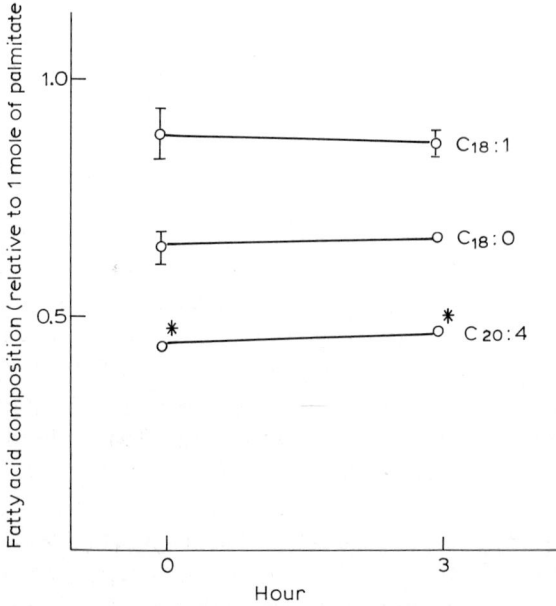

Fig. 16. Change in fatty acid composition of brain homogenate after 3 hours of oxygenation. Three fatty acids in the brain homogenate were measured before and after incubation by the method described in "Materials and methods".

id peroxidation was not sufficient to give rise to detectable changes in fatty acid composition.

(6) Change in protein moiety and -SH groups

It has been observed that membrane lipid peroxidation affects a variety of cell components including proteins, amino acids and nucleic acids (Desai and Tappel, 1963; Roubal and Tappel, 1966; Tappel, 1973; Mukai and Goldstein, 1976). -SH groups in biological materials including glutathione, proteins and cysteine are considered to be especially vulnerable to oxidative damage. Thus, the time-dependent decrease in the content of -SH groups may be expected during the oxygenation of brain homogenate. As expected, more than half of the intitial content of -SH groups disappeared during 2 hours (Fig. 17). This observation naturally lead us to study possible damage to protein molecules. As shown in Fig. 18, high molecular weight protein complexes were formed following lipid peroxidation (indicated by thin arrow). At the same time, some protein bands (indicated by thick arrow) faded gradually, while others became more prominent (Koster and Slee, 1980, 1983). These electrophoretic observations suggest that high molecular weight protein complexes may form by aggregation at the expense of lower molecular proteins. However, there were no totally eliminated bands.

(7) Possible formation of radical species

To investigate the possible generation of free radicals during the oxygenation of brain homogenate,

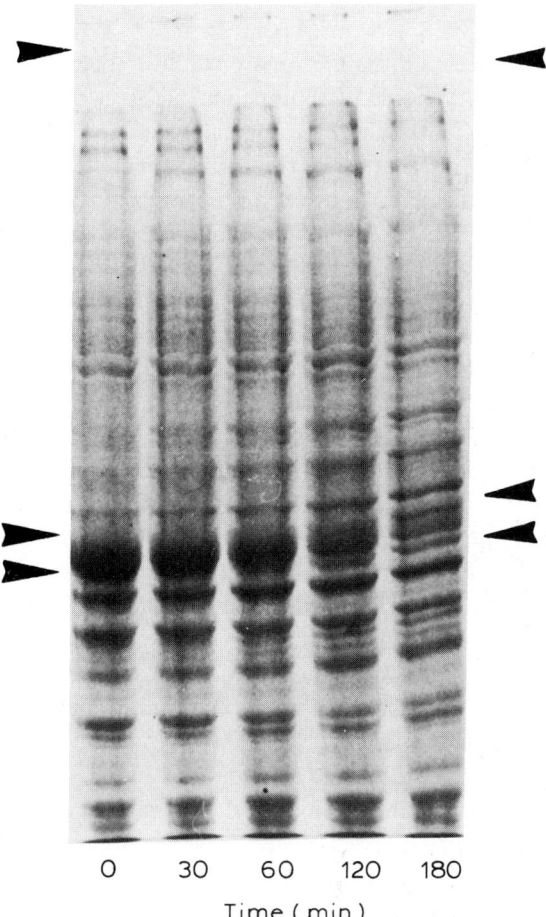

Fig. 17. Profile of SDS-polyacrylamide gel electrophoresis for brain proteins. An aliquot of brain homogenate was taken at the time cited, treated as described in "Materials and methods" and each 90 μg of the protein was applied on the gel for electrophoresis. High molecular weight protein complexes (0); somewhat degraded proteins (180).

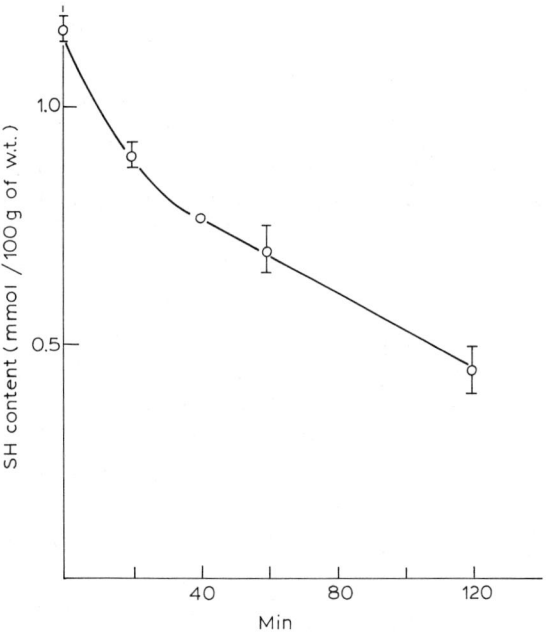

Fig. 18. Time course change in SH content during the oxygenation of homogenate. SH content of brain homogenate was measured at the time indicated. Values are expressed as mean ± SD ($n = 4$). W.T., wet tissue.

0.25 M α-phenyl-N-tert.-butylnitrone (PBN, a spin trap) and 5% alcohol were added to the homogenate, followed by continuous flushing with 100% O_2. An aliquot of the mixture was taken at the time cited for the ESR spectrometry. If alcohol is attacked by certain reactive free radicals, but not by ascorbate free radical, it would be easily converted to the carbon-centered radical (for example, CH_3CHOH) which could react with PBN to produce PBN-alcohol adduct (Pryor, 1976). As shown in Fig. 19, strong doublet signals of a well known ascorbate radical ($g = 2.0054$) (Lagercrantz, 1964; Laroff et al., 1972) were detected at the un-oxygenation and early oxygenation stage, but gradually disappeared and were replaced with new signals with a hyperfine splitting constant of $a^H = 16.1$ and $a^H = 3.3$, which can be assigned to the PBN-alcohol radical adduct. Under the same experimental conditions save that PBN and alcohol were omitted, the molar ratio of ascorbate/dehydroascorbate in the brain homogenate decreased gradually and reversed with increasing time (Fig. 19, right column). These results suggest that ascorbate at physiological concentration, even though it can be involved in lipid peroxidation, appears to protect against the formation of a water-soluble radical (such as alcohol radical) by its reduction activity. At present, it is not known which radical species generated in the oxygenated brain homogenate attacks the alcohol.

Discussion

Most free radicals are highly reactive species, because they possess an unpaired electron in their molecular orbitals. Free radical reactivity and its resulting alternation of membrane function is currently considered to be one of the important factors contributing to development of brain edema and irreversible ischemic brain injury (Siesjö, 1981). Demopoulos and Flamm have proposed that in the intraischemic period (electron depletion) hydrogen abstraction from inner mitochondrial membrane lipid occurs by coenzyme Q semiquinone radical (Demopoulos et al., 1977). On the other hand, Kogure has suggested that activation of O_2 is essential for initiation of post-ischemic lipid peroxidation by demonstrating little or no TBARS formation under 100% N_2 (Kogure et al., 1982). In the present experiments, the rat brain surface emitted weak light promptly after embolization which lasted at least 4 hours, indicating the generation of excited species from an early stage of reoxygenation around multiple ischemic areas. Earlier, it was demonstrated by autoradiographic technique that blood is sufficiently re-supplied to infarcted cerebral hemisphere even 5 min after embolization in the same model (Kogure et al., 1974). Therefore, it is considered that chemiluminescence from the surface of rat brain is closely related to re-oxygenation of injured brain tissues.

Chemiluminescence is well known to accompany lipid peroxidation (Sugioka and Nakano, 1976). When brain homogenate in Tris-HCl buffer (pH

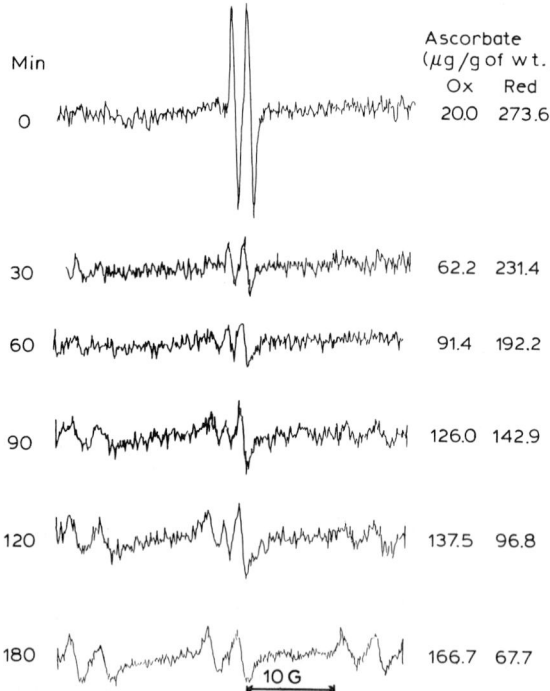

Fig. 19. ESR spectra obtained from oxygenated brain homogenate. The incubation mixture contained 0.25 M PBN, 5% alcohol (v/v) and brain homogenate in 0.1 M Tris-HCl buffer. The incubation was started by flushing with O_2. The right column of the figure shows the time course change of ascorbate (RED) and dehydroascorbate (OX). W.T., wet tissue.

7.4) was exposed to O_2, it also emitted light which would be terminated in the presence of an inhibitor of lipid peroxidation, di-*tert*-butylhydroquinone. Furthermore, both, increases in TBARS and luminescence during oxygenation of brain homogenate provided evidence that lipid peroxidation actually occurred in brain homogenate. Active oxygen species, such as hydroxy radical (·OH), singlet molecular oxygen ($^1O_2$) and iron-O_2 complex ($Fe^{2+}O$, $Fe^{3+}...O_2^-$ complex) are considered to be initiators and stimulators of lipid peroxidation. Even though it is unknown which active oxygen species is an initiator of the lipid peroxidation in the present system, metal ion, especially iron (probably in the ferrous state), plays a key role in the development of lipid peroxidation, since there was complete inhibition of chemiluminescence and TBARS formation by EDTA or desferrioxamine (data not shown). Sugioka et al. have demonstrated that iron-ADP complex, but not ·OH is essential for adriamycin-induced lipid peroxidation (Sugioka et al., 1983). Gutteridge also emphasized the significance of non-protein bound iron salt or chelate in neuronal ceroid lipofuscinosis and certain degenerative disorders (Gutteridge et al., 1979). Non-protein bound iron in ferric state would be reduced to ferrous state for initiating lipid peroxidation. The present experiments obtained with brain homogenate suggest that NADPH-dependent cytochrome P-450 reductase is an enzyme able to catalyze the reduction of endogenous iron, which can, of course, also be done by ascorbate in a non-enzymatic process.

The chemiluminescence spectrum obtained with oxygenated brain homogenate was quite different from that obtained from transition of $^1O_2$ pair (Nakano et al., 1975), but closely resembled that for excited indole analogs (Vladimirov et al., 1970). The mechanism for the generation of excited indole analogs and chemiluminescence in the present system are considered to be as follows: (a) lipid peroxyl radicals, generated during lipid peroxidation, abstract hydrogen from an -NH group at the indole ring of tryptophan residue in protein; (b) the resulting radical catches H^+, yielding an indole cation radical; (c) the cation radical catches an electron (probably solvated electron), yielding an excited indole species in the triplet state; (d) the excited species emit light with a wavelength 550–580 nm during its return to the ground state (Vassilev, 1963).

If the above mechanism is correct, a close interaction of lipid and protein would be required for generation of excited species resulting in both, changes to fatty acid composition of the brain lipids, and to the structure of proteins. The structural damage, however, may be only minimal. This assumption can be supported from the following findings: (a) there was no substantial change in the fatty acid composition of the brain homogenate after flushing with O_2; (b) there was no significant generation of chemiluminescence in the lipid fraction after separation from the brain homogenate, even though O_2 was introduced; (c) there was no significant change in the electrophoretic pattern of brain protein after oxygenation of the brain homogenate. On the other hand, the NADPH-dependent microsomal phospholipid peroxidation system or its reconstituted system emits light in the visible region which has been ascribed to $^1O_2$ pair and excited carbonyl (Sugioka and Nakano, 1976). In this case, substantial lipid peroxidation with the greater changes in polyunsaturated fatty acids occurs, probably before interacting with microsomal protein. Thus, it is obvious that chemiluminescence spectra should be different in each system dependent on the extent to which lipid peroxidation occurs.

Part III. Involvement of radioligand binding for cholinergic muscarinic receptors in an ascorbate-induced lipid peroxidation

Finally, little is known of the effect of lipid peroxidation, or the products resulting from it, on neurotransmission in the central nervous system. But it has been observed that ascorbate in vitro decreases the binding of radioligands to certain neurotransmitter acceptors (Dunlap et al., 1979; Cox et al., 1980; Leslie et al., 1980). It has been proposed that the ascorbate-induced loss of receptor binding activity may result from the peroxidation of lipid membranes (Heikkila et al., 1982; Muakkahssah-Kelly et al., 1982, 1983).

Present work reports that the ascorbate-induced loss of receptor binding, as well as lipid peroxidation, is dependent on the concentration of ascorbate used and the nature of buffer ions present.

Materials and methods

Wistar strain male rats (body weight approximately 250 g) were decapitated and the forebrain rapidly removed. The forebrain was homogenized in 10 vols. of 0.32 M sucrose using a Potter type homogenizer (1000 rpm, 5-dance). The homogenate was centrifuged at $1000 \times g$ for 10 min at 4°C. The resulting supernatant was centrifuged at $17500 \times g$ for 20 min at the same temperature. The pellet obtained was then resuspended in 50 mM Tris-HCl buffer (pH 7.4) and the suspension was again centrifuged at $17500 \times g$ for 20 min at 4°C to obtain a washed pellet (crude mitochondrial fraction). The washed pellet was resuspended in 50 mM Tris-HCl buffer (pH 7.4) or in 50 mM Na-K phosphate buffer (pH 7.4) with the aid of a sonic oscillator. The buffer suspension was incubated with various concentrations of ascorbate (0, $10^{-5}, 10^{-4}, 10^{-3}, 10^{-2}$ M) and 4 nM [^{3}H]QNB (quinuclidinyl benzilate: 33.2 Ci/mmol, New England Nuclear) for 30 min at 37°C. The reaction was initiated by the addition of ascorbate. At the end of incubation time, thiobarbituric acid reactive substances (TBARS) in the medium were measured by the method of Ohkawa et al. (Ohkawa et al., 1979). At the same time, specific [^{3}H]QNB binding was measured.

The brain homogenate (crude mitochondrial fraction) in 50 vols. of Tris-HCl buffer (pH 7.4) was incubated with or without 0.5 mM ascorbate. Then they were centrifuged at $17500 \times g$ for 20 min and washed three times with 50 mM Tris-HCl buffer (pH 7.4). The washed pellet was used for the assay of [^{3}H]QNB-binding parameters (B_{max}, K_d). The [^{3}H]QNB-binding assay was carried out according to the modified method of Yamamura and Snyder (Yamamura and Snyder, 1974). For [^{3}H]QNB-binding assay, 1 ml of 50 mM Na-K phosphate buffer mixture containing [^{3}H]QNB (0.1–1.5 nM) and rat brain homogenate (about 0.1 mg protein) were incubated for 60 min at 25°C. Specific binding was calculated by subtracting non-specific binding from total binding. Non-specific binding was measured in the presence of 10 μM atropine sulfate. The binding reaction was terminated by rapid filtration using a Whatman GF/B filter, and it was washed three times with 3 ml of ice-cold buffer. After drying, the filters were placed in vials containing 10 ml of ACS II (Amersham), and the radioactivity was assayed by liquid scintillation spectrometer (Aloka LSC 900). Protein was determined by the method of Lowry et al. (Lowry et al., 1951) using bovine serum albumin as a standard.

To test the effects of metal-chelating reagents and scavengers of oxygen radicals, the brain homogenate in 50 mM Tris-HCl buffer (pH 7.4) (containing about 1 mg protein) was incubated with 0.5 mM ascorbate and with one of the active oxygen scavengers or metal-chelating reagents. Then they were used for the measurement of TBARS. Active oxygen scavengers used in these experiments were dimethylfuran (10^{-5} M), sodium benzoate (50 mM), catalase (20 μg/ml), superoxide dismutase (8×10^{-7} M), desferrioxamine (10^{-5} M) and EDTA (1 mM).

To neglect the contamination of metal ion from blood, crude mitochondrial fractions obtained from both, 0.15 M KCl-perfused rat forebrain and non-perfused, were incubated with or without 0.5 mM ascorbate in the Tris-HCl buffer (pH 7.4) at 37°C. They were assayed for TBARS.

Results and discussion

As shown in Fig. 20, [^{3}H]QNB-binding activity for rat brain membrane pellet was strikingly suppressed by ascorbate in the range of $10^{-4} \sim 10^{-3}$ M. However, concentrations of ascorbate above or below this (10^{-2} M, 10^{-5} M) did not suppress binding. The same figure also shows that the [^{3}H]QNB-binding activity loss is almost parallel to the increase of TBARS expressed as malondialdehyde (MDA) formation. The "U-shaped" pattern of loss of

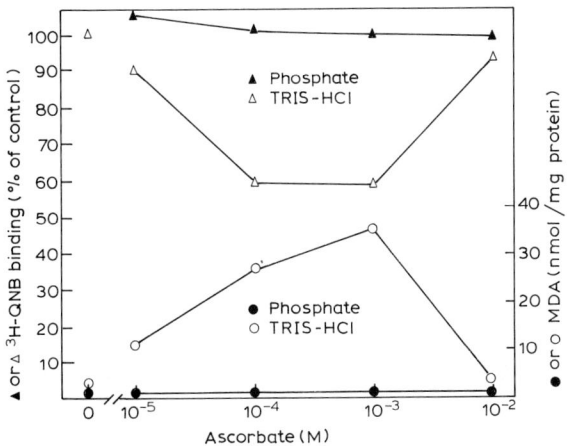

Fig. 20. Effect of ascorbate on the specific binding of [^{3}H]QNB and on the lipid peroxidation in brain homogenates. The experimental conditions are described in "Materials and methods". Each experiment was repeated three to five times in triplicate. Standard deviations are less than 10%.

[^{3}H]QNB-binding resembled that previously reported with [^{3}H]spiperone or [^{3}H]serotonin (Heikkila et al., 1982; Muakkahssah et al., 1982). However, neither loss of [^{3}H]QNB-binding activity nor MDA formation was observed at any concentration of ascorbate in a phosphate buffer.

To examine the participation of active oxygen species and transition metal(s) on the ascorbate-induced TBARS formation, each of the active oxygen scavengers (dimethylfuran for singlet oxygen, sodium benzoate for ·OH, catalase for H_2O_2, superoxide dismutase for ·O_2^-), or metal-chelating reagents (EDTA or desferrioxamine) was added to the system, prior to the initiation of the reaction. TBARS was measured after 30 min following addition of ascorbate (Table 1). Only EDTA or desferrioxamine was substantially inhibitory towards ascorbate-induced formation of TBARS. EDTA, at the same concentration, also completely protects against the loss of [^{3}H]QNB-binding activity induced by ascorbate (data not shown).

It has been reported that exogenously added Fe and ascorbate cause a peroxidative cleavage of phospholipid in isolated hepatic microsomes (Nakano et al., 1975) and that lipid peroxidation is actively dependent on the presence of suitable transition metals (Gutteridge et al., 1979). Ascorbate is known to reduce ferric ion (Fe^{3+}) to the ferrous state which can lead to the formation of perferryl ion (a powerful initiator of lipid peroxidation) in the presence of O_2.

In the present work, the ascorbate-induced lipid peroxidation, monitored by the formation of TBARS was remarkably inhibited by the addition of metal-chelating reagents such as EDTA and des-

TABLE 1

Effects of some active oxygen scavengers or metal-chelating reagents on the TBARS (MDA) formation

	MDA (nmol/mg protein)	% of MDA formation
Control	1.62 ± 0.11	
Ascorbate (0.5 mM)	13.92 ± 0.34	(100)
Ascorbate + dimethylfuran (10^{-5} M)	11.84 ± 0.25[a]	(84.8)
Ascorbate + sodium benzoate (50 mM)	11.72 ± 0.76[a]	(84.2)
Ascorbate + catalase (20 µg/ml of reaction mixture)	11.24 ± 0.13[a]	(80.2)
Ascorbate + superoxide dismutase (8×10^{-7} M)	10.95 ± 0.49[a]	(78.7)
Ascorbate + desferrioxamine (10^{-5} M)	0.88 ± 0.44[a]	(6.3)
Ascorbate + EDTA (1 mM)	0.68 ± 0.10[a]	(4.9)

The data represent mean ± SD. $n = 4$, [a]$p < 0.005$.

ferrioxamine. But there is only little inhibition (Table 1) by a variety of active oxygen scavengers. This indicates that some active oxygen species exist in the incubation medium, but only oxygen-metal complex has powerful catalyzing effects on lipid peroxidation among them. The damage by ascorbate in Tris-HCl buffer was completely abolished by the replacement of Tris-HCl buffer with a phosphate buffer. This may suggest a complete chelation of free Fe^{3+} by phosphate. Thus, non-phosphate-chelated iron in the tissue preparation (probably as an Fe^{2+} species) may play an important role in the ascorbate-induced lipid peroxidation.

Judging from a good correlation seen between lipid peroxidation and loss of [^{3}H]QNB-binding activity in the presence of ascorbate, it seems likely that peroxidative damage to membranes causes the loss of receptor binding. However, Muakkassah-Kelly et al. (1983) reported a direct effect of ascorbate on the decrease of the [^{3}H]serotonin-binding to the rat cortical membranes. In our experiments, however, ascorbate caused no loss of [^{3}H]QNB-binding without formation of TBARS in the presence of 1 mM EDTA (data not shown). Thus, ascorbate-induced loss of [^{3}H]QNB-binding is considered to be secondarily mediated by membrane damage resulting from lipid peroxidation. Neurotransmitter receptors (ligand-binding sites) are thought to be buried or to float in the lipid bilayer membrane (Singer and Nicholson, 1972) and their biological functions to have a close relationship with boundary lipid membrane. It has been shown that iron-ascorbate-induced lipid peroxidation decreases membrane fluidity in the liver microsomes and mitochondria (Dobretsov et al., 1977), probably due to loss of unsaturated fatty acids such as arachidonic acid and docosahexaenoic acid from membrane phospholipids. Similar changes also occur in rat brain cortical membranes (Rehncrona et al., 1980).

Fig. 21 shows the scatchard plots of [^{3}H]QNB-binding assay. It shows that 0.5 mM ascorbate pretreated rat brain homogenate decreases in B_{max} (0.9 ± 0.1 pmol/mg protein; $p<0.01$), but not in K_d (37.9 ± 8.1 fM; p = N.S.) as compared with as-

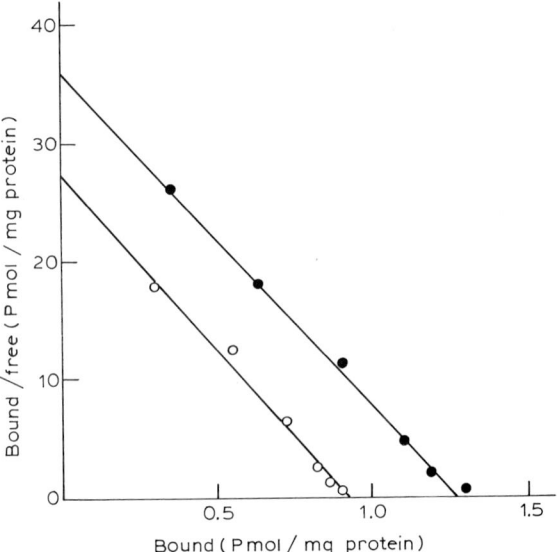

Fig. 21. Scatchard plots of [^{3}H]QNB binding for rat forebrain homogenate. The experimental conditions are described in "Materials and methods". Plots are typical results of four separate experiments. ●–●, control (without ascorbate); ○–○, ascorbate-treated homogenate.

corbate non-treated control (B_{max} = 1.3 ± 0.1 pmol/mg protein, K_d = 36.2 ± 6.6 fM). Thus, loss of [^{3}H]QNB-binding activity due to ascorbate occurs as a function of decreasing B_{max} (receptor quantity), but not as a function of K_d (receptor quality). Peroxidation of membrane lipids is thought to cause conformational changes in receptor proteins and thereby decrease the radioligand binding properties. Binding of [^{3}H]QNB to recep-

TABLE 2

TBARS (MDA) formation from perfused rat forebrain or non-perfused forebrain (nmol/mg protein)

	Perfused brain	Non-perfused brain
Control	1.48 ± 0.11[a]	1.61 ± 0.20[d]
Ascorbate (0.5 mM)	15.35 ± 0.87[b]	14.93 ± 0.69[e]
Ascorbate + EDTA (1 mM)	0.55 ± 0.10[c]	0.73 ± 0.17[f]

The data represent mean ± SD. n = 4
[a×b×c,d×e×f]: $p < 0.01$, [a×d,b×e,c×f]: p = N.S.

tors is so selective that it is easily influenced by a slight conformational change of the receptor protein arising from damage by boundary lipid peroxidation. These conformational changes result in a complete blocking for binding of each ligand. Since each binding of ligands thus follows the law of all or none, ascorbate-induced loss of binding occurred as decreasing the B_{max} but not influencing the K_d. This type of binding activity loss is found to be irreversible without regard to the washing to exclude ascorbate (Fig. 21).

Table 2 shows that there is no significant difference of ascorbate effect on the TBARS formation between perfused brain and non-perfused brain. These results indicate that metal ions (probably Fe^{2+}), which catalyze the lipid peroxidation in the Tris-HCl buffer, are not provided from the contaminated blood during the sampling processes but come from intrinsic ones.

References

Balentine, J.D. (1977) Experimental pathology of oxygen toxicity. In: F.F. Jobsis (Ed.), *Oxygen and Physiological Function*. Professional Information Library, Dallas, TX, pp. 311–378.

Coleman, R. (1973) Membrane-bound enzymes and membrane ultrastructure. *Biochim. Biophys. Acta*, 300: 1–30.

Cox, B.M., Leslie, F.M. and Dunlap, C.E. III. (1980) The use of ascorbate as a probe of opioid receptor structure: evidence for two independent mechanisms of receptor destruction by ascorbate. *J. Recept. Res.*, 1: 329–354.

Demopoulos, H., Flamm, E., Seligman, M., Power, R., Pietronigro, D. and Ransohoff, J. (1977) Molecular pathology of lipids in CNS membranes. In: F. F. Jobsis (Ed.), *Oxygen and Physiological Function*. Professional Information Library, Dallas, TX, pp. 491–508.

Desai. I.D. and Tappel, A.L. (1963) Damage to proteins by peroxidized lipids. *J. Lipid Res.*, 4: 204–207.

Dobretsov, G.E., Borchevskaya, T.H., Petrov, V.A. and Vladimilov, Yu.A. (1977) The increase of phospholipid bilayer rigidity after lipid peroxidation. *FEBS. Lett.*, 84: 125–128.

Duffy, T E., Nelson, S.R. and Lowry, O.H. (1972) Cerebral carbohydrate metabolism during acute hypoxia and recovery. *J. Neurochem.*, 19: 959–977.

Dunlap, C.E. III, Leslie, F.M., Rado, M. and Cox, B.M. (1979) Ascorbate destruction of opiate stereospecific binding in guinea pig brain homogenate. *Mol. Pharmacol.*, 16: 105–119.

Flamm, E.S., Demopoulos, H.B., Seligman, M.L., Poser, R.G. and Ransohoff, J. (1978) Free radicals in cerebral ischemia. *Stroke*, 9: 445–447.

Folbergrová, J., Ljunggren, B. and Siesjö, B.K. (1974) Influence of complete ischemia on glycolytic metabolites, citric acid cycle intermediates, and associated amino acids in rat cerebral cortex. *Brain Res.*, 80: 265–279.

Folch, J., Lees, M. and Sloane-Stanley, G.H. (1957) A simple method for isolation and purification of total lipids from animal tissue. *J. Biol. Chem.*, 226: 497–509.

Glavind, J., Hartmann, S., Clemmenson, J., Jessen, K.E. and Dam, H. (1952) Studies on the role of lipoperoxides in human pathology, *Acta Pathol. Microbiol. Scand.*, 30: 1–6.

Grassetti, D.R. and Murray, J.F. (1967) Determination of sulfhydryl groups with 2,2′ or 4,4′-dithiopyridine. *Arch. Biochem. Biophys.*, 119: 41–49.

Gutteridge, J.M.C., Richmond, R. and Halliwell, B. (1979) Inhibition of the iron-catalysed formation of hydroxyl radicals from superoxide and of lipid peroxidation by desferrioxamine. *Biochem. J.*, 184: 469–472.

Gutteridge, J.M.C., Rowley, D.A. and Halliwell, B. (1981) Superoxide-dependent formation of hydroxyl radicals in the presence of iron salts. *Biochem. J.*, 199: 263–265.

Gutteridge, J.M.C., Westermarck, T. and Santavouri, P. (1983) Iron and oxygen radicals in tissue damage: implications for the neuronal ceroid lipofuscinosis. *Acta Neurol. Scand.*, 68: 365–370.

Heikkila, R.E., Cabbot, F.S. and Manzino, L. (1982) Inhibitory effects of ascorbic acid on the binding of [³H]dopamine antagonists to neostriatal membrane preparations: relationship to lipid peroxidation. *J. Neurochem.*, 38: 1000–1006.

Inaba, H., Shimizu, Y., Tsuji, Y. and Yamagishi, A. (1979) Photon counting system of extra-weak chemi- and bioluminescence for biochemical applications. *Photochem. Photobiol.*, 30: 169–175.

Inaba, H., Yamagishi, A., Takyu, C. et al. (1982) Development of an ultra-high sensitive photon counting system and its application to biochemical measurements. *Opt. Laser Eng.*, 3: 125–130.

Janzen, E.G. (1980) A critical review of spin trapping in biological systems. In: W.A. Pryor (Ed.). *Free Radicals in Biology*, Vol. 4. Academic Press, New York, pp. 115–154.

Kasha, M. and Khan, A.U. (1970) The physics, chemistry and biology of singlet molecular oxygen. *Ann. NY Acad. Sci.*, 171: 5–23.

Kobayashi, S., Sugioka, K., Nakano, M., Takyu, C., Yamagishi, A. and Inaba, H. (1980) Excitation of indole acetate in myeloperoxidase-H_2O_2 system: possible formation of indole acetate cation radical. *Biochem. Biophys. Res. Commun.*, 93: 967–973.

Kogure, K., Busto, R., Scheinberg, P. and Reinmuth, O.M. (1974) Energy metabolites and water contents in rat brain during the early stage of development of cerebral infarction.

Brain, 97: 103–114.

Kogure, K., Morooka, H., Busto, R. and Scheinberg, P. (1979) Involvement of lipid peroxidation in postischemic brain damage. *Neurology*, 29: 546.

Kogure, K., Watson, B.D., Busto, R. and Abe, K. (1982) Potentiation of lipid peroxides by ischemia in rat brain. *Neurochem. Res.*, 7: 437–454.

Koster, J.F. and Slee, R.G. (1980) Lipid peroxidation of rat liver microsomes. *Biochim. Biophys. Acta*, 620: 489–499.

Koster, J.F. and Slee, R.G. (1983) Lipid peroxidation of human erythrocyte ghosts induced by organic hydroperoxides. *Biochim. Biophys. Acta*, 752: 233–239.

Krebs, H.A. (1972) The Pasteur effect and the regulations between respiration and fermentation. *Essays Biochem.*, 8: 2–34.

Laemmli, U.K. (1970) Cleavage of structural proteins during the assembly of the head of the bacteriophage T4. *Nature*, 27: 680–685.

Lagercrantz, C. (1964) Free radical in the auto-oxidation of ascorbic acid. *Acta Chim. Scand.*, 18: 562.

Laroff, G.B., Fessenden, R.W. and Schuller, R.H. (1972) The electron spin resonance spectra of radical intermediates in the oxidation of ascorbic acid and related substances. *J. Am. Chem. Soc.*, 94: 9062–9073.

Leslie, F.M., Dunlap, C.E. III and Cox. B.M. (1980) Ascorbate decreases ligand binding to neurotransmitter receptors. *J. Neurochem.*, 34: 219–221.

Lowry, O.H., Rosebrough, N.J., Farr, A.L. and Randall, R. (1951) Protein measurement with the Folin phenol reagent. *J. Biol. Chem.*, 193: 265–275.

May, H.E. and McCay, P.B. (1968) Reduced triphosphopyridine nucleotide oxidase catalyzed alternations of membrane phospholipid. *J. Biol. Chem.*, 243: 2288–2295.

Morton, R.K. (1955) Methods of extraction of enzymes from animal tissues. In: S.P. Colowick and N.O. Kaplan (Eds.), *Methods in Enzymology*. Academic Press, New York, pp. 25–51.

Muakkahssah-Kelly, S.F., Anderson, J.W., Shih, J.C. and Hochstein, P. (1982) Decreased [^{3}H]serotonin and [^{3}H]spiperone binding consequent to lipid peroxidation in rat cortical membranes. *Biochem. Biophys. Res. Commun.*, 104: 1003–1010.

Muakkahssah-Kelly, S.F., Anderson, J.W., Shih, J.C. and Hochstein, P. (1983) Dual effects of ascorbate on serotonin and spiperone binding in rat cortical membranes. *J. Neurochem.*, 41: 1429–1439.

Mukai, F.H. and Goldstein, B.P. (1976) Mutagenicity of malondialdehyde, a decomposition product of peroxidized polyunsaturated fatty acids. *Science*, 191: 868–869.

Nakano, M., Noguchi, T., Sugioka, K., Fukuyama, H. and Sato, H. (1975) Spectroscopic evidence for the generation of singlet oxygen in the reduced nicotinamide dinucleotide phosphate-dependent microsomal lipid peroxidation system. *J. Biol. Chem.*, 250: 2404–2406.

Noguchi, T., Takayama, K. and Nakano, M. (1977) Conversion of 2,5-dimethylfuran to 2-hydroxy-5-hydroperoxy-2,5-dimethyldihydrofuran, a true $^1O_2$-derived reaction in aqueous $^1O_2$ generating systems. *Biochem. Biophys. Res. Commun.*, 78: 418–423.

Norberg, K. and Siesjö, B.K. (1975) Cerebral metabolism in hypoxia. II. Citric acid cycle intermediates and associated amino acids. *Brain Res.*, 86: 45–54.

Ohkawa, H., Ohnishi, N. and Yagi, K. (1979) Assay for lipid peroxides in animal tissues by thiobarbituric acid reaction. *Analyt. Biochem.*, 95: 351–358.

Pryor, W.A. (Ed.) (1976) *Free Radicals in Biology*. Academic Press, New York.

Pryor, W.A. (1976) The role of free radical reaction in biological systems. In: W.A. Pryor (Ed.), *Free Radicals in Biology*, Vol. 1. Academic Press, New York, pp. 1–49.

Pryor, W.A., Stanley, J.P., Blair, E. and Cullen, G.B. (1976) Autoxidation of polyunsaturated fatty acids. *Arch. Environ. Health*, 33: 201–210.

Rehncrona, S., Smith, D.S., Akerson, B., Westerberg, E. and Siesjö, B.K. (1980) Peroxidative changes in brain cortical fatty acids and phospholipids, as characterized during Fe^{2+} and ascorbic acid stimulated lipid peroxidation in vitro. *J. Neurochem.*, 34: 1630–1638.

Roe, J.H., Mills, M.B., Oesterling, M.J. and Damron, C.M. (1948) The determination of diketo-l-gulonic acid, dehydro-l-ascorbic acid, and l-ascorbic acid in the same tissue extract by the 2,4-dinitrophenyl hydrazine method. *J. Biol. Chem.*, 174: 201–208.

Roubal, W.T. and Tappel, A.L. (1966) Damage to proteins, enzymes and amino acids by peroxidizing lipids. *Arch. Biochem., Biophys.*, 113: 5–8.

Siesjö, B.K. (1978) Glycolytic events. In: *Brain Energy Metabolism*. John Wiley and Sons, Chichester, pp. 511–512.

Siesjö, B.K. (1981) Cell damage in the brain: a speculative synthesis. *J. Cereb. Blood Flow Metabol.*, 1: 155–185.

Siesjö, B.K. (1981) Adverse factors affecting neuronal metabolism: relevance to the dementias. In: P. J. Roberts (Ed.), *Biochemistry of Dementia*. John Wiley and Sons Ltd., Chichester, pp. 91–120.

Singer, S.J. and Nicolson, D.L. (1972) The fluid mosaic model of the structure of cell membranes. *Science*, 175: 720–731.

Sugioka, K. and Nakano, M. (1976) A possible mechanism of the generation of singlet molecular oxygen in NADPH-dependent microsomal lipid peroxidation. *Biochim. Biophys. Acta*, 423: 203–216.

Sugioka, K. and Nakano, M. (1982) Mechanism of phospholipid peroxidation induced by ferric iron-ADP-adriamycin co-ordination complex. *Biochim. Biophys. Acta*, 713: 333–343.

Sugioka, K., Nakano, H., Noguchi, T., Tsuchiya, J. and Nakano, M. (1981) Decomposition of unsaturated phospholipid by iron-ADP-adriamycin co-ordination complex. *Biochem. Biophys. Res. Commun.*, 100: 1251–1256.

Sugioka, K., Nakano, H., Nakano, M., Tero-Kubota, S. and Ikegami, Y. (1983) Generation of hydroxyl radicals during the enzymatic reductions of the Fe^{3+}-ADP-phosphate-adriamycin and Fe^{3+}-ADP-EDTA systems. *Biochim. Biophys. Acta,* 753: 411–421.

Sundt, T.M., Grant, W.C. and Garcia, J.H. (1969) Registration of middle cerebral artery flow in experimental infarction. *J. Neurosurg.,* 31: 311–322.

Svingen, B.A., Burge, J.A., O'Neal, F.O. and Aust, S.D. (1976) The mechanism of NADPH-dependent lipid peroxidation. *J. Biol. Chem.,* 254: 5892–5899.

Tappel, A.L. (1973) Lipid peroxidation damage to cell components. *Fed. Proc.,* 32: 1870–1874.

Van Deenen, L.L.M. (1966) Phospholipids and biomembranes. *Prog. Chem. Fats Other Lipids.,* 8: 1–127.

Vladimirov, Y.A., Roshchupkin, D.I. and Fesenko, E.E. (1970) Photochemical reactions in amino acid residues and inactivation of enzymes during UV-irradiation. A review. *Photochem. Photobiol.,* 11: 227–246.

Waltz, A.G. (1969) Red venous blood. Occurrence and significance in ischemic and nonischemic cerebral cortex. *J. Neurosurg.,* 31: 141–148.

Welsh, F.A., Durity, F. and Langfitt, T.W. (1977a) The appearance of regional variations in metabolism at a critical level of diffuse cerebral oligemia. *J. Neurochem.,* 28: 71–79.

Welsh, F.A., O'Conner, M.J. and Langfitt, T.W. (1977b) Regions of cerebral ischemia located by pyridine nucleotide fluorescence. *Science,* 198: 951–953.

Williamson, J.R., Clark, J.B. and Nicklas, W.J. (1971) Control of glycolysis and oxidative metabolism in tissues. In: B.K. Siesjö and S.C. Sørensen (Eds.), *Ion Homeostatis of the Brain.* Munkgsgaard, Copenhagen, pp. 381–416.

Yagi, K. (Ed.) (1982) *Lipid Peroxide in Biology and Medicine.* Academic Press, New York.

Yamamura, H.I. and Snyder, S.H. (1974) Muscarinic cholinergic binding in rat brain. *Proc. Natl. Acad. Sci. USA,* 71: 1725–1729.

Yoshida, S., Inoh, S., Asano, T., Sano, K., Kubota, M., Shimazaki, H. and Ueta, N. (1980) Effect of transient ischemia of free fatty acids and phospholipids in the gerbil brain: lipid peroxydation as a possible cause of post-ischemic injury. *J. Neurosurg.,* 53: 323–331.

Yoshimoto, T., Yamamoti, S., Sugioka, K., Nakano, M., Takyu, C., Yamagishi, A. and Inaba, H. (1980) Studies on the tryptophan-dependent light emission by prostaglandin hydroperoxidase reaction. *J. Biol. Chem.,* 225: 10199–10204.

Subject Index

Acetyl CoA, 115
Acid-base homeostasis, 121
Acidosis
    tissue, 9
Action potential, 63–64, 66
Adenosine
    A1 receptor, 77
Adenylate cyclase, 171
Amino acid, 198
    influx, 201
Aminoacyl-tRNA, 198
γ-Aminobutyric acid (GABA), 66–67, 76
    -ergic neurons, 53
AMPA (α-amino-3-hydroxy-5-methyl-4-isoazolepropionic acid), 73
Amygdaloid nucleus, 70
Anoxia, 42, 51
Antiport = ion exchange system, 123, 126, 146
    Cl^-/HCO_3^-, 159
    Na^+/H^+, 159
Arachidonic acid, 79, 227
Aspartate
    N-methyl-D-aspartate, 71, 73
ATP, 33
ATPase, 212
    calcium-, 171
    Na^+/K^+, Mg^{2+}, 214
Autoradiography, 197–198, 208
    deoxyglucose method, 25
    light-microscopic, 200
    receptor, 90
Axon, 185
    terminal, 187
    transport, 187

Barbiturate, 9
Base
    deficit, 122
    excess, 122
BB concentration, see Buffer
Boundary (Border) zone, 19, 208

Brain
    edema, 231
    immature, 108
Brain injury
    acidosis promoted, 145
Buffer
    buffer base (BB) concentration, 122, 124
    capacity, 127–128, 130
    sources and sinks for H^+ = H^+ buffer mechanism, 126, 163
    strong acid, 122
    strong anions, 124
    strong cations, 123
    strong ion difference (SID), 125
    subicular regions, 70

Calcium (Ca^{2+}), 36, 54, 64–65, 79, 169
    activated neutral protease (CANP), -μCANP, -mCANP, 185, 191–193
    activated proteolysis, 193
    antagonist, 93
    ATP-dependent Ca^{2+}-sequestration, 102
    ATPase, 104
    buffering protein, 79
    calmoldulin-dependent protein phosphorylation, 12
    concentration, 116
    conductivity, 66–67
    cytoplasmic, 170
    dependent degradation of NF, 192
    dependent protease, 107
    entry blocker, 79, 89–90
    entry blocker (-PN200-110, -D600, -D888), 90–94
    extracellular, 61
    free, 187
    influx, 193
    intracellular, 11, 112, 116, 170
    overload, 101
    uniporter, 99
    voltage-dependent calcium channels (VDCC), 89, 91–93
Calcium-dependent protease, 113
Calcium transport, 97, 107–108, 111, 113
    anaerobic mitochondria, 101

pyruvate-supported 108, 112–114
pyruvate carboxylase, 14
Calmodulin, 168–169, 171
CANP, see Calcium
cAMP, see Cyclic
Caudate nucleus, 74, 76
CBF
   hydrogen clearance method, 25
   local, 32
   regional, 32
Cell injury
   irreversible, 170
Cell volume regulation, 146
Cerebro spinal fluid, 71
cGMP, see Cyclic
Chemiluminescence, 246
Chloride, 80
Choline
   CDP, 219
   acetyl transferase (CAT), 34
Cholinomimetics, 75
Chromatography
   SDS-polyacrylamide, 202
CMRGlc, 60
   local, 32
   regional
Columnar pattern, 30
Cyclic
   AMP, 80
   GMP, 80
Cytochrome
   P-450 reductase, 248
Cytoskeleton
   neuronal, 185
Cytotoxic, 169
   effects, 75

Delayed neuronal death = delayed neuronal damage, 45, 47, 50, 52, 54, 56, 59
   hippocampus, 4
Dendrite, 185
Denervation, 111
   hippocampus, 107
Dentate gyrus, 70
Deoxyglucose (2-DG), 30, 60, 71
   method, 25
Diazepam, 173
Dichloracetate, 108
Diglycerides, 212
1,4-Dihydropyridine, 89–94
Diletiazem, 89, 94
Donnan
   double Donnan hypothesis = pump-leak hypothesis, 146

ECoG = electrocorticogram, 202
EEG, 36
Electrode
   calcium, 109
   hydrogen (H^+), 155
Electrophoresis
   SDS-polyacrylamide, 174
Energy failure, 8
Entorhinal cortex, 111–113
Epileptic seizures, 140, 142
ESR spectrometry, 252
Ethanolamine
   plasmalogen, 216
Excitotoxicity, 53

Fatty acids, 212, 227
   polyunsaturated fatty acid (PUFA), 227
Forebrain ischemia, rat, 46
Free fatty acids (FFA), 212
Free radical, see also Radical, 80, 112, 237, 252

Gerbil 42, 45, 59
   global ischemia, 32
Glia -oligodendro, 206
Glucose (CMRGlc), 60
   3-O-methyl-D-, 60
Glutamate, 71, 36
   GABA-, 34
   GAD-, 34
   L-, 112
Glycogen
   metabolism, 171
Gradient
   proton electrochemical, 108
Granule cell, 208

Hippocampus, 41–42, 111
   Ammon's horn, 41
   CA1 (Sommer's sector), 41–42, 44–47, 49–52, 54–55, 59, 61, 70, 201, 206–207
   CA1N, 59, 61, 63, 65–67, 77
   CA2, 41, 44–45, 201
   CA3, 41, 44–46, 54, 201, 206
   CA4, 41, 44, 46, 52
   H2 sector, 32
   selective vulnerability, 39
Homeostasis, H^+, 158
Hydrogen
   clearance method, 25
Hyperglycemia, 160
Hypermetabolism, 9
Hypoxia-ischemia, 29
Hypoglycemia, 71, 140
   brain damage, 69

Hypoperfusion
  secondary, 24–26

Immunoblot, 192–193
Immunoreactive fragment, 192
Immunocytochemistry, 43
Indole analogs, 253
Insulin, 116
Iodoantipyrine (^{14}C-labelled), 60
Ion
  bicarbonate, 155
  hydrogen, 155
  perferryl, 255
  membrane ion exchange, 121
  transport, Na^+/Ca^{2+} exchange, 102
Ischemia, 41–42, 51, 69, 143, 198
  complete, 160
  incomplete, 162
  cell change, 40, 45, 47, 51–52
  ischemic cell damage = ischemic neuronal change, damage, 39–42
  reactive change, 40
  stroke, 56

Ketone bodies, 115
Kinase, 108
  cAMP-dependent, 187
  glycogen synthase, 171, 177
  myosin light chain, 177
  phosphorylase, 171, 177

Lactate, 33
  acidosis, 160
Lateral septal nucleus, 77
Limbic system, 70
Lipid
  protein interaction, 245
  peroxidation, 237, 257

Maturation phenomenon, 3, 40
Methionine adenosyl transferase (MAT), 199, 201
Microfilament, 116
Microtubules, 107, 116, 170, 185–187
  associated proteins (MAPs), 177, 185
Microvacuolation, 40
Mitochondria, 107–108, 111, 113
Mongolian gerbil, see Gerbil
Monkey, 202, 208
Monoclonal antibodies, 192

NADH
  fluorescent photography, 241
  fluorescence, 21–23, 25, 30
Neurofilament (NF), 170, 185
  degradation, 186
  intermediate, 186, 189
  protease, 186, 187
  proteolysis, 192
  protofilament, 186
  subunit, 186
Neuron-specific enolase (NSE), 43
  anti-NSE antibody, 43
Neuronal activity
  spontaneous (SNA), 60, 64, 66–67
Neurotransmitter, 172
Neutral red, 60–61
No-reflow phenomenon, 5, 22
Noradrenaline, 78

Ouabain, 103
Oxalate
  pyroantimonate stain, 79
Oxidative phosphorylation, 108
Oxygen
  -iron complex, 253
  -metal complex, 249
  radicals, 231
  singlet molecular, 253

Pathoclisis, 42
Pathway
  commissural, 112
  perforant, 112
  septo-hippocampal, 112
  Schäffer commissural, 110
PDH, see Pyruvate
Pentobarbital, 55
Perforant pathway, 72
pH
  antiport, 126
  Base Deficit/Base Excess, 122
  buffer base (BB) concentration, 122
  buffer base, see Buffer, sources and sinks for H^+
  buffer capacity, 127–128, 130
  epileptic seizures, 140, 142
  hypoglycemia, 140
  ischemia, 140, 143
  membrane ion exchange, 121
  sources or sinks for H^+, 126
  strong acid, 122
  strong anions, 123
  strong cations, 123
  strong ion differences (SID), 125
Phenothiazine, 171
Phenylalkylamine drug receptor, 92–93
Phenytoin, 172
Phosphatase, 108
Phosphodiesterase, cyclic nucleotide, 171

Phospholipase, 170
  A_2, 227
  C-phosphatidylinositol-specific, 227
Phospholipid
  lyso-, 212
  membrane, 230
Phosphorylation, 186, 189, 193, 202
  α-PDH-, 110
  PDH-, 111
  protein, 169, 199
  resuscitation, 3
Post-ischemic hypoperfusion syndrome, 7
Potassium, extracellular, 61, 64–65
Prostaglandin E_2, $F_{2\alpha}$, 215
Protease = calcium-activated neutral protease (CANP), 189
Protein
  synaptic vesicle, 202
  synthesis, 197–198, 200, 202, 207–208
  turnover, 197–199, 204
  biosynthesis, 11
  kinase, 169
Proteolysis, 185
  calcium activated, 185
Purkinje cell, 30, 71, 206, 208
Pump leak hypothesis, 147, see also Donnan
Pyramidal cell, 206–207
  layer, 201
Pyruvate dehydrogenase (PDH), 108
  activity, 113
  kinase, 109
  phosphatase, 109

Quinuclidinyl benzilate (QNB), [^{3}H]QNB-binding activity, 254
Quisqualate (QA), 73

Radical
  alkoxy, (ROO·), 238
  alkyl (R·), 238
  hydroxy, 253
Rat, 31, 46
  forebrain ischemia, 46
  hippocampus, 47
  neonate, 113
Receptor
  phenylalkylamine drug receptor of VDCC, 89
  interactions, agonist, 138

autoradiography, 90
adenosine A1, 77
Reperfusion, 22, 162
Respiration, mitochondrial, 148
Resuscitation, postischemic, 3

Schäffer collaterals, 72
Schäffer-commissural pathways, 110
Seizure, 71
Selective vulnerability, 3, 29, 339, 41–42, 47, 53, 59, 69, 208
-SH groups, 251
Somatically evoked potentials (SEP), 202
Spinal cord, injuries, 211
Status epilepticus, 71
Striatum, 72
Strong acid, 122
Strong anions, 124
Strong cations, 123
Strong ion difference (SID), 125
Subicular regions, 70
Substantia nigra, 70
Synapse
  presynaptic afferents, 116
  synaptic activation, 108
  synaptic junction, 172
  synaptic vesicle, 172-173
Synthesis, RNA, 207

Thalamus, 70, 76
Thromboxane B_2, 213
Transmitter, excitatory, 116
Trifluoperazine, 173
Tubulin, 189
  β-, 174
  kinase, 174

VDCC, see Calcium
Verapamil, 89, 92–93
  [^{3}H]demethoxy- (D888), 89
Veratridine, 103
Vincristine, 179
Vulnerability, metabolic, 20, 21

Watershed lesions, 29–30

Xanthine oxidase, 233